# Radiology On-Call
# Survival Guide

# Radiology On-Call Survival Guide

## Brian Funaki, M.D.

Fellow, Section of Angiography and Interventional Radiology, Department of Radiology, University of Chicago Pritzker School of Medicine, Chicago

## Martin J. Lipton, M.D.

Professor and Chairman, Department of Radiology, University of Chicago Pritzker School of Medicine, Chicago

Little, Brown and Company

Boston　New York　Toronto　London

**Library of Congress Cataloging-in-Publication Data**

Funaki, Brian.
      Radiology on-call survival guide / Brian Funaki, Martin J. Lipton.
         p.   cm.
      Includes bibliographical references and index.
      ISBN 0-316-28237-5
      1. Radiology, Medical--Handbooks, manuals, etc.  I. Lipton,
Martin J.  II. Title
      [DNLM: 1. Radiology--handbooks.  2. Diagnostic Imaging--handbooks.
      3. Internship and Residency--handbooks.    WN 39 F979r 1996]
      R896.7.F86  1996
      616.07'57--dc21
      DNLM/DLC
      for Library of Congress                  96-45213
                                              CIP

Printed in the United States of America
RRD-VA

Editorial: Tammerly J. Booth, Joanne S. Toran
Copyeditor: Elizabeth Willingham
Indexer: Elizabeth Willingham
Production Supervisor: Mike Burggren
Editorial and Production Services: Silverchair Science + Communications
Cover Designer: Mike Burggren

# Contents

# Preface

Radiology has been one of the medical specialties affected the most dramatically by the advent of "managed care" and the decrease in hospital stays and increase in outpatient procedures. These changes have affected both the intensity of care and the patient mix of many medical centers. At the same time, technology has progressed at a breakneck pace, so that radiology residents must not only become familiar with all forms of digital radiology but also be capable of performing magnetic resonance imaging, magnetic resonance angiography, computed tomography, color Doppler ultrasound, nuclear medicine studies, and interventional procedures. Many centers, such as the University of Chicago, have a pediatric hospital as well as obstetric and gynecology units that also must be the responsibility of the residents on call.

The complexity and volume of work confronting radiology residents on call has escalated for two additional reasons. First, the practice of emergency medicine requires radiology residents to assess, under pressure, the continuous flow of trauma patients requiring prompt attention and to deliver excellent service within an increasingly competitive environment. Second, in many hospitals the transplant service requires the skills of radiology residents. For example, the decision to take an adult or infant transplant recipient back to the operating room may rest on the precision and confidence displayed in identifying vascular continuity with the latest ultrasound machines.

These increasing pressures coincide with those of medicolegal issues and the increasing sensitivity and demands of regulatory agencies. Decision-making skills learned during residency become the basis for the standards of practice of radiologists in the future, and this responsibility can also weigh heavily.

Equally important are the skills residents require in interacting with people. The manner and style of interacting with colleagues, the ability to discuss a problem concerning patient care in a calm, intelligent way, and knowing what crucial questions to ask are increasingly important during resident call. In any given clinical situation, it is vital to select the procedure that can be done most comfortably with the best outcome. Patient outcome analysis is becoming an important field in radiology, and residents need to understand what each diagnostic modality can offer to yield the quickest and safest result.

This handbook was written as a response to the difficulties and fears experienced by radiology residents during their hours on call at the University of Chicago Hospitals. No pocket reference could be found that addresses the questions so frequently asked by residents on call. This text is designed to answer those questions directly and succinctly. The emphasis is on practical application skills, and these guidelines have been tested and verified using our own subspecialty faculty, fellows, and residents. All our current residents have received a copy of this handbook in the form of handouts and have then contributed to the recommendations and accuracy of these pages. We have used as a guide, whenever possible, the recommendations of the *American College of Radiology Standards*.*

This handbook is designed to be carried in the pocket by residents during their time on call and referred to frequently. It contains many useful tips and some well-delineated details regarding procedures, techniques, equipment, drug dosages, and methods of administration. We hope it will help in preparing residents for exciting and rewarding careers in radiology.

Finally, a word of caution. This text is not intended to be a substitute for obtaining help when in doubt or whenever further advice is needed. Residents should follow rules that can be stated simply as follows: show up on time and be willing and available at all times, seek faculty help early and whenever in serious doubt, document what you do, always act with professional dignity and integrity, and remember the patient's well being and care is your first responsibility. We wish you well and hope this handbook will make your radiology path easier and safer.

B.F.
M.J.L.

---

*American College of Radiology, 1891 Preston White Drive, Reston, VA 20911. Copyright 1995.

# Acknowledgments

This handbook has been used in various forms for the past 3 years by the radiology residents on call at the University of Chicago Hospitals. In large part, this book is a reflection of knowledge I have acquired from the attendings and fellow residents. In particular, I thank the following people for their suggestions, comments, and guidance: Fred Winsberg, Jordan Rosenblum, Jeffrey Leef, Arunas Gasparaitis, Geraldine Newmark, Craig Hackworth, Tamar Ben-Ami, Mark Glazer, George Szymski, John Fennessy, Sherri Sachs, Douglas Seeb, Robert Kao, Matthew Difazio, Michele Semin, Catherine Boyle, and Yong Hahn. Special thanks to Dr. Charles Lerner for the original idea and framework of the on-call manual and to my father, Dr. Clarence Funaki, for his overall grasp, insight, and general knowledge of radiology.

B.F.

# Radiology On-Call
# Survival Guide

## Notice

The indications and dosages of all drugs in this book have been recommended in the medical literature and conform to the practices of
the general medical community. The medications described do not
necessarily have specific approval by the Food and Drug
Administration for use in the diseases and dosages for which they
are recommended. The package insert for each drug should be con-
sulted for use and dosage as approved by the FDA. Because standards for usage change, it is advisable to keep abreast of revised
recommendations, particularly those concerning new drugs.

# Contrast Reactions

It is estimated that 5–10% of patients experience adverse reactions to administration of iodinated contrast media. (Fewer patients experience adverse reactions to nonionic contrast.) A life-threatening reaction is seen in one of every 1,000–2,000 administrations; the vast majority (>90%) occur within 30 minutes of injection. Your responsibility is to recognize a contrast reaction and stabilize the patient until more experienced personnel are available. Call for a **code** if you need to give any drug with the exception of diphenhydramine (Benadryl). If the patient is a child, be sure to ask for the **pediatric code** team. Be sure to **legibly** document in the chart exactly what reaction occurred and what treatment was given. It is also worthwhile to follow up on the patient in 1–2 hours if possible.

I. **Nonionic contrast** causes a lower overall incidence of contrast reactions.
  A. **Indications for using nonionic contrast**
    1. Previous reaction to contrast (consider premedication)
    2. Known allergy to iodine or shellfish
    3. Asthma (especially if on medication)
    4. Myocardial instability or congestive heart failure (CHF)
    5. Risk of aspiration or severe nausea and vomiting
    6. Difficulty communicating or inability to give history
    7. Taking beta blockers
    8. Small children at risk for electrolyte imbalance or extravasation
    9. Renal failure with diabetes, sickle cell disease, or myeloma
    10. At physician discretion or patient request
    11. Neonates
  B. **Metformin hydrochloride (Glucophage),** an oral anti-hypertensive medication used in the treatment of non–insulin-dependent diabetes mellitus, should be withheld for at least 48 hours before and 48 hours after administration of IV contrast. The drug may potentiate acute renal failure that can be caused by iodinated contrast.
II. **General premedication regimen**
  A. **Methylprednisolone:** 32 mg PO at 12 and 2 hours before procedure
  B. **Diphenhydramine:** 50 mg PO 1 hour before procedure
III. **Equipment. The proper medications and equipment to treat an allergic contrast reaction must be easily accessible!** A **code box** containing the essential medications for contrast reactions as well as the following equipment should be immediately available:
  A. Oxygen
  B. Bag ventilation device
  C. Stethoscope
  D. Blood pressure cuff
  E. IV fluids (normal saline or Ringer's lactate—*not* D5 ½ normal saline)

**IV. Reactions and treatment.** The manifestations of an adverse contrast reaction are limited. Be aware that epinephrine is given **SQ** at a concentration of 1:1000 but **IV** at a concentration of 1:10,000. Since the dose is the same (0.1 mg), the injected amount of **epinephrine IV is 1 ml** while the injected amount of **SQ epinephrine is 0.1 ml.** Another important note is that when IV fluids are needed, normal saline or Ringer's lactate should be given rather than D5 ½ normal saline. **Pediatric doses** are given in the following table:

| Age | Weight (lbs) | Epinephrine (mg) | Atropine (mg) |
|---|---|---|---|
| Newborn | 7 | 0.03 | 0.06 |
| 1 mo | 10 | 0.04 | 0.08 |
| 3 mos | 13 | 0.06 | 0.12 |
| 6 mo | 17 | 0.08 | 0.16 |
| 9 mos | 20 | 0.09 | 0.18 |
| 1 yr | 22 | 0.10 | 0.20 |
| >1 yr | | Adult dose | |

**A. Vomiting or coughing** may be the first indication of a more severe reaction. No treatment is necessary unless symptoms progress.

**B. Urticaria (hives): Anaphylactoid**
  1. **Signs and symptoms:** multiple raised, red, pruritic papules
  2. **Treatment.** Unless severe, no treatment is necessary.
     a. **Observation.** Patients should be observed carefully since hives may precede a more severe reaction.
     b. **Diphenhydramine,** 50 mg PO (pediatric dose: 1.25 mg/kg IM or IV). Diphenhydramine can cause drowsiness and exacerbate hypotension; it should not be given to outpatients who will be driving.

**C. Facial or laryngeal angioedema**
  1. **Signs and symptoms:** face and neck soft-tissue swelling with stridor (patient may be sitting up holding his or her neck).
  2. **Treatment**
     a. **Epinephrine,** 1:1000 0.1 ml (0.1 mg) SQ q15min. The pediatric dose is 0.01 mg/kg IV slow push over 3–5 minutes.
     b. **Oxygen,** 2–6 liters/minute
     c. **Diphenhydramine,** 50 mg IM
     d. **Cimetidine,** 300 mg PO or IV
     e. **Ice pack** if affected area is accessible

**D. Bronchospasm: Idiosyncratic/non–dose dependent**
  1. **Signs and symptoms:** wheezing
  2. **Treatment**
     a. **Albuterol,** 2 breaths
     b. **Oxygen,** 2–6 liters/minute
     If persistent:
     c. **Epinephrine,** 1:1000 0.1 ml (0.1 mg) SQ q15min. The pediatric dose is 0.01 mg/kg IV slow push over 3–5 minutes.

**d. IV:** keep vein open.
E. **Generalized anaphylaxis**
1. **Signs and symptoms:** constellation of tachycardia (>100 beats per minute), shortness of breath, sneezing, facial swelling, hives, watery eyes
2. **Treatment**
   a. **Epinephrine,** 1:10,000 1 ml (0.1 mg) IV slow push (0.2 ml/min) q15min
   b. **Oxygen,** 2–6 liters/minute
   c. **Elevate feet** with pillows.
   d. **IV fluids:** normal saline or Ringer's lactate
F. **Pulmonary edema**
1. **Signs and symptoms:** shortness of breath without stridor or wheezing
2. **Treatment. Do not give epinephrine.** May give 20–40 mg IV furosemide (Lasix).
G. **Hypotension** (systolic BP <70) **with bradycardia** (<50 beats per minute): **Vagal reaction**
1. **Signs and symptoms:** patient feels faint, cool and diaphoretic to touch, moist skin
2. **Treatment**
   a. **Elevate feet** with pillows.
   b. **IV fluids:** normal saline or Ringer's lactate if hypotension persistent
   c. **Atropine,** 1 mg IV push up to 2–3 mg (1-mg vial). **Do not** give low dose as this may exacerbate hypotension (pediatric dose, 0.02 mg/kg; minimum pediatric dose, 0.1 mg; maximum dose for child, 1 mg; maximum dose for adolescent, 2 mg).
H. **Hypotension** (systolic BP <70) **with tachycardia/normocardia: Volume depletion**
1. **Signs and symptoms:** patient feels faint, has "racing" heart
2. **Treatment**
   a. **Elevate feet** with pillows.
   b. **IV fluids:** normal saline or isotonic Ringer's lactate (not D5 ½ normal saline)
   c. **Oxygen,** 2–6 liters/minute
V. **Contrast extravasation** is an uncommon, albeit not rare, event. Most commonly, it occurs during power injection of IV contrast during CT scanning. If the amount of extravasation is small (<5 ml), usually no treatment is necessary. For larger volumes of extravasation:
A. **Treatment**
1. Elevation of extremity
2. Ice packs for 15 minutes to 1 hour three times per day for 1–3 days
3. Observation for 2–4 hours
4. Plastic surgery consultation if:
   a. Volume exceeds 30 ml ionic or 100 ml nonionic contrast
   b. Skin blistering
   c. Altered tissue perfusion (decreased capillary refill over or distal to site)
   d. Increasing pain over several hours
   e. Change in sensation distal to site

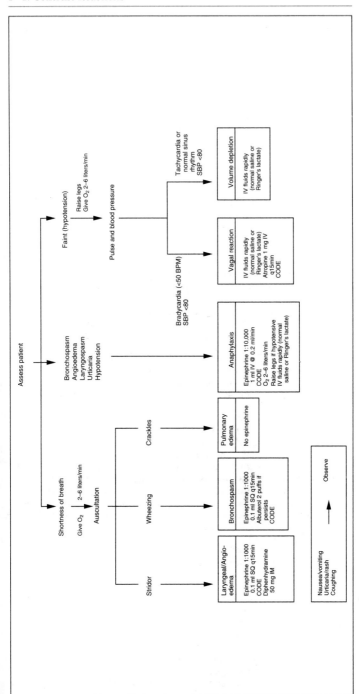

Assess patient

**Shortness of breath** — Give O₂ 2–6 liters/min — Auscultation

- Stridor → Laryngeal/Angio-edema
  - Epinephrine 1:1000 0.1 ml SQ q15min
  - CODE
  - Diphenhydramine 50 mg IM
- Wheezing → Bronchospasm
  - Epinephrine 1:1000 0.1 ml SQ q15min
  - Albuterol 2 puffs if persists
  - CODE
- Crackles → Pulmonary edema
  - No epinephrine

**Bronchospasm / Angioedema / Laryngospasm / Urticaria / Hypotension** → Anaphylaxis
- Epinephrine 1:10,000 1 ml IV @ 0.2 ml/min
- CODE
- O₂ 2–6 liters/min
- Raise legs if hypotensive
- IV fluids rapidly (normal saline or Ringer's lactate)

**Faint (hypotension)** — Raise legs / Give O₂ 2–6 liters/min — Pulse and blood pressure

- Bradycardia (<50 BPM) SBP <80 → Vagal reaction
  - IV fluids rapidly (normal saline or Ringer's lactate)
  - Atropine 1 mg IV q15min
  - CODE
- Tachycardia or normal sinus rhythm SBP <80 → Volume depletion
  - IV fluids rapidly (normal saline or Ringer's lactate)

Nausea/vomiting / Urticaria/rash / Coughing → Observe

B. **Document** both the type of contrast and volume extravasated in the medical chart.

C. **Follow up** with daily phone calls until symptoms resolve.

# References

Bush WM Jr. Contrast media reactions: Recognition and response. RSNA Categorical Course in Genitourinary Radiology 1994, Pp 29–37.

Cohan RH, Ellis JH, Garner WL. Extravasation of radiographic contrast material: Recognition, prevention and treatment. *Radiology* 200:593, 1996.

Dachman AH. New contraindication to intravascular iodinated contrast material. *Radiology* 197:545, 1995.

McClennan BL. Adverse reactions to iodinated contrast media. Recognition and response. *Invest Radiol* 29(Suppl 1):S46.

# Plain Film Evaluation

## Cervical Spine

I. **Clinical history**
   A **Mechanism:** usually motor vehicle accidents or falls
   B. **Age of patient:** usually less than 40 years old
   C. **Location:** most occur in the lower cervical spine (C3–7).
   D. **Number:** average of two injuries per patient
II. **Imaging**
   A. **Plain films.** Our preference is a five-view evaluation of the cervical spine. The most inferior aspect of C7 must be included on the examination.
      1. Anteroposterior (AP)
      2. Lateral
      3. AP open mouth
      4. Left oblique
      5. Right oblique
   Other helpful views include:
      6. **Swimmer's view:** to visualize C7
      7. **Pillar view:** to visualize the posterior elements
      8. **Flexion-extension views**
   B. **CT.** In positive or questionable cases, obtain a noninfused CT (most patients will be receiving a head CT anyway).
      1. 3-mm cuts through the area(s) in question
      2. 1.5-mm cuts through the odontoid; these will allow two-dimensional reconstruction if necessary.
III. **Interpretation**
   A. **Plain films**
      1. **Contour lines.** Four contour lines depicted below should be traced when analyzing a lateral view of the C-spine. In most fractures, one or more of these lines will be disrupted. Also, check for the "ring of C2" because some odontoid fractures not well visualized on the lateral view will disrupt this ring.

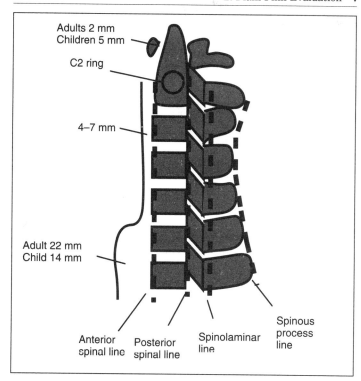

Adults 2 mm
Children 5 mm

C2 ring

4–7 mm

Adult 22 mm
Child 14 mm

Anterior spinal line

Posterior spinal line

Spinolaminar line

Spinous process line

2. **Posterior cervical line.** The anterior aspects of the spinous processes of C1–3 should fall within 2 mm of this line. Disruption occurs in upper cervical spine fractures but also may be a normal finding in 5–10% of the population.

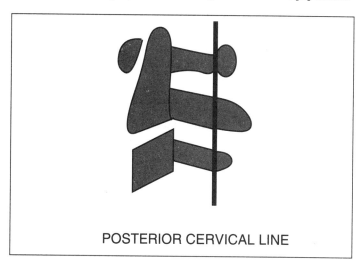

POSTERIOR CERVICAL LINE

**3. Open mouth odontoid view** is used to assess the lateral masses of C1 and odontoid.

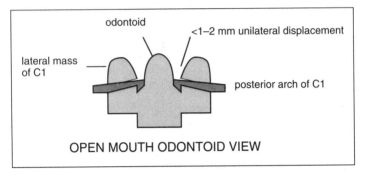

odontoid

<1–2 mm unilateral displacement

lateral mass of C1

posterior arch of C1

OPEN MOUTH ODONTOID VIEW

**4. Ancillary signs.** There are several ancillary signs that suggest significant ligamentous or bony injury. The presence of one or more of these signs (even in the absence of an obvious fracture) should prompt further evaluation with CT.

**a. Prevertebral soft tissues**

**(1) Findings.** Displacement or bulging of prevertebral fat stripe is evidence of hematoma even in the absence of measurable widening of the tissues. The apparent absence of bony injury with a central cord syndrome is consistent with a **hyperextension-dislocation** injury.

**(2) Pitfalls**

i. **Nasogastric or endotracheal tube placed.** Swelling should be noted but interpreted with caution.

ii. **Infants.** Soft-tissue prominence can occur in infants imaged during exhalation. In an infant with prevertebral soft-tissue swelling and no evidence of bony or ligamentous injury, repeat the lateral view during inspiration with the neck positioned in mild extension.

iii. **Mediastinal hematoma** (i.e., aortic laceration) can cause prevertebral soft-tissue swelling due to blood dissecting cephalad.

**b. Widening of facet joint**

**c. Widening of interspinal joint**

**d. Focal kyphosis**

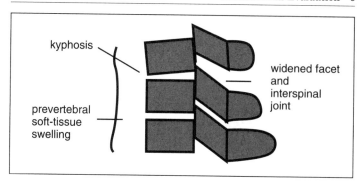

5. **Pitfalls.** Be cognizant of common anatomic variants that can simulate pathology.
   a. **Os odontoideum (unfused odontoid)** may be confused with odontoid fracture (look for smooth, well-corticated borders).

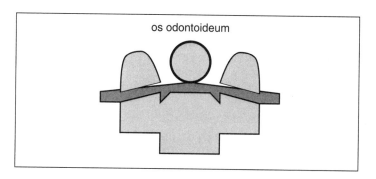

   b. **Incomplete posterior arch of C1** may be confused with a Jefferson fracture.
   c. **Accessory ossicles at C1** may be confused with fracture fragments.
   d. **Congenital fusion** of vertebral bodies
   e. **Vertical pseudofracture of odontoid** is due to superimposition of the front teeth.

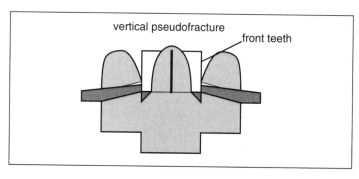

**f. Horizontal pseudofracture of odontoid** is due to Mach effect of the posterior arch of C1.

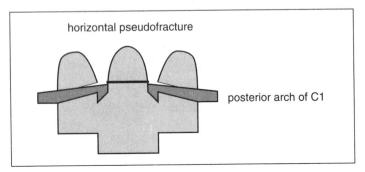

horizontal pseudofracture

posterior arch of C1

**g. Ligamentous laxity of C1–3** (especially in children) may simulate subluxation. Use the posterior cervical line.

6. **Fractures.** It is critically important to be familiar with the appearance of all of the possible C-spine fractures. The following lists injuries categorized by mechanism:

a. **Hyperflexion injuries**
- Flexion tear drop*
- Bilateral locked facets*
- Hyperflexion sprain-anterior subluxation
- Simple wedge compression
- Burst
- "Clay shoveler's"

b. **Hyperextension injuries**
- Hyperextension fracture subluxation*
- Hangman's fracture*
- Extension tear drop*
- Linear avulsion from anterior longitudinal ligament
- Atlas fractures
- Neural arch
- Crush fracture of pillars and lamina

c. **Vertical compression injuries**
- Jefferson fracture of C1*
- Occipital condyle
- Burst fractures of lower C-spine

d. **Lateral hyperflexion injuries**
- Odontoid*
- Transverse process
- Uncinate process
- Pillar
- Vertebral body compression

e. **Flexion-rotation injuries**
- Unilateral locked facet

*Unstable injuries, due to ligamentous injury.

**B. CT images** can often be confusing, especially if the patient is positioned obliquely in the scanner.
  1. **Checklist**
      a. **Scout view,** a "free" lateral view of the cervical spine
      b. **Complete "ring"** at each vertebral body level
      c. **Cord** free of bone fragments
      d. **Transverse foramen** fractures may cause damage to the vertebral artery.

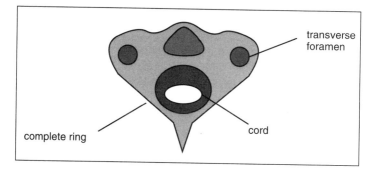

  2. **Pitfalls**
      a. **Uncovertebral joints:** when imaged axially, can appear as linear defects in the vertebral body simulating fractures.

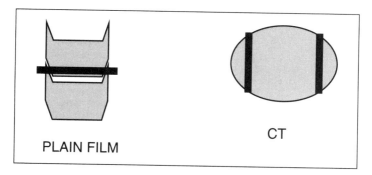

      b. **Vertebral venous plexus:** exits the posterior aspect of the vertebral body and can rarely mimic a fracture (most prominent in the lumbar spine).
      c. **Disk space.** If the patient is positioned obliquely in the scanner, degenerative changes can rarely mimic a fracture of the vertebral body.

# Intensive Care Unit Radiography

## I. Clinical history
### A. Check lung status.
Most ICU patients receive routine chest x-rays (CXRs) (at least daily), and often, little or no clinical information is provided. In general, the after-hours evaluation of these studies should be directed toward detection of findings that will acutely affect patient management. Although in many cases the ICU physician will review all films on his or her patient, never assume that an abnormality, no matter how obvious, has been detected. Always **telephone** the physician taking care of the patient.
### B. Rule out pneumothorax.
Commonly, after any central venous line is placed, a portable CXR is obtained to exclude line placement complication.

## II. Checklist
### A. Tubes and wires
### B. Lungs
### C. Heart
### D. Abdomen

## III. Interpretation
### A. Tubes, wires, and devices
**1. Endotracheal tube (ETT).** Be aware of different types of ETTs (e.g., double-lumen versus single-lumen tubes) used in your hospital. Remember that the metallic inner reinforcer in some tubes ends approximately 2 cm proximal to the true end of tube.

**a. Preferred location**
(1) The distal tip should be approximately 5–7 cm above the carina when the head and neck are in neutral position (i.e., bottom of the mandible at the level of C6–7).
(2) The ETT moves (1–2 cm) in the same direction as the chin (i.e., moves caudal with downward chin tilt).

**b. Complications**
(1) **Too high:** cuff in hypopharynx or at vocal cords, which can result in air leak, aspiration, and gastric distention.
(2) **Too low:** usually in right mainstem bronchus, causing left lung collapse and right lung hyperinflation.
(3) **In esophagus:** gastric distension; tube may appear lateral to trachea on right posterior oblique view.
(4) **Overinflation of cuff** (>1.5× tracheal diameter): predisposes to tracheal necrosis and stenosis

**2. Chest tube**
**a. Preferred location.** Both the side hole and end hole should be in the pleural space.

**b. Complications**
(1) **Side hole in subcutaneous tissue:** marked subcutaneous emphysema
(2) **Terminates in lung:** rare complication. Commonly, when the tube appears to terminate in

the lung, the tip is actually in a pleural fissure (usually of no consequence).

**3. Nasogastric tube**
  **a. Preferred location:** in the stomach with the side hole distal to the gastroesophageal junction
  **b. Complications**
    **(1) Too high:** may cause aspiration pneumonia.
    **(2) In trachea and bronchi:** position should always be checked before feeding is initiated.

**4. Transvenous pacemaker**
  **a. Preferred location.** Tip should be in right ventricular (RV) apex.
  **b. Complications**
    **(1) Perforated septum:** tip too far lateral (usually minimal consequences)
    **(2) In coronary sinus or vein:** tip pointed posterior and cephalad

**5. Central lines.** Be cognizant of variations in venous anatomy such as a left-sided or double superior vena cava (SVC).
  **a. Preferred location:** tip in distal SVC near the right atrium (RA).
  **b. Complications**
    **(1) Catheter embolus (sheared tip) to right heart or pulmonary artery:** often best seen on lateral view.
    **(2) Terminates in improper location**
      **i.** May terminate in brachiocephalic veins or azygous vein (usually no immediate consequence, although repositioning may be necessary for optimal functioning).
      **ii.** Rarely, the catheter (or guide wire used for insertion) may perforate the vessel and result in hemorrhage.

**6. Swan-Ganz catheter:** central venous catheter that allows measurement of left heart pressure when "wedged" in the peripheral pulmonary capillary bed.
  **a. Preferred location:** in the proximal left or right pulmonary artery (catheter may appear discontinuous at the intracardiac portion due to heart motion).
  **b. Complications**
    **(1) Peripheral pulmonary termination:** may cause hemorrhage or infarct.
    **(2) Improper course:** may loop on itself and terminate in different vessels.
    **(3) Partially inflated balloon:** may incite thrombosis.

**7. Intra-aortic balloon pump:** balloon measuring 26–28 cm in length that is inflated during diastole, increasing perfusion to coronary arteries.
  **a. Preferred location:** should terminate immediately distal to left subclavian artery. The tip is marked with a radiopaque rectangle (approximately $1 \times 3$ mm in size).
  **b. Complications:** may terminate in aortic arch or great vessel, predisposing to cerebral embolism or dissection.

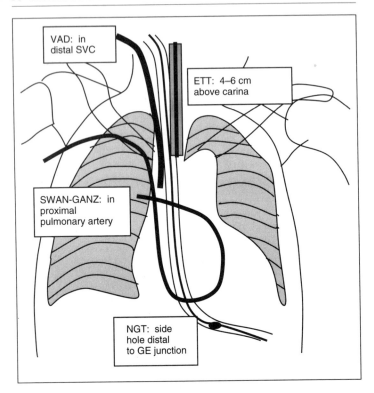

| Device | Preferred location of tip |
|---|---|
| Endotracheal tube | 5–7 cm cephalad to carina<br>Cuff: less than width of trachea |
| Chest tube | Pleural space |
| Nasogastric tube | Stomach with side hole distal to gastroesophageal junction |
| Transvenous pacemaker | RV apex |
| Central line | Junction of SVC and RA |
| Swan-Ganz catheter | Main right or left proximal pulmonary artery |
| Intra-aortic balloon pump | Distal to left subclavian artery |

**B. Thorax**
   1. **Supine pneumothorax:** air in pleural space that is often loculated anteriorly in bedridden patients
      **a. Findings**
         (1) **Anteromedial (earliest location):** sharp delineation of mediastinal contours, outline of medial diaphragm under cardiac silhouette
         (2) **Subpulmonic**
            i. Costophrenic angle on side of pneumothorax unusually deep ("deep sulcus sign")
            ii. May see lucent upper abdominal quadrant or sharp diaphragm despite left lower lobe infiltrate

   **(3) Apical/lateral (least common):** absence of lung markings peripheral to a sharp border

   **(4) "Tension":** shift of mediastinum and diaphragm away from affected side. May occur in patients on ventilators.

  **b. Pitfall: Skin folds**

   **(1)** They produce a density difference in lung field without a sharp border.

   **(2)** They run in pairs or three at a time.

   **(3)** Apparent lung margins extend beyond the lung field with lung markings peripheral to apparent pleural line.

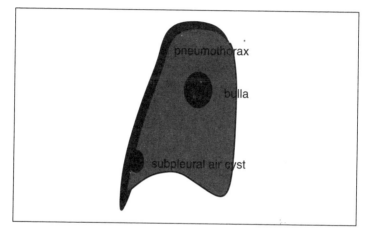

 **2. Bullae:** cystic collection within lung parenchyma due to destruction of alveoli. **Findings include:**

  **a. Faint lung markings** in affected area

  **b. Spherical shape**

  **c. Coexistent signs of emphysema**

 **3. Subpleural air cyst (bleb):** cystic air collection in visceral pleura (usually basilar) due to high ventilatory pressures. Commonly ruptures into pleural space creating **pneumothorax.**

 **4. Pneumatocele:** central cystic air collection commonly seen in children after staphylococcal pneumonia or trauma.

 **5. Pneumomediastinum:** air in mediastinum often due to positive pressure ventilation, asthma, childbirth, or esophageal rupture. Occasionally leads to pneumothorax.

  **a. Findings**

   **(1) Subcutaneous emphysema** in neck

   **(2) Air** surrounding trachea and mainstem bronchi

  **b. Pitfalls**

   **(1) Pneumopericardium:** air extends only to top of pericardium (very rare)

   **(2) Large hiatal hernia**

 **6. Opacification in hemithorax**

  **a. Collapse/atelectasis:** volume loss, rotation, and

mediastinal shift (trachea + pulmonary artery) toward **affected** side (check ETT). The radiograph may appear rotated to the side of collapse; this is due to loss of volume on that side, not poor positioning.

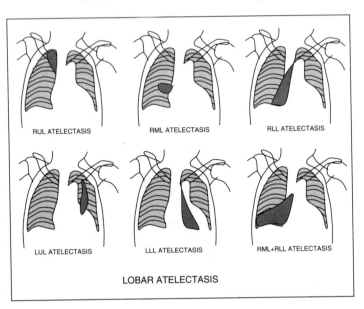

RUL ATELECTASIS

RML ATELECTASIS

RLL ATELECTASIS

LUL ATELECTASIS

LLL ATELECTASIS

RML+RLL ATELECTASIS

LOBAR ATELECTASIS

b. **Pleural effusion**. Mediastinal shift toward **unaffected** side; lateral decubitus views may be helpful.
   (1) **Findings**
      i. Gentle, sloping upward curve at the costophrenic angle (small effusions)
      ii. Abnormal lateral displacement of diaphragmatic apex (subpulmonic)

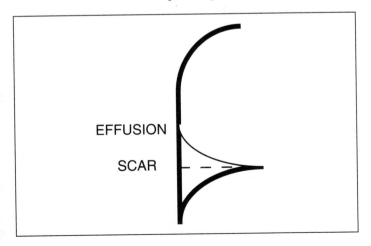

EFFUSION

SCAR

**(2) Pitfall.** Scars have a horizontal orientation.
   **c. Tumor**
   **d. Pneumonectomy**
**C. Abdomen**
   **1. Pneumoperitoneum:** air in peritoneal space usually due to ruptured hollow viscus or recent abdominal surgery.
   **a. Findings**
   **(1) Rigler's sign:** both sides of bowel wall visualized. Need approximately 1 liter of intraperitoneal air.
   **(2) Triangle sign:** gas between three bowel loops or two bowel loops and parietal peritoneum
   **(3) Hyperlucent liver**
   **(4) Hepatic edge sign:** air outlining inferior portion of liver
   **(5) Anterior superior oval:** oblong air collection anterior to the liver
   **(6) Ligamentum teres sign:** sharply defined vertical slit or oval at the porta hepatis
   **(7) Doge hat sign:** triangle-shaped air collection in Morison's (hepatorenal) pouch
   **b. Pitfalls**
   **(1) Postoperative air** usually resolves within **7–10 days** but may persist 2–4 weeks in very thin patients.
   **(2)** Rigler's sign may be mimicked by abundant omental or mesenteric fat or meteorism (air swallowing resulting in multiple dilated gas-filled loops apposing each other).
   **(3)** Air under the right hemidiaphragm occurs on an **upright** chest radiograph, **not** a portable radiograph.
   **c. Follow-up**
   **(1)** Perform left side down decubitus plain film centering on the liver to achieve horizontal beam. Do **not** request "upright" portable film.
   **(2)** Air usually collects between the right lateral liver margin and lateral hemidiaphragm. In patients with wide hips, it may collect in the right pelvis.

# Selected Readings

### Cervical Spine

Clark WM, Gehweiler JA, Laib R. Twelve significant signs of cervical spine trauma. *Skel Radiol* 3:201, 1979.

Harris JH Jr, Edeiken-Monroe B. *The Radiology of Acute Cervical Spine Trauma* (2nd ed). Baltimore: Williams & Wilkins, 1987.

Keats TE. *Atlas of Normal Roentgen Variants That May Simulate Disease*. Chicago: Year Book, 1988.

### Intensive Care Unit Radiography

Cho KC, Baker SR. Extraluminal air: Diagnosis and significance. *Radiol Clin North Am* 32:829, 1994.

Goodman LR, Putman CE. *Critical Care Imaging* (3rd ed). Philadelphia: Saunders, 1992.

Proto AV, Tocino I. Radiographic manifestations of lobar collapse. *Semin Roentgen* 15:117, 1980.

Tocino IM. Pneumothorax in the supine patient: Radiographic anatomy. *Radiographics* 5:557, 1985.

# Ultrasound

## Basic Vascular Ultrasound

I. **Clinical history.** In general, the on-call indications for vascular studies are:
   A. Rule out deep venous thrombosis (DVT).
   B. Rule out hepatic artery thrombosis in liver transplant.
   C. Rule out renal transplant rejection.
   D. Rule out abdominal aortic aneurysm (AAA).
II. **Basic Doppler principles.** A general understanding of Doppler principles is necessary to optimize the technical parameters needed to perform vascular studies competently. In rudimentary terms, a transducer sends out a pulse that interacts with moving blood at a particular distance from the transducer. By the Doppler principle, the frequency of the original signal is altered, producing the Doppler frequency shift. This pulse is reflected back and received by the transducer. This frequency shift is then depicted as velocity information on the screen.

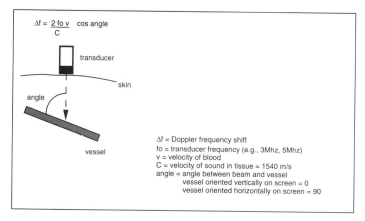

$$\Delta f = \frac{2\,f_0\,v}{C}\ \cos\ \text{angle}$$

transducer

skin

angle

vessel

$\Delta f$ = Doppler frequency shift
$f_0$ = transducer frequency (e.g., 3Mhz, 5Mhz)
$v$ = velocity of blood
$C$ = velocity of sound in tissue = 1540 m/s
angle = angle between beam and vessel
     vessel oriented vertically on screen = 0
     vessel oriented horizontally on screen = 90

This equation states that the Doppler frequency shift (which, in turn, is calculated to blood velocity) depends on the frequency of the transducer and angle between the beam and vessel. To increase the Doppler frequency shift and thereby increase sensitivity to low flow, **use the highest frequency transducer possible** and either **attempt to image vessels oriented vertically** (cos angle approaches 1) or use a **stand-off pad** to change the insonating angle.

The **pulse repetition frequency** (PRF) is the number of times a signal is sent out and received in 1 second. A PRF of 5 kHz means that 5000 pulses are sent out per second with 200-$\mu$sec intervals between pulses. Similarly, a PRF of 8 kHz means that 8000 pulses are sent out per second and there is a

125-$\mu$sec interval between pulses. **There is no relationship between the transducer frequency and PRF.** To obtain unambiguous velocity information, the pulse must travel to the vessel, then back to the transducer before the next pulse is sent out. Since the speed of sound in tissue is 1540 m/sec, a pulse will make a 1-cm round trip (2 cm total distance) in 13 $\mu$sec. A PRF of 5 kHz allows each pulse to travel a total of 200 $\mu$sec/13 $\mu$sec/cm or 15 cm (round trip) before the next pulse will be sent. Therefore, when interrogating a vessel using a PRF of 5 kHz, a vessel must be no farther than 15 cm from the transducer to gain unambiguous velocity information. If a vessel farther than 15 cm away from the probe is interrogated, "aliasing" or wrap-around artifact occurs. If the PRF is increased, the time interval between pulses is decreased. Therefore, the distance between transducer and vessel for which unambiguous velocity information can be obtained is also decreased.

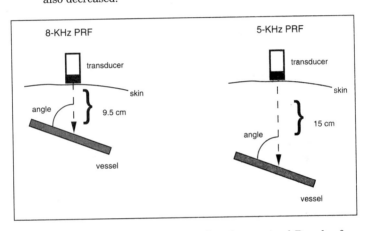

The following equation states that the maximal Doppler frequency shift (velocity scale) that can be depicted without aliasing is equal to ½ the pulse repetition frequency. Therefore, **to increase the velocity scale, PRF should be increased; to decrease the velocity scale, PRF should be decreased.** Alternatively, if the direction of flow is known, the **baseline** can be moved. When imaging deeper vessels, by necessity, the PRF must be decreased (as described above) and the velocity scale also decreases.

maximal $\Delta f$ = ½ PRF

maximal $\Delta f$ = velocity scale

PRF = pulse repetition frequency

For example, if you image a vessel with blood flowing at a velocity of 80 cm/sec with a 5-MHz probe at an angle of 60 degrees:

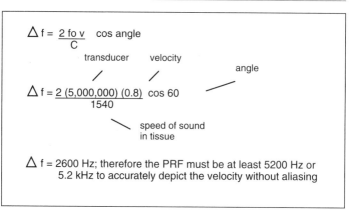

$$\Delta f = \frac{2\ f_0\ v}{C}\ \cos\ \text{angle}$$

transducer    velocity

angle

$$\Delta f = \frac{2\ (5,000,000)\ (0.8)}{1540}\ \cos\ 60$$

speed of sound
in tissue

$\Delta f$ = 2600 Hz; therefore the PRF must be at least 5200 Hz or
5.2 kHz to accurately depict the velocity without aliasing

III. **Technical parameters.** The nomenclature on different
machines varies; however, all follow the same general principles. You should become familiar with the equipment in your
institution.
A. **The velocity scale** is the range of velocities derived for a
given pulse repetition frequency. Flow **toward** the transducer is red on color Doppler and above the line on pulsed
Doppler, and flow **away** from the transducer is blue on
color Doppler and below the line on pulsed Doppler. Both
the scale (to a maximum value) and baseline can be adjusted as necessary.

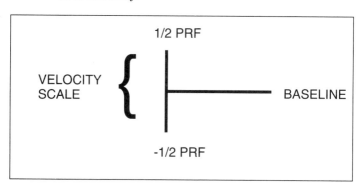

1/2 PRF

VELOCITY
SCALE                              BASELINE

-1/2 PRF

B. **Output (power)** increases the power of the pulse sent
from the transducer.
C. **Gain** amplifies the returning signal and noise depicted on
the screen. Separate switches control gray-scale gain, color
gain, and pulsed Doppler gain.
D. **The wall filter** is the threshold control to eliminate low-
frequency shift information (low velocity cut-off).
E. **The insonating angle** should be aligned parallel to the
vessel of interest. Best measurements are made when the
angle is less than 60 degrees.

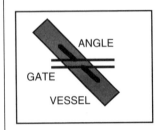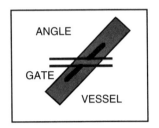

CHANGING ANGLE TO ALIGN WITH
VESSEL ORIENTATION

**F. The sample size** is the size of the area being interrogated.

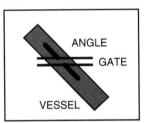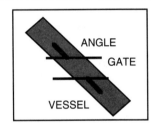

CHANGING SAMPLE VOLUME TO FIT
VESSEL SIZE

**G. The resistive index** (RI) is calculated as

$$\frac{\text{peak systolic velocity} - \text{peak diastolic velocity}}{\text{peak systolic velocity}}$$

or more simply

1 – diastolic velocity/systolic velocity

In vessels with high resistance, the diastolic flow will decrease relative to the systolic flow. This will, in turn, **increase** RI.

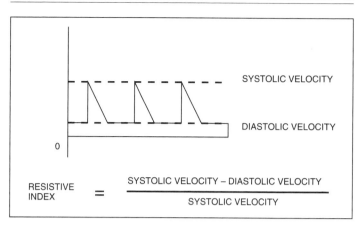

$$\text{RESISTIVE INDEX} = \frac{\text{SYSTOLIC VELOCITY} - \text{DIASTOLIC VELOCITY}}{\text{SYSTOLIC VELOCITY}}$$

## IV. Scanning strategies

### A. The general sequence for interrogating a vessel is as follows:

1. Use color Doppler to establish the location and direction of flow in the vessel of interest.
   a. Increase **gain** until background noise is visible, then reduce slightly.
   b. Decrease **wall filters** to lowest setting.
   c. Adjust the **steering angle** (ATL) or use a stand-off pad as needed.
2. Use **pulsed Doppler** to obtain waveform and velocity measurements.
   a. Move **gate** to vessel of interest.
   b. Align **angle** with vessel.
   c. Adjust **sample volume** if needed.
   d. Obtain **spectrum.**
   e. Adjust **baseline** and **velocity scale.**
   f. Freeze image.
3. Calculate RI if needed.

### B. For **Acuson 128XP/10**

1. "D color"
2. "D PW"
   a. Use trackball to move gate to vessel of interest.
   b. Toggle "angle" button to align the insonating angle parallel with the vessel.
   c. Toggle "scale" to set velocity range.
   d. Toggle "baseline" to optimize waveform depiction.
   e. "Freeze" image.
3. Calculate RI.
   a. "Calc/Select"
   b. Button number 4 (three times) to switch to RI
   c. Button number 3 (measure)
   d. Use trackball to move line to systolic (highest) peak of tracing.
   e. Button number 3 (enter)
   f. Button number 4 (maximal)
   g. Use trackball to move line to diastolic peak of tracing.
   h. Button number 3 (enter)

**C. For Sequoia 512**
1. "D Color"
2. "PW"
   a. Use trackball to move gate to vessel of interest.
   b. Use "angle" button to align the insonating angle parallel with the vessel.
   c. Toggle "scale" to set velocity range.
   d. Toggle "baseline" to optimize waveform depiction.
   e. "Freeze" image.
3. Calculate RI.
   a. "Calipers on/off," then move to systolic peak with trackball.
   b. "Add caliper," then move to diastolic peak with trackball.
   c. RI will automatically be displayed.

**D. For Quantum Quad 2000**
1. "Color flow"
2. "Spectrum"
   a. Use trackball to move gate to vessel of interest.
   b. Use knob to align insonating angle parallel with vessel.
   c. Button number 4 (sample vol), then knob to change sample volume (if needed).
   d. Button number 1 (spec & image) or button number 2 (spec only).
   e. "Select" twice to change velocity range.
   f. "Baseline," then use knob to optimize waveform depiction.
   g. Freeze image.
3. Calculate RI.
   a. "Marker"
   b. Use trackball to move line to systolic (highest) peak of tracing.
   c. Button number 1 (toggle)
   d. Use trackball to move line to diastolic peak of tracing.
   e. Button number 2 (Pourcelot's ratio)

**E. For ATL Ultramark 9**
1. "Color": "Steering angle" if needed
2. "DOP"
   a. Use trackball to move gate to vessel of interest.
   b. Toggle "angle/angle correction" to align insonating angle parallel with vessel.
   c. Toggle "sample size" to change sample volume.
   d. "DOP"
   e. Toggle "velocity range" as appropriate.
   f. Toggle "baseline" as appropriate.
   g. Freeze image.
   h. Press "additional DOP Fx."
   i. Press "split screen."
3. Calculate RI.
   a. "Calc"
   b. "Peaks"
   c. Use trackball to move line to systolic (highest) peak of tracing.
   d. "Set"
   e. Use trackball to move line to diastolic peak of tracing.
   f. "Enter"

**F.** For **Siemens Sonoline Elegra**
1. "Color": move trackball as needed.
2. Doppler
    **a.** Use trackball to move gate to vessel of interest.
    **b.** Toggle "angle correct" to align insonating angle parallel with vessel.
    **c.** Toggle "sample size" to change sample volume.
    **d.** "Update."
    **e.** Toggle "scale" as appropriate.
    **f.** Toggle "baseline" as appropriate.
    **g.** Freeze image.
3. Calculate RI.
    **a.** "RI" on touchscreen.
    **b.** "Caliper/next," then use trackball to systolic peak of tracing.
    **c.** "Caliper/next," then use trackball to diastolic peak of tracing.
**G.** For **GE Logiq 700 MR**
1. "CF"; move trackball as needed.
2. "PW"
    **a.** Use trackball to move gate to vessel of interest.
    **b.** Toggle "angle correct" to align insonating angle parallel with vessel.
    **c.** Toggle "sample size" to change sample volume.
    **d.** "Update."
    **e.** Toggle "scale" as appropriate.
    **f.** Toggle "baseline" as appropriate.
    **g.** Freeze image.
3. Calculate RI.
    **a.** "Caliper," then use trackball to systolic peak of tracing and press "set."
    **b.** "Caliper," then use trackball to diastolic peak of tracing and press "set."
    **c.** "Calc," then toggle on "Resis Index" on small screen.
**H.** Because different institutions use different machines, we provide a generalized scanning strategy in each section with an area to take notes. One of the most difficult things to remember when you begin taking call is which buttons to press to perform the correct function (especially at 3:00 A.M.). Before taking call, fill in the blanks with the appropriate information and refer to the section as needed.
**V. Pitfalls**
**A. Aliasing.** Artifact in which the highest velocity of a waveform tracing misplaced on the velocity scale and the waveform is seen at both the top and bottom of the scale. This occurs when the Doppler frequency shift is greater than ½ PRF.

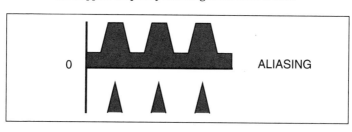

Adjust either the velocity range (increase PRF) or baseline to optimize waveform depiction or use a lower-frequency transducer (decreases magnitude of Doppler shift).

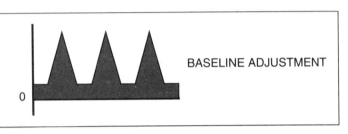

BASELINE ADJUSTMENT

0

**B. Insonating angle.** The best velocity information is achieved from vessels that are oriented vertically on the screen. The insonating angle should always be less than 60 degrees to obtain meaningful velocity information. Velocity information from vessels oriented horizontally is suspect.

**C. Sample volume.** With large sample volumes, vessel detection is improved; however, spectral broadening occurs since many different velocities are being sampled at once (due to laminar flow in a vessel). Thus, large sample volumes degrade the signal-to-noise ratio. Increasing the sample volume is done when searching for a vessel that may not be apparent on color flow imaging. For example, in imaging the hepatic artery in liver transplants, a "blind" search can be done by increasing the sample volume and slowly moving the gate along the portal vein in the expected course of the hepatic artery.

# Aortic Ultrasound

**I. Clinical history**

  **A. Pulsatile abdominal mass: rule out abdominal aortic aneurysm (AAA).** An **AAA** is enlargement of the aortic lumen to a diameter of greater than 3 cm. They are usually **infrarenal**, fusiform, and the result of atherosclerotic disease. Typically they enlarge at a rate of about 0.2 cm per year.

  **B. Indications for surgery**
   **1.** Size greater than 4–5 cm
   **2.** Pain
   **3.** Rapid increase in size
   **4.** Distal emboli
   **5.** Renal obstruction or hemorrhage
   If an aneurysm is **suprarenal**, etiologies other than atherosclerotic disease such as trauma, syphilis, or infection must also be considered.

**II. Imaging**

  **A.** Begin with a 3.5-MHz probe and attempt to follow the aorta from the diaphragm until it bifurcates in the lower abdomen. This is best done by using a **coronal** approach. Use color flow to distinguish between the aorta and inferior vena cava as necessary. Remember to keep the insonating angle less than 60 degrees by either scanning at an angle or using a stand-off pad.

**B.** In some patients, bowel gas will obscure the infrarenal aorta. If this occurs, proceed to CT.

**C.** If an aneurysm is seen, document the following:
   **1.** Location, length, and maximal diameter
   **2.** Extent of mural thrombus and calcification
   **3.** Patent channel (use color flow Doppler)
   **4.** Periaortic hemorrhage, masses, or lymph nodes—it is important not to confuse adenopathy with an aneurysm because both can appear hypoechoic
   **5.** Extension into the iliac arteries (1 cm normal diameter) or proximal aorta

**D.** On color flow images, an aneurysm may appear as swirling pixels of red, white, and blue in a "yin-yang" configuration (although this classically suggests a pseudoaneurysm). Using pulsed Doppler, a holosystolic waveform with or without turbulence is seen.

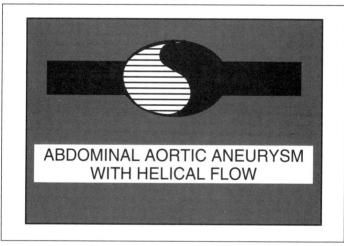

ABDOMINAL AORTIC ANEURYSM
WITH HELICAL FLOW

**E.** If the study is abnormal, perform a renal ultrasound to rule out hydronephrosis, which will affect the surgical decision-making process (there is increased risk at surgery if hydronephrosis is present).

**F.** Take images with size measurements of the proximal (normal ≤ 3 cm), mid (normal ≤ 2 cm), and distal (normal ≤ 1 cm) aorta if the study is normal.

## Ultrasound for Appendicitis

**I. Clinical history.** Common signs and symptoms include fever, right lower quadrant pain, nausea and vomiting, and leukocytosis.

## II. Imaging
### A. Plain films.
Always obtain plain films first. Other entities such as bowel obstruction may have similar presentations or coexist with appendicitis.

### B. Ultrasound scanning strategy
1. Ask the patient to point with one finger to the point of maximal tenderness.
2. Begin scanning the lateral right mid-abdomen in the transverse plane with a 5- or 7-MHz linear transducer.
3. Scan caudally, gradually increasing compression toward the point of maximal tenderness. (This helps push bowel gas away from the right lower quadrant.)

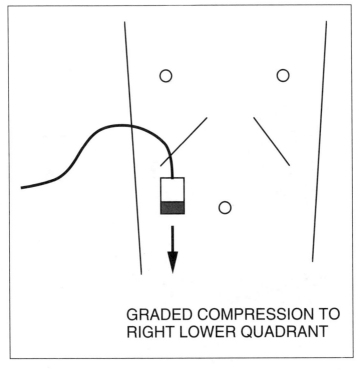

GRADED COMPRESSION TO
RIGHT LOWER QUADRANT

4. The appendix lies at the cecal tip. An abnormal appendix appears as a "bull's-eye" with an echogenic submucosal band surrounded by anechoic outer wall. Occasionally, a loop of bowel can be confused with an enlarged appendix; remember that **peristalsis** does not occur in the appendix. (It may not be possible to demonstrate the entire appendix on one image since it is curved in multiple planes.)
5. Scanning more caudally will demonstrate the psoas and iliac muscles and the external iliac artery and vein.
6. A retrocecal appendix can usually be visualized by scanning coronally and transversely using a lateral approach.

### III. Interpretation
#### A. Plain films
1. An appendicolith (occurs in 10% of cases of acute appendicitis) with abdominal pain has a greater than 90% probability of acute appendicitis (often with gangrene and perforation).
2. A localized right lower quadrant ileus ("sentinel loop")
3. Usually **no free air**

#### B. Ultrasound
1. Noncompressible tubular structure with a blind end measuring 6 mm or more (outer wall to outer wall) in diameter
2. Mural wall thickness 2 mm or more
3. Appendicolith
4. Periappendiceal abscess: loss of submucosal layer of appendix with surrounding complex fluid collection

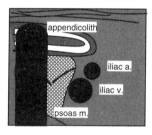 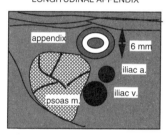

TRANSVERSE APPENDIX    LONGITUDINAL APPENDIX

**VARIABLE POSITIONS OF THE APPENDIX
ON A TRANSVERSE IMAGE OF THE RLQ**

#### C. Pitfalls
1. Inspissated stool mimicking an appendicolith
2. Grossly enlarged appendix (1.5–2.0 cm) mimicking bowel
3. Hydrosalpinx
4. Focal appendicitis: the body of the appendix may appear normal with inflammation localized to the distal tip.

# Ultrasound-Guided Aspiration

### I. Clinical history
#### A. Mark ascites for diagnostic paracentesis. When looking for free fluid in the abdomen, remember that the most dependent portions of the peritoneal cavity (in supine position) are the hepatorenal recess (Morison's pouch) and pelvic cul-de-sac. If fluid is not seen in either of these two regions, there probably is not enough ascites (if there is any at all) to tap or the fluid is loculated.
#### B. Mark effusion for diagnostic thoracentesis.

## II. Imaging
### A. Abdomen
1. Use either a 3.5- or 5.0-MHz sector probe and place the patient in the position that will be used for paracentesis.
2. Scan the entire abdomen and pelvis, searching for a pocket of fluid amenable to tap. There should be no bowel or other organs between the fluid and abdominal wall. If a suitable collection is found, measure the depth to abdominal structures (e.g., bowel) and give the clinical service an estimate of the overall size of the collection. This can be done by multiplying length × width × height × 0.5 (volume of a prolate ellipse).
3. Mark the skin surface.

### B. Thorax
1. Review the CXR to determine size and location of pleural effusion.
2. Use a 5-MHz **linear transducer** and apply the probe directly to the chest. (A sector scanner that allows scanning through the ribs can also be used but may be limited due to its narrow near field of view and because the pleural space is frequently obscured by near-field artifact.)
3. Use the ribs as landmarks, and when fluid is seen, measure the distance from the skin surface to fluid (i.e., thickness of subcutaneous tissues and muscle). The underlying lung should always be seen moving (with respect to fluid) with respiration.
4. If no fluid is seen using the direct approach, use a 3.5-MHz sector scanner and scan cranially from the abdomen through the liver or spleen. Even if fluid is seen using this approach, there may not be enough for thoracentesis.

### C. Pitfalls.
Effusions may be echogenic or contain septations, making them difficult to differentiate from solid tissue. In general, if the suspicious area moves and changes shape with respiration, it can be safely aspirated.

---

# Ultrasound for Ectopic Pregnancy

## I. Clinical history
### A. Ruling out ectopic pregnancy
1. **Signs and symptoms:** adnexal mass, bleeding, and pain 3–5 weeks after last menstrual period. This classic triad occurs in less than 50% of women with ectopic pregnancies.
2. Any clinically stable patient at risk for ectopic pregnancy should be considered for ultrasound.
3. Death occurs in 1 per 5000 women with ectopic pregnancies.

### B. Risk factors.
Any process that results in tubal scarring increases the risk for ectopic pregnancy. A history of pelvic inflammatory disease is found in about half of women with ectopic pregnancies. Other risk factors include prior ectopic pregnancy, fertility drugs, intrauterine device in place, in vitro fertilization, and prior tubal surgery.

C. **Pregnancy test results.** Never search for an ectopic pregnancy without a pregnancy test since a negative test excludes pregnancy. There are several types of pregnancy tests.
   1. **Enzyme-linked immunosorbent assay (ELISA)** (qualitative) is rapid and sensitive and does not require specialized personnel to perform.
   2. **Radioimmunoassay (RIA)** (quantitative) for measuring serial beta-human chorionic gonadotropin ($\beta$-hCG) levels. (These are critical if ultrasound findings are equivocal.) To further confuse matters, two available standards for quantifying $\beta$-hCG levels are used. It is imperative to know which standard your hospital is using. The older **Second International Standard (SIS) levels** are approximately one-half the newer **International Reference Preparation (IRP) levels** (i.e., 1000 mIU/ml SIS = 2000 mIU/ml IRP).

II. **Imaging**
   A. **Overall strategy**
      1. If the patient's bladder is full, begin scanning the pelvis transabdominally with a 3.5-MHz transducer.
      2. Attempt to **document an intrauterine pregnancy (IUP)**. If an IUP is not seen, look for signs of an ectopic gestation.
      3. If your findings are equivocal or the bladder is empty, proceed to an endovaginal examination. (For medicolegal reasons, if you are a man, make sure that a woman observer accompanies you into the room during the examination.) An endovaginal examination allows detection of an IUP approximately 1 week earlier than an abdominal examination. A gestational sac should be seen endovaginally with $\beta$-hCG levels of 1000 mIU/ml SIS (2000 mIU/ml IRP) and transabdominally with $\beta$-hCG levels of 1800 mIU/ml SIS (3600 mIU/ml IRP).
      4. See the table on page 32.
   B. **Important facts**
      1. Gestational age = menstrual age – 2 weeks (most ultrasound measurements are given in menstrual age).
      2. Mean sac diameter = (length + weight + height) ÷ 3. The gestational sac grows 1.1 mm/day in normal pregnancies.
      3. $\beta$-hCG appears 8 days after conception and doubles every 2–3 days up to 8 weeks. Low or slow-rising levels are consistent with ectopic pregnancy. $\beta$-hCG and mean sac diameter increase proportionally—discordance suggests demise.
      4. You must see the embryo transabdominally when the gestational sac is greater than 25 mm. You must see the yolk sac when the gestational sac is greater than 20 mm.
      5. A crown–rump length of more than 5 mm with no identification of cardiac activity (endovaginally) is diagnostic of fetal death.

III. **Interpretation**
   A. **Intrauterine pregnancy**
      1. **Uterus**
         a. **Decidua-chorionic sac sign (or "double decidual sac sign)**
            (1) Represents chorion and decidua parietalis

| Menstrual age (wks) | β-hCG (SIS) | Gestational sac size (mm) | Yolk sac | Crown–rump length (mm) | Heartbeat |
|---|---|---|---|---|---|
| 5 | 1000 | 3 | | | Begins |
| 5.5 | 2000 | 6 | +endovaginal | | |
| 6 | 5000 | 10 | | 3 | ±endovaginal |
| 6.5 | 10,000 | 15 | | 6 | +endovaginal |
| 7 | 20,000 | 20 | | 10 | |

(2) Should be more than 2 mm thick

(3) If the mean sac diameter is less than 10 mm, this finding may not yet be visible transabdominally.

**b. Gestational sac**

(1) Round or oval hypoechoic area in uterine fundus

(2) Low resistive index color flow adjacent to site

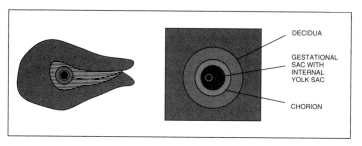

DECIDUA

GESTATIONAL SAC WITH INTERNAL YOLK SAC

CHORION

**c. Yolk sac**

(1) Small round hypoechoic area within the gestational sac

(2) Normally present if gestational sac is 8 mm or more endovaginally or 20 mm or more transabdominally

(3) Appearance precedes embryo by 1.0–1.5 weeks.

**d. Embryo**

(1) Ill-defined echogenic blob adjacent to the yolk sac

(2) Normally present if gestational sac is 18 mm or more endovaginally or 25 mm or more transabdominally

(3) Fetal heart activity normally present if embryo is 5 mm or more endovaginally or 10 mm or more transabdominally

**e. Doppler.** Peak systolic velocity of endometrial arteries greater than 20 cm/s is commonly seen with IUP.

2. **Adnexa.** Corpus luteum cyst: hypoechoic or anechoic cyst in an ovary

B. **Ectopic pregnancy.** The only sign that is absolutely diagnostic of an ectopic pregnancy is a live extrauterine embryo (i.e., there is cardiac activity). An extrauterine gestational sac with a yolk sac is also generally considered diagnostic of ectopic pregnancy. Either of these findings occur in approximately one-third of ectopic pregnancies. Most radiologists believe that absence of an IUP with β-hCG levels greater than 1000 in the proper clinical setting is diagnostic of ectopic pregnancy. The following are other signs suggestive of ectopic gestation:

1. **Uterus. Pseudogestational sac:** only a single layer of decidua seen without adjacent increased blood flow; may represent abnormal IUP.

2. **Adnexa**

**a. Adnexal ring**

(1) Hypoechoic area adjacent to the ovary (usually between the cornu of the uterus and ovary) containing the yolk sac or embryo.

      **(2)** Surrounded by increased color flow with a resistive index less than 0.3 ("ring of fire")—directly proportional to β-hCG levels.

      **(3)** A corpus luteum cyst may be difficult to distinguish from an adnexal ring. To differentiate the two, apply gentle, firm pressure on the suspected ring with either the probe or your hand to determine if it is separate from the ovary. If the ring glides over the surface of the ovary ("sliding organ sign"), it is separate from the ovary and does not represent a corpus luteum cyst. The diagnosis of an ectopic pregnancy is favored.

    **b. Hematosalpinx:** enlarged, echogenic tube

**3. Cul-de-sac: Free fluid**

    **a.** Nonspecific finding

    **b.** If echogenic, it more likely represents blood and has a greater specificity for ectopic pregnancy

    **c.** May be seen with intact, rupturing, or aborting ectopic pregnancy

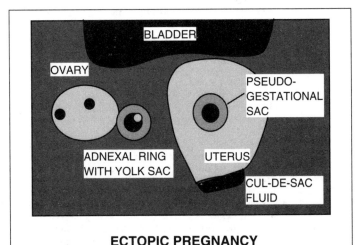

**ECTOPIC PREGNANCY**

**C. Indeterminate study**

    **1.** No definitive evidence of the findings discussed above with positive β-hCG

    **2.** May represent normal early IUP, small ectopic pregnancy, or abnormal or aborted IUP

    **3.** Recommend follow-up with serial β-hCG levels and ultrasound or laparoscopy

**IV. Pitfalls**

**A. Coexisting ectopic and intrauterine pregnancy**

    **1.** Occurs in approximately 1 in 30,000 pregnancies in women **without** risk factors.

    **2.** In women with risk factors for ectopic pregnancy (e.g., fertility drugs) the risk is approximately 1 in 5000 pregnancies.

**B. Uterine blood flow.** Increased blood flow with low RI can occur with tubo-ovarian abscess, corpus luteum cyst, or fibroids.

**C. Overdistended bladder:** can push fluid out of cul-de-sac

**D. Cornual pregnancy**
   1. Implantation in the interstitial portion of the tube may mimic an intrauterine pregnancy.
   2. There is a high risk of bleeding and death with rupture.
   3. The **"line sign"** consists of the endometrial lining extending to the border of the ectopic pregnancy.

**E. Decidual cysts:** anechoic, thin-walled endometrial cysts that may simulate IUP

**F. Ectopic pregnancy mimics**
   1. Tubo-ovarian abscess
   2. Mesenteric cysts: not thin-walled
   3. Pedunculated fibroids: hypoechoic, occasionally calcified
   4. Bowel: peristalsis
   5. Ovarian cysts

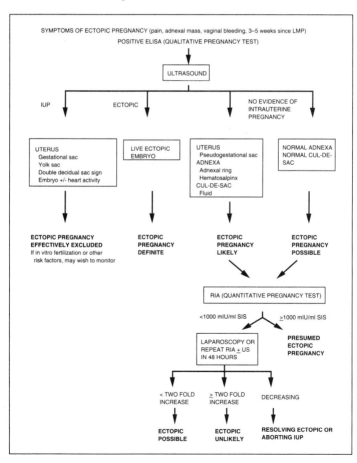

# Gallbladder Ultrasound

I. **Clinical history**
   A. **The patient's last meal.** Fasting for a minimum of 6–8 hours is required. Usually, the gallbladder can be seen and stones excluded even if a patient has had a recent meal; however, the gallbladder may be partially or completely contracted, so wall thickness cannot be used as an indicator of acute cholecystitis.
   B. **History of abdominal surgery.** Always check the abdominal plain film for cholecystectomy clips in the right upper quadrant. Do not be surprised if either the referring physician or the patient does not realize a cholecystectomy has already been performed.

II. **Scanning strategy**
   A. Place the patient supine and use a 3.5- or 5-MHz probe scan from a low intercostal or subcostal approach.
   B. The gallbladder will be a hollow viscus in the region of the portal vein origin that does not show color flow.
   C. The common bile duct (CBD) is usually found directly anterior to the portal vein. Use color flow to distinguish between the hepatic artery and the CBD.
   D. Take at least 6–12 images. Remember to take both longitudinal and transverse images of the gallbladder as well as to scan the patient in several positions (supine, sitting, left lateral decubitus). Occasionally, a stone will not be visualized until different positions are used.

III. **Interpretation**
   A. **Acute cholecystitis**
      1. **Ultrasonic Murphy's sign**
         a. Exquisite tenderness directly over the gallbladder only, not elsewhere
         b. Very high positive predictive value (>90%) for acute cholecystitis in a patient with gallstones
      2. **Wall thickness/vascularity**
         a. Normal is less than 2–3 mm (fasting)
         b. The most common cause of wall thickening in a fasting patient is liver disease, not acute cholecystitis. Other causes include congestive heart failure (CHF), renal disease, chemotherapy, and AIDS.
      3. **Pericholecystic fluid collection:** indicative of acute cholecystitis with perforation and abscess
   B. **Common bile duct obstruction**
      1. **Common bile duct**
         a. Normal is less than 6 mm from outer wall to outer wall
         b. Enlargement implies obstruction (partial or complete) that has been present for at least 24 hours.
         c. Possible etiologies: common duct stone, stricture, pancreatic disease/neoplasm, papilla of Vater lesion
      2. **Intrahepatic bile duct dilatation**
         a. "Double barrel" sign (portal vein branches and dilated bile ducts)
         b. Absence of color flow in large intrahepatic tubular structures (bile ducts)
         c. Indicates a more chronic (>1 week) obstruction

**C. Cholelithiasis (calculi):** echogenic foci that produce shadowing when located at the focal spot
**D. Sludge (concentrated bile)**
  **1.** Bile stasis usually due to prolonged fasting or obstruction
  **2.** Moves slowly with positional change
**E. Acalculous cholecystitis** (diagnosis of exclusion)
  **1.** Usually in bedridden patients with severe intercurrent illnesses such as burns, trauma, or AIDS
  **2.** High incidence of gallbladder perforation with gangrene
  **3.** Findings may be absent or similar to acute cholecystitis (e.g., wall thickening or pericholecystic fluid)

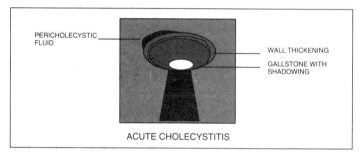

ACUTE CHOLECYSTITIS

**IV. Pitfalls**
  **A. Ringdown artifact** ("comet tail" or "dirty shadowing") from air in the duodenum adjacent to the gallbladder can be confused with acoustic shadowing from gallstones.
  **B. Hepatic fluid collection** (biloma, abscess, or cyst) can be confused for the gallbladder.
  **C. Emphysematous cholecystitis** produces marked acoustic shadowing that can be confused for a gallbladder filled with stones. A plain film may show gas in the gallbladder wall.
  **D. A single calculus** impacted in the gallbladder neck can cause acute cholecystitis and be difficult to visualize.
  **E. Wall-echo-shadow triad.** If the gallbladder is filled with stones, the only finding may be shadowing behind the gallbladder (i.e., anechoic region in the gallbladder fossa). The wall-echo-shadow (WES) complex may also be seen.

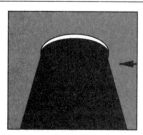

WALL-ECHO-SHADOW TRIAD

See the section on hepatobiliary scan in Ch. 7.

# Liver Transplant Ultrasound

I. **Clinical history: Elevation of liver enzymes after transplant. Assess the patency of the vessels.** The crux of this examination lies in demonstrating the presence or absence of flow in the hepatic artery, which thromboses in 3–10% of transplant recipients. The hepatic artery is necessary to sustain the biliary ductal anastomosis. If it is occluded, the patient is taken to the operating room; if not, he or she is usually monitored.

II. **Overall scanning strategy**
   A. Use either a 3.5- or 5-MHz probe and start to scan immediately to the right superior aspect of the intersection of the patient's incision. (If the transplanted organ is a left lateral segment, the hilum will be found at the transected edge at the right.)

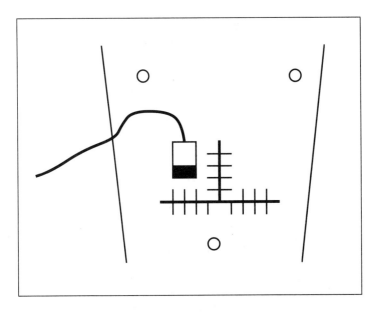

   B. Use color Doppler to find the portal vein.
   C. The hepatic artery runs parallel to the portal vein and is frequently quite large in transplant patients. If the artery is not seen immediately, try "fishing" for it with Doppler by enlarging the sample volume and slowly moving the gate along the portal vein. Listen for the characteristic sound of arterial flow and watch for an arterial Doppler waveform.
   D. Take images with waveforms of the portal vein, hepatic artery, and three branches of the hepatic vein.

III. **Tips**
   A. **General examination.** Many of these examinations are done portably. Make sure you know *where* the patient is

located. If the machine is not equipped with an optical disk, remember to bring film cassettes and gel with the machine.

1. Load the film and turn on the machine.

2. Scan the right upper quadrant and locate the porta hepatis.

3. Magnify the area of interest. Activate an "area of interest" box. Change the size or position of the box as necessary. Once you have the area desired in the box, enlarge the area.

4. Activate color flow. The portal vein should be the largest red vessel. Since the hepatic artery flows in the same direction as the portal vein, it will also appear red but may be "pulsatile" since flow varies with the cardiac cycle.

5. Activate pulsed Doppler and move the gate to the area of interest (hepatic artery); toggle on to see the waveform. The insonating angle should be less than 60 degrees. If the hepatic artery waveform is not seen, hit "toggle off" to see color flow or disable pulsed Doppler waveform function altogether. (Most machine functions are "toggle on–toggle off.")

6. Once the hepatic artery waveform is seen, several parameters may need to be adjusted before freezing the image.

   a. **Gate:** enlarges or decreases sample size. A large gate is better when searching for the vessel and a small gate is better once the vessel is found.

   b. **Scale:** changes the velocity scale by adjusting the PRF. Change this parameter if the waveform is either too large (aliasing) or too small compared to scale.

   c. **Baseline:** moves the zero position up or down on the velocity scale.

Once these parameters are correct (i.e., the waveform fills the template without aliasing), freeze the image.

7. Scroll back as needed and label the image (e.g., hepatic a.). _____

8. Expose the film. Many machines are equipped with a filming system using an optical disk. _____ _____

9. If the machine is equipped with a portable color printer, take a color image. If your gray-scale images do not turn out well (not an uncommon occurrence when you first start residency), you will have a color image of the hepatic artery and will not have to repeat the most difficult part of the exam. Repeat the above steps to obtain waveforms of the portal vein (get left, right, and middle if possible) and three branches of the hepatic vein. Remember to angle the transducer cephalad to visualize the hepatic veins as they enter the inferior vena cava. _____

B. "Last ditch" effort
1. If nothing resembling the hepatic artery is seen on color images, try "fishing" for it as follows: _____
   a. Find the porta hepatis and enlarge the area. _____
   b. Activate the pulsed Doppler, then increase the size of the **gate** as wide as possible. _____
   c. Slowly move the gate along the portal vein. **Listen** and watch for the arterial waveform superimposed on the portal vein tracing. _____

2. If the artery is found, decrease the size of the gate to obtain a better tracing (i.e., eliminate the unwanted waveform from the adjacent portal vein). _____

3. Print the image. _____

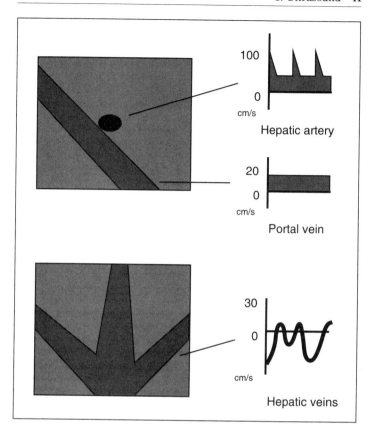

100
0
cm/s
Hepatic artery

20
0
cm/s
Portal vein

30
0
cm/s
Hepatic veins

## IV. Pitfalls
A. A **pulsus parvus-tardus waveform** (which may occur distal to any arterial stenosis) can be confused with portal venous flow. In this manner, a stenotic, patent hepatic artery may be confused with the portal vein and lead one to mistakenly believe that the hepatic artery is occluded.
B. ICUs tend to be very well lit. Ambient light creates an annoying glare on the monitor. Ask the ICU personnel to turn off as many lights as possible and resist the temptation to turn up the gray-scale gain because this will result in overexposed images ("snowstorm" effect).

# Lower Extremity Venous Doppler Ultrasound

## I. Clinical history
A. **Patient with a swollen, hot, painful leg.** An emergency deep venous thrombosis (DVT) study should be performed on a patient who has unilateral leg symptoms **in**

the absence of pulmonary symptoms. If the patient has pulmonary symptoms, proceed directly to a ventilation-perfusion (V̇/Q̇) scan.

**B. Risk factors for DVT** include cancer, trauma, prolonged immobilization, leg injury, hypercoagulable states, and oral contraceptives.

**C. Bilateral symptoms.** In patients with bilateral symptoms (in the absence of trauma), the yield of lower extremity ultrasound is very low and probably should not be performed emergently.

## II. Anatomy

**A. Deep veins:** common femoral vein, superficial femoral vein, deep femoral vein (profunda), popliteal, anterior tibial, peroneal, posterior tibial

**B. Superficial veins:** greater and lesser saphenous

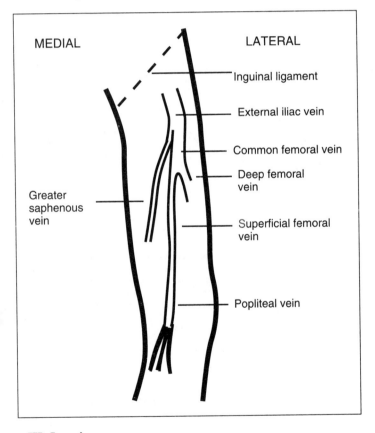

## III. Imaging

**A.** Both **duplex Doppler compression ultrasound (DDCU)** and **color Doppler imaging (CDI)** are very sensitive and specific for evaluation of suspected lower extremity DVT; they should be considered complementary exams. The American College of Radiology recommends DDCU as the single most appropriate study for suspected DVT. At our institution residents are taught to use CDI as the initial study, with DDCU reserved for equivocal areas. On call we frequently use both techniques.

**B.** Concentrate your efforts on the **CFV** and **popliteal vein.** If these appear normal, DVT elsewhere in the deep venous system is unlikely.

**C. Color Doppler imaging**

  **1.** Place the patient supine with the head slightly **above** the level of the legs. This will help distend the leg veins.

  **2.** Abduct and externally rotate the leg of interest.

  **3.** Use a 5-MHz linear probe and scan the common femoral vein from the inguinal ligament inferiorly to the superficial femoral vein and finally to the popliteal vein until the trifurcation in the calf. Use Doppler waveforms to differentiate vein from artery if necessary.

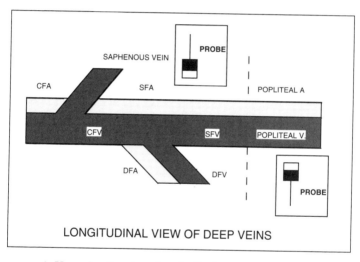

LONGITUDINAL VIEW OF DEEP VEINS

  **4.** Use color flow in a longitudinal orientation with or without Doppler waveforms. In a normal study, obtain images of the CFV, bifurcation, SFV, and popliteal vein at minimum. Our personal preference is to take longitudinal color pictures with Doppler waveforms (with Valsalva and calf augmentation) of these areas.

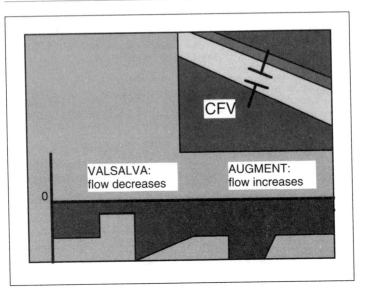

5. If a DVT is identified, take images of the abnormal area and attempt to document the proximal extent of the clot.

**D. Duplex Doppler compression ultrasound**

1. Compress at 1-cm intervals in the transverse plane from the CFV to the popliteal vein. The vein should be easily compressible (i.e., both walls of the vein should coapt before the accompanying artery) in all areas except at the adductor canal, where color flow imaging may need to be used.

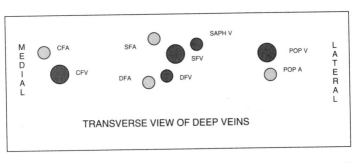

TRANSVERSE VIEW OF DEEP VEINS

2. Attempt to augment flow by squeezing the patient's calf or having the patient plantarflex, then dorsiflex the foot ("gas pedal maneuver").

3. If a DVT is identified, take images of the abnormal area and attempt to document the proximal extent of the clot.

**IV. Interpretation**

**A. Normal study**

1. Color flow fills vein.

   **2.** Vein is compressible.
   **3.** Normal respiratory variation and augmentation. Velocity is extremely variable—from 1–20 cm/s.
**B. Acute DVT**
   **1. Vein not compressible**
      **a.** If the accompanying artery is compressed but the vein is not, this is diagnostic of a DVT.
      **b.** Often, the clot will expand the vein.
   **2. No evidence of color flow.** In (Hunter's) adductor canal near the knee, neither the SFV or artery may be compressible in many patients who do not have DVT; thus, color flow may need to be used.
   **3. Visualized thrombus:** may be hypoechoic, hyperechoic, or virtually anechoic. Acute thrombus tends to be anechoic to hypoechoic and increases in echogenicity over time.
   **4. Doppler waveform**
      **a.** Absence of normal respiratory phasic variation or no change with Valsalva maneuver suggests a thrombus cephalad to probe.
      **b.** Absence of augmentation with calf compression is suggestive of thrombus lower in the extremity (i.e., between the probe and the calf).
**C. Chronic DVT**
   **1.** Vein with thickened, irregular walls and/or irregular, narrowed lumen
   **2.** Numerous adjacent venous collateral vessels
**V. U of C examination.** These are done with the Quantum Quad 2000.
   **1.** Select 5-MHz linear transducer. Attach stand-off pad to probe with gel if needed, then turn on machine.                                             _____
   **2.** Select exam type ("extremities").                                             _____
   **3.** Type in patient information.                                             _____
   **4.** Turn on color printer and adjust as necessary.                                             _____
   **5.** Begin scanning in the groin and proceed inferiorly. Find the CFV where it bifurcates into the DFV and SFV using a medium flow setting                                             _____
   **6.** Freeze and print the image in either gray-scale or color.                                             _____
   **7.** Perform compression, augmentation, and Valsalva as necessary.                                             _____
   **8.** Activate pulsed Doppler.                                             _____
   **9.** Move gate to the artery of interest, then align the gate parallel to this artery (the angle should be less than 60 degrees; this is shown in the upper right-hand corner of the screen of most machines).
   **10.** Toggle on pulsed Doppler to obtain a waveform.                                             _____
   **11.** If the waveform exceeds the

velocity scale (aliasing), several adjustments can be made.

**a. Baseline** _____

**b. Velocity scale** _____

Once the waveform fits the velocity scale, freeze the image. Perform compression, augmentation, and Valsalva as necessary.

12. Label the image (e.g., L CFV). _____

13. Print the image. _____

## VI. Pitfalls

A. **Color flow is not seen or does not completely fill the vein.** Try the following maneuvers:
1. "Gas pedal maneuver"
2. Compress above the level of the probe.
3. Squeeze the calf.
4. Increase gain.
5. Decrease PRF.
6. Increase the field of view.

Be careful not to artifactually fill a vein containing thrombus with color; if color flow extends beyond the wall of the vessel, increase the flow setting (PRF) or decrease the gain.

B. **Wrong color in the vessels**
1. Change the flow direction.
2. Remember that the artery has momentary flow reversal during diastole and will briefly appear blue (exacerbated by CHF).

C. **No flow in adductor canal**
1. Scan the popliteal vein using Doppler waveforms.
2. Ask the patient to hold his or her breath, then exhale. The waveform should not change if there is occlusive thrombus cephalad to the probe.

D. **Scanning the popliteal fossa**
1. The patient can be turned prone or the leg simply flexed at the knee. It may be helpful to scan in the transverse plane if longitudinal images are confusing.
2. Remember that on longitudinal images, in the thigh, the SFV is **below** the SFA. At the knee, the probe is moved from an anterior to posterior orientation so the popliteal vein appears on **top** of the popliteal artery.

# Ultrasound for Pelvic Pain

## I. Clinical history

A. **Young woman with negative β-hCG and pelvic pain.** The most common etiologies of pelvic pain in a young woman with a negative pregnancy test include pelvic inflammatory disease (PID), ovarian torsion, appendicitis, and hemorrhagic ovarian cyst.

## II. Imaging

A. If the patient's bladder is full, begin scanning the pelvis transabdominally with a 3.5-MHz transducer.

**B.** If your findings are equivocal or the bladder is empty, proceed to an endovaginal examination. (For medicolegal reasons, if you are a man, make sure a woman observer accompanies you into the room during the exam.)

## III. Interpretation

**A. Pelvic inflammatory disease.** Adnexal and cervical motion tenderness is common.

1. Endometritis: fluid in the endometrial canal
2. Uterine enlargement with ill-defined contour
3. Pyosalpinx
4. Tubo-ovarian abscess: complex fluid collection with or without gas in the adnexal region

**B. Ovarian torsion** presents with acute onset of pain. Dermoids are found in approximately 50% of cases. Other risk factors include ovarian hyperstimulation due to infertility drugs, pregnancy, and youth.

1. Ovary
   a. Enlargement
      (1) Length × height × width × 0.5 (volume of prolate ellipse)
      (2) Normal: 2.5–22.0 cc
      (3) Torsion: 26–440 cc (average diameter approximately 8 cm)
      (4) Compare to normal side.
   b. Contains scattered small peripheral cysts (follicles)
   c. Commonly located in the midline
2. Free fluid (50%)
3. Doppler imaging is a controversial topic. Neither the positive nor negative findings are well established but may be helpful in conjunction with other findings. Comparison of side-to-side intraovarian blood flow should be performed. The absence of flow on the symptomatic side with normal flow on the contralateral side strongly suggests torsion.

**C. Hemorrhagic cysts** usually occur in younger women (<40 years) and commonly present with pain.

1. Highly variable appearance
   a. Fluid and debris
   b. Septations
   c. Hyperechoic clot
   d. Free fluid
2. Consider malignancy in older women.

## OVARIAN LESIONS

### NORMAL OVARY

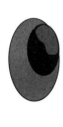

Follicles
2 x 3 x 4 (<15 cm³)

### FUNCTIONAL CYST

F/U 6 weeks

### SEPTATED CYST

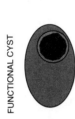

F/U 6 weeks

### HEMORRHAGIC CYST

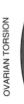

Rapidly changing
Acoustic enhancement
Common in younger patients
May have ANY appearance
F/U 6 weeks

### ENDOMETRIOMA

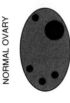

Fluid fluid level
Swirling low level echoes
Bright speckles

### DERMOID/TERATOMA

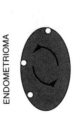

May contain calcium/hair/fat
Differential shadowing/echogenicity
Usually excised
Rokitansky nodule

### OVARIAN TORSION

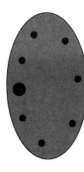

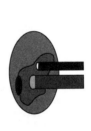

Enlarged (>25–440 cm³)
Peripheral follicles

# Placental Ultrasound

**I. Clinical history**

   **A. Second- and third-trimester bleeding or pain. Placenta previa** occurs in approximately 0.5% of pregnancies and usually presents with painless vaginal bleeding in the second or third trimester. It is an indication for cesarean section because vaginal delivery may result in extensive hemorrhage. **Placental abruption** occurs when the placenta separates from the uterus. It is usually painful and may or may not have associated vaginal bleeding. Abruption can be a life-threatening event for both mother and fetus. Both placental abruption and placenta previa are more common with older age, multiparity, and prior cesarean sections.

**II. Imaging**

   **A.** Place the patient in a supine or Trendelenburg position and scan transabdominally with a 3.5-MHz probe. Gentle traction on the fetal head may be necessary in some near-term pregnancies.

   **B.** The bladder should be only partially full. Overfilling can artificially elongate the cervical canal (normal <3.5 cm), causing a normal placenta to appear to be near or over the internal cervical os.

   **C.** Note the location of the placenta (anterior, posterior, or fundal) in the uterus.

   **D.** Transperineal ultrasound technique may be helpful in difficult cases.

     **1.** Empty bladder.

     **2.** Place a 3.5-MHz probe directly on the perineum over the labia minora.

     **3.** The cervical canal will be oriented vertically on the screen.

   **E.** Gentle endovaginal scanning can also be performed.

**III. Interpretation**

   **A. Placenta previa:** placenta implanting over the cervical os. The fetus is often in a transverse lie.

     **1.** Low-lying placenta: placenta within 2 cm of os

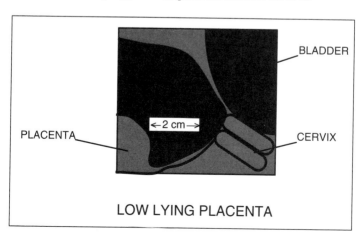

LOW LYING PLACENTA

**2.** Marginal placenta: placenta ends at margin of os without covering it

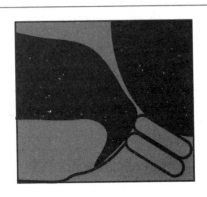

**MARGINAL PLACENTA**

**3.** Partial placenta previa: implantation on one side of os covering os

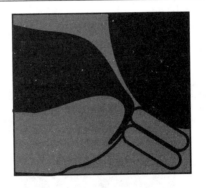

**PARTIAL PLACENTA PREVIA**

**4.** Complete placenta previa: implantation on both sides of os

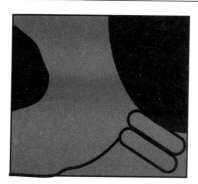

## COMPLETE PLACENTA PREVIA

5. **Pitfalls.** Several common conditions mimic placenta previa.
   a. **Full bladder**
      (1) Can efface the anterior myometrium and elongate the cervical canal, mimicking the appearance of a placenta previa in a normal pregnancy.
      (2) The normal cervical canal length should be less than 3.5 cm.
      (3) Have the patient partially empty the bladder and rescan.
   b. **Placental contraction**
      (1) Contraction of the lower uterine segment can mimic the placenta or lift the edge of the placenta, mimicking a placenta previa.
      (2) The normal placenta thickness approximately equals maternal age in weeks (<4 cm thick at term).
      (3) Wait 30 minutes and rescan.
      (4) Other causes of a large placenta include Rh incompatibility, maternal anemia, maternal diabetes, and in utero infection.
   c. **Second trimester**
      (1) A "pseudo–placenta previa" commonly occurs in the second trimester. As the pregnancy progresses, this situation resolves. Resolution may be due to differential growth rates of the lower myometrium and placenta.
      (2) If the placenta is implanted on both sides of the cervical os (i.e., complete placenta previa), the condition will not resolve and cesarean section is indicated.
B. **Placental abruption:** bleeding between the placenta and uterus that is associated with preterm labor and delivery. Hematomas larger than 60 ml are associated with

increased fetal mortality. An estimate of the size of the hematoma can be made by multiplying length × width × height × 0.5 (volume of prolate ellipse).

1. Retroplacental abruption
   a. Arterial hemorrhage
   b. Can be asymptomatic but usually is painful
   c. If separation of more than 30% of the placenta occurs, fetal hypoxia can result.
   d. Associated with cocaine abuse
   e. Occasional vaginal bleeding
2. Subchorionic hemorrhage
   a. Venous hemorrhage
   b. Vaginal bleeding common
   c. Usually asymptomatic and without significance if small
   d. Common early presentation (<20 weeks' gestation)

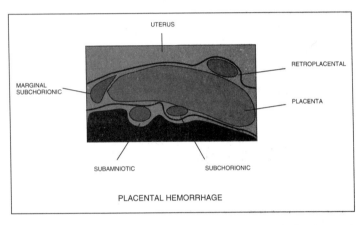

PLACENTAL HEMORRHAGE

3. **Pitfalls.** Many conditions can mimic or hide placental abruption.
   a. False-negative studies
      (1) Blood may be isoechoic with the placenta.
   b. False-positive studies (mimics)
      (1) Leiomyoma (fibroid): need to compare with previous studies
      (2) Uterine contraction: wait for 30 minutes and rescan.
      (3) Chorioangioma
      (4) Mole
      (5) Normal vascular structures (maternal lakes, marginal sinuses, basal veins): use color Doppler imaging. Multiple sonolucent placental masses are usually insignificant.

# Renal Ultrasound

I. **Clinical history**
   A. **Choosing between CT, ultrasound, or excretory uro-**

**gram (IVU).** There is no general consensus regarding the imaging evaluation of suspected renal colic. The three popular modalities—IVU, noninfused helical CT, and ultrasound (with or without abdominal radiograph)—have comparable sensitivities and specificities for renal obstruction. Traditionally, IVU was the study of choice and still provides the best overall anatomic evaluation of the urinary tract if intervention is planned. Ultrasound is generally the study of choice for pregnant women and children since exposure to ionizing radiation is eliminated. Recently, noninfused helical CT has been used and may provide the most rapid information with the added benefit of visualization of other abdominal and pelvic structures.

**B. History of renal disease.** Medical renal disease from any cause can result in small echogenic kidneys with a loss of definition of the central sinus fat complex.

**C. Contrast allergy.** If the patient has a contrast allergy, perform a noninfused helical CT examination or ultrasound instead of the IVU.

**D. BUN and creatinine.** Elevation of either is not an absolute contraindication to IVP; however, a creatinine above 1.5 mg/dl is associated with higher risk of acute tubular necrosis. Again, suggest a noninfused helical CT or ultrasound examination.

## II. Imaging

**A. General examination**

1. Place the patient in a supine position and scan with a 3.5-MHz probe.
2. Use a subcostal or low costal approach to visualize the right kidney (using the liver as an acoustic window).
3. The left kidney is more difficult to demonstrate; turn the patient on his or her right side and scan through the flank or back, using the spleen as an acoustic window if possible.
4. Use color Doppler with or without Doppler waveforms to distinguish large vessels from dilated calyces.
5. Scan the kidneys in both the transverse and longitudinal direction and obtain appropriate size measurements.
6. Attempt to visualize the ureter (especially if there is hydronephrosis).
7. Scan the bladder in both the longitudinal and transverse planes. Use color Doppler to scan ureteric "jets" as they flow into the bladder. Small calculi are occasionally seen at the ureterovesical junction.

**B. Renal transplant examination**

1. Turn on the machine. _____
2. Select a 3-MHz sector probe. _____
3. Select "abdominal" application. _____
4. Type in patient information. _____
5. Load film if necessary. Make sure you know which side of the machine the camera faces.
6. Begin scanning the left or right iliac fossa for the trans- _____

planted kidney. Adjust the field of view as necessary.

7. Select a window to obtain a small area of color flow. Scan the iliac fossa for the anastomosis with the internal iliac artery and vein and obtain an image of this area. _____

8. Next, switch to a 5-MHz probe. Select an arcuate or segmental artery (i.e., one in the middle of the kidney) and activate pulsed Doppler. _____

9. Move the gate to the artery of interest, then align the gate parallel to this artery (the angle should be less than 60 degrees; this is shown in the upper left-hand corner of the screen of most machines). _____

10. Toggle on pulsed Doppler to obtain a waveform. _____

11. If the waveform exceeds the velocity scale (aliasing), several adjustments can be made:
    **a. Baseline**
    **b. Velocity scale**
    Once the waveform fits the velocity scale, freeze the image. _____

12. Label the image (e.g., L transplant kidney). _____

13. Print the image. _____

14. Measure the size of the kidney and any area of interest. _____

15. To calculate resistive index:
    **a.** Toggle on marker function. _____
    **b.** Mark the end-diastolic velocity and end-systolic velocity. _____
    **c.** Calculate. _____
    **d.** Label the image (e.g., intrarenal RI). _____
    **e.** Print the image. _____

## III. Interpretation
### A. Hydronephrosis
1. **Anechoic dilated central echo complex.** Polycystic kidneys can also have this appearance; however, the cysts will not coalesce centrally. Vascular structures appear hypoechoic; color Doppler will differentiate dilated calyces from vessels.
2. If **hydronephrosis** is seen, have the patient void; back pressure from the bladder can cause a mild hydro-

nephrosis (especially in infants). Hydronephrosis that is worse after voiding suggests reflux. Also, never forget that hydronephrosis can occur without obstruction (e.g., chronic reflux).

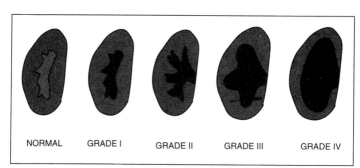

| NORMAL | GRADE I | GRADE II | GRADE III | GRADE IV |

**B. Pregnancy**
 1. "Physiologic" hydronephrosis
 2. Right kidney affected twice as commonly as left kidney
**C. Calculi**
 1. Check kidneys, bladder, and ureters (if possible).
 2. Look for acoustic shadowing—remember to keep focal spot on suspected calculus.
 3. Most calculi less than 3 mm are impossible to detect by ultrasound.
**D. Perinephric fluid**
 1. Ruptured calyx
 2. Abscess
 3. Hemorrhage
**E. Transplant**
 1. **Lymphoceles**
   a. Usually arise within 1–3 weeks after transplantation and are located medial or inferior-lateral to the lower pole of the kidney
   b. May contain septations and/or debris
 2. **Urinomas**
   a. Usually arise within 1–2 weeks after transplantation
   b. Located near the lower pole of the transplant or in the region of the bladder
 3. **Rejection**
   a. RI greater than 0.80 (peak systolic – end diastolic/peak systolic)
   b. Pulsatility index (PI) greater than 1.65 (peak systolic – end diastolic/mean)
   c. Elevation of PI or RI is **not** a specific sign of rejection. Other causes of an increased PI or RI include severe acute tubular necrosis, renal vein obstruction, pyelonephritis, extrarenal compression, ureteric obstruction, chronic rejection, cyclosporine toxicity, and hemolytic-uremic syndrome.
**IV. Pitfalls**
 **A. False-positive:** hydronephrosis without obstruction
   1. Postobstructive dilatation

    **2.** Vesicoureteral reflux
    **3.** Schistosomiasis
  **B. False-negative.** Obstruction without hydronephrosis; sonography may be normal in up to 50% of patients with acute obstruction.
    **1.** Within 3 hours of onset of obstruction
    **2.** Forniceal rupture with decompression
    **3.** Decreased urine output due to dehydration
    **4.** Intrarenal pelvis
    **5.** Distal obstruction

# Testicular Ultrasound

**I. Clinical history**
  **A. Time course of swelling and pain.** In acute torsion, the testicle is salvageable for approximately 6–8 hours after the event. Occasionally, spontaneous detorsion occurs and the patient will describe sudden relief of pain.
  **B. History of trauma**
  **C. Most recent sexual intercourse.** In the acute nontraumatic, painful testicle, the differential diagnosis is torsion versus infection.
  **D. Choice of Doppler ultrasound or nuclear medicine scan.** Ultrasound has generally replaced the nuclear medicine scan as the initial study of choice in suspected torsion because it is faster and equally or more sensitive. However, be aware that some physicians still prefer nuclear medicine studies, especially if the patient is prepubertal and flow is not seen on color Doppler imaging. While not yet firmly established, "power Doppler imaging" may play an important role in the evaluation of the acute testicle in the near future.

**II. Imaging.** Gray-scale images are generally unhelpful in distinguishing between torsion and epididymitis. Epididymal enlargement, the presence of a hydrocele, and abnormal testicular echotexture occur in both entities. Thus, differentiation depends on Doppler imaging of the **intratesticular** arteries. Remember that capsular flow will be increased in both torsion and infection and is therefore useless in differentiating the two entities.

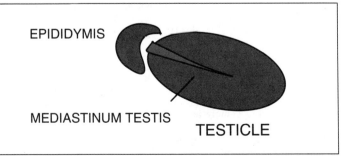

EPIDIDYMIS

MEDIASTINUM TESTIS    TESTICLE

Position the patient supine and place a towel over the thighs and under the scrotum to support the testicles. The room should be kept warm and warm gel should be used.

1. Select a 7-MHz linear probe. _____
2. Load film if necessary.
3. Turn on the machine and select _____
   "small parts" exam.
4. Type in patient information. _____
5. Select color flow at lowest _____
   threshold and wall filter settings
   (this is done automatically on
   most machines).
6. Adjust the gain by turning it so _____
   that background noise is just
   visible then turn down slightly.
7. Select a window to obtain a _____
   small area of color flow.
8. Find intratesticular artery and _____
   activate pulsed Doppler. Move
   gate to the artery of interest,
   then align the gate parallel to
   this artery (the angle should be
   less than 60 degrees; this is
   shown in the upper left-hand
   corner of the screen of most
   machines).
9. Toggle on pulsed Doppler to _____
   obtain a waveform. If you can't
   obtain a waveform, increase the
   sample volume.
10. If the waveform exceeds the _____
    velocity scale (aliasing), several
    adjustments can be made:
    a. **Baseline**
    b. **Velocity scale**
    Once the waveform fits the
    velocity scale, freeze the image.
11. Label the image (e.g., L testicle). _____
12. Print the image. _____

III. **Interpretation**
   A. **Testicular intraparenchymal flow**
      1. Normal velocity 10–12 cm/s
      2. Absent flow = torsion
      3. Increased flow = infection or spontaneous detorsion
      4. Partial torsion can occur where arterial flow with decreased velocity and blunted acceleration will be found (i.e., instead of having a rapid upslope on waveform, a blunted curve is seen—the so-called **parvustardus** waveform). Diastolic velocity appears increased relative to systolic velocity, resulting in a **decreased RI**. (These are findings seen distal to any significant arterial stenosis.)

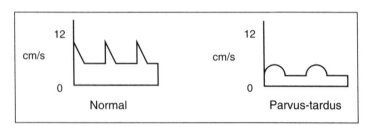

| | |
|---|---|
| 12 cm/s  0  Normal | 12 cm/s  0  Parvus-tardus |

**B. Peritesticular fluid collection**
  1. Hydrocele
  2. Hematocele
  3. Abscess
**C. Epididymis**
  1. Hypoechoic = infection or torsion
  2. Enlargement = infection or torsion
See the nuclear medicine testicular scan in Ch. 7.

---

# References

### Basic Vascular Ultrasound

Curry TS, Dowdey JE, Murry RC. *Christensen's Physics of Diagnostic Radiology* (4th ed). Philadelphia: Lea & Febiger, 1990.

### Aortic Ultrasound

Gooding GAW. The Abdominal Great Vessels. In CM Rumack, SR Wilson, JW Charboneau (eds), *Diagnostic Ultrasound*. St. Louis: Mosby–Year Book, 1991.

### Ultrasound for Appendicitis

Abu-Yousef MM, Phillips ME, Franken EA Jr. et al. Sonography of acute appendicitis: A critical review. *Crit Rev Diagn Imaging* 29:381, 1989.

Yacoe ME, Jeffrey RB Jr. Sonography of appendicitis and diverticulitis. *Radiol Clin North Am* 32:899, 1994.

### Ultrasound-Guided Aspiration

McGahan JP. Ultrasound-Guided Aspiration and Drainage. In CM Rumack, SR Wilson, JW Charboneau (eds), *Diagnostic Ultrasound*. St. Louis: Mosby–Year Book, 1991.

### Ultrasound for Ectopic Pregnancy

Atri M, Ledric C, Gillett P, et. al. Role of endovaginal sonography in the diagnosis and management of ectopic pregnancy. *Radiographics* 16:755, 1996.

Cadkin AV, McAlpin J. The decidua-chorionic sac: A reliable sonographic indicator of intrauterine pregnancy prior to detection of a fetal pole. *J Ultrasound Med* 3:539, 1984.

Filly RA. Ectopic Pregnancy. In PW Callen (ed), *Ultrasonography in Obstetrics and Gynecology* (3rd ed). Philadelphia: Saunders, 1994.

Frates MC, Laing FC. Sonographic evaluation of ectopic pregnancy: An update. *AJR Am J Roentgenol* 165:251, 1995.


## Gallbladder Ultrasound

Laing FC. The Gallbladder and Bile Ducts. In CM Rumack, SR Wilson, JW Charboneau (eds), *Diagnostic Ultrasound*. St. Louis: Mosby–Year Book, 1991.

Rosenthal SJ, Cox GG, Wetzel LH, Batnitzky S. Pitfalls and differential diagnoses in biliary sonography. *Radiographics* 10:285, 1990.


## Lower Extremity Venous Doppler Ultrasound

Knighton RA, Priest DL, Zwiebel WJ, et al. Techniques for color flow sonography of the lower extremity. *Radiographics* 10:775, 1990.

Lewis BD, James EM, Welch TJ, et al. Diagnosis of acute deep venous thrombosis of the lower extremities: Prospective evaluation of color Doppler flow imaging versus venography. *Radiology* 192:651, 1994.


## Ultrasound for Pelvic Pain

Helvie MA, Silver TM. Ovarian torsion: Sonographic evaluation. *J Clin Ultrasound* 17:327, 1989.

Moore L, Wilson SR. Ultrasonography in obstetric and gynecologic emergencies. *Radiol Clin North Am* 32:1005, 1994.

Rosado WM Jr, Trambert MA, Gosink BB, Pretorius DH. Adnexal torsion: Diagnosis using doppler sonography. *AJR Am J Roentgenol* 159:1251, 1992.


## Placental Ultrasound

Crane S, Chun B, Acker D. Treatment of obstetrical hemorrhagic emergencies. *Curr Opin Obstet Gynecol* 5:675, 1993.

Townsend RR. Ultrasound Evaluation of the Placenta and Umbilical Cord. In PW Callen (ed), *Ultrasonography in Obstetrics and Gynecology* (3rd ed). Philadelphia: Saunders, 1994.

Spirit BA, Gordon LP. The Placenta. In CM Rumack, SR Wilson, JW Charboneau (eds), *Diagnostic Ultrasound*. St. Louis: Mosby–Year Book, 1991.


## Renal Ultrasound

Kriegshauser JS, Carroll BA. The Urinary Tract. In CM Rumack, SR Wilson, JW Charboneau (eds), *Diagnostic Ultrasound*. St. Louis: Mosby–Year Book, 1991.

Haddad MC, Sharif HS, Shahed MS et al. Renal colic: Diagnosis and outcome. *Radiology* 184:83, 1992.


## Testicular Ultrasound

Feld R, Middleton WD. Recent advances in sonography of the testis and scrotum. *Radiol Clin North Am* 30:1033, 1992.

# Computed Tomography

## General Considerations

Because CT will be the imaging modality of choice for a large proportion of on-call exams, it is important to be familiar with its indications, artifacts, and limitations. Remember that even with very competent technicians, responsibility for the study, including safety, quality assurance, and interpretation, is the physician's (i.e., the radiology resident on call).

I. **Indications.** In general, and especially at night, resist requests for "scan of whole body from head to toe because we don't have a clue as to what's going on." Common indications for CT scan include:

A. Brain evaluation in trauma or suspected stroke

B. Spine, thorax, abdomen, pelvic trauma

C. Aortic dissection

D. Nontraumatic acute abdomen

II. **Imaging**

A. **Accessories**. Remove as many nonessential artifact-producing entities from the field of view as possible. These include:

1. Arms
2. Wires
3. ECG leads
4. Tubes
5. Back boards

B. **Bowel contrast**

1. Unless there is a medical reason to the contrary, all patients should receive 800–1000 ml of either barium or 3% Hypaque/dilute gastrografin (mix one capful of full-strength gastrografin in a cup of water) at least 15–30 minutes (if possible) before scanning (1–2 hours is preferable).

2. For colonic pathology, administer
   a. Glucagon (1 mg IV)
   b. Rectal contrast or air insufflation

3. Children

| Weight (kg) | Gastrografin (ml) | Added water (ml) |
|---|---|---|
| 0–5 | 3.5 | 120 |
| 5–7 | 4.5 | 180 |
| 7–10 | 7.0 | 240 |
| 10–15 | 8.0 | 300 |
| 15–20 | 10.5 | 360 |
| 20–25 | 11.5 | 420 |
| 25–35 | 15 | 540 |
| 35–45 | 18.5 | 660 |
| 45–50 | 21 | 780 |
| >50 | 24 | 900 |

Give three-fourths of a dose 1 hour before the study and the remainder on the CT table.

C. **IV contrast.** In general, use nonionic contrast for emergent studies. All studies should be performed with flow-controlled injection, which requires a 20-gauge or larger IV. Be sure to check the IV site. Avoid contrast extravasation into the soft tissues! If the IV is questionable, start a new one.
  1. Avoid giving IV contrast to any nondialysis patient with a creatinine level higher than 1.5 mg/dl.
  2. In dialysis patients, tell the clinical service the patient must be dialyzed the following day.
  3. Do **not** power-inject through central lines or implantable venous access devices. A recent study demonstrated that both Hickman and Leonard catheters could be safely used with a power injector **in vitro**. In vivo studies have not yet been performed.
  4. Consider decreasing the contrast dose if the patient has only one kidney.
  5. The children's dose is 2–3 ml/kg of Omnipaque 240.
  6. Give a larger dose if the patient weighs more than 75 kg.
  7. Scan delay
    a. Nonhelical scanner: if normal cardiac output 45 sec (70 sec if patient has congestive heart failure [CHF])
    b. Helical scan: if normal cardiac output 70 sec (95 sec if patient has CHF)
  8. **Contraindication.** Metformin hydrochloride (Glucophage) is a medication used by some diabetics that is eliminated from the body by the kidneys. Any patient at risk for contrast-induced renal failure should either discontinue the drug for several days before and after the study or not receive IV contrast.
  9. The gauge of the IV may dictate the maximum injection rate: 22 g is less than or equal to 2 ml/sec.
D. **Tampon.** If possible, have women insert a tampon before scanning to help delineate pelvic anatomy.
E. **Artifacts**
  1. Metal—e.g., wires, leads, and bullets
  2. High-density barium: from recent fluoroscopic GI examination
  3. Motion
F. **Maneuvers to decrease artifacts**
  1. Decompress stomach with nasogastric tube, then withdraw tube into esophagus before scanning.
  2. Raise arms.
  3. Use large field of view.
  4. Remove ECG leads.
G. **Pitfalls: Air injection.** If air is inadvertently injected into the patient (may be seen in the heart or pulmonary arteries), place him or her in the left lateral (left side down) decubitus position to keep the air in the right heart.
III. **Interpretation.** If possible, always check the scan while the patient is still on the table. This will allow rescanning of questionable areas.
A. Resist the temptation to read the study off the monitor. It is very difficult to read scans from a monitor (especially when surrounded by a group of frantic clinicians pointing to every anatomic structure on the screen and asking, "What's that?") If pressured by members of the clinical service, tell

them you will give a "wet reading," but your final reading
will be available only after the hard copies are printed.
**B.** Obtain thin cuts or additional cuts of suspicious areas as
necessary.
**C.** In suspected renal trauma, obtain delayed scans 30 minutes after infusion.
**D.** Consider rectal contrast or air insufflation for lower GI
pathology.

# Aortic Dissection

**I. Clinical history**
   **A.** Twice as common as rupture of an abdominal aortic
   aneurysm
   **B.** Usually occurs in men in their 60–70s
   **C.** Classically, patients present with tearing chest pain radiating to the back.
   **D.** Predisposing conditions include hypertension, bicuspid
   aortic valve, connective tissue disease, and pregnancy.
**II. Choice of diagnostic study.** At our institution, an emergent CT exam for aortic dissection can be performed more
   quickly than an MRI exam. Since the sensitivity and specificity are similar for both imaging modalities, in patients
   referred to the radiology department at night, CT is usually
   our study of choice. However, if the patient has a contrast
   allergy or will be followed with serial exams (e.g., the
   patient has Marfan's syndrome), an MRI exam should be
   considered. In a stable patient, MRI is considered by many
   to be the modality of choice for evaluating suspected aortic
   dissection.

| Modality | Strengths | Weaknesses |
|---|---|---|
| Transthoracic echocardiography | Assesses aortic valve, hemoperi-cardium, left ventricular function<br>Can be done portably | Cannot evaluate entire aorta |
| Transesophageal echocardiography | Assesses aortic valve, hemoperi-cardium, left ventricular function<br>Can be done portably | Blind spots: behind the trachea, below the diaphragm |
| CT | Images the entire aorta and adja-cent organs<br>Widely available | Cannot assess aortic valve or left ven-tricular function<br>Requires contrast |
| MRI | Assesses entire aorta, branch vessels, and valves | May not be toler-ated by very ill patients |

| Modality | Strengths | Weaknesses |
|---|---|---|
| | | Other contraindications: pacemakers, many patient monitoring devices |
| Aortography | Gold standard | Invasive<br>Requires contrast |

## III. Imaging
### A. Chest radiograph
1. Excludes other etiologies such as pneumothorax and rib fractures
2. Comparison films are extremely helpful.

### B. Preinfused CT study
1. Perform on a helical scanner if possible.
2. Scan of the chest and abdomen (10-mm cuts with 5-mm spacing) to iliac arteries

### C. Determining scan delay
1. Place a region of interest box in the descending aorta approximately 2 cm below the arch (at the level of the pulmonary arteries) or at the level of interest dictated by the noninfused study.
2. Administer a 20-ml test bolus of nonionic contrast at 3 ml/sec for 20 sec.
3. Do 1 scan every 2 sec at this level between 5 and 30 sec in the arch or between 5 and 15 sec in the abdomen to generate a time-density curve. Time is plotted on the X-axis and density on the Y-axis. Determine scan delay by subtracting time to early peak (>100 Hounsfield units [HU]) from the time of initial bolus, then subtract 5 sec.

### D. Infused CT study
1. Perform the scan by administering 150 ml of nonionic contrast at 3 ml/sec.
2. Do one 10-mm slice per second (pitch = 1) from 2 cm above the arch through the pelvis.
3. A single breath hold through the chest will give the best images. If this is not possible, scan for 10 sec, breath for 6 sec, then scan for 10 sec, and so on
4. Thin cuts may be needed at the origins or the celiac axis, superior mesenteric artery, and renal arteries in type B dissections.

## IV. Interpretation
### A. Chest radiograph
1. Widened superior mediastinum (>8 cm)
2. Superior extension of the left mediastinal stripe above the aortic arch forming an apical cap
3. Right paratracheal widening
4. Left pleural effusion
5. Inward displacement of atherosclerotic calcifications (>6 mm)
6. Tracheal (endotracheal tube) or esophageal (nasogastric tube) deviation to the right
7. Inferior displacement of left mainstem bronchus

## B. Classification

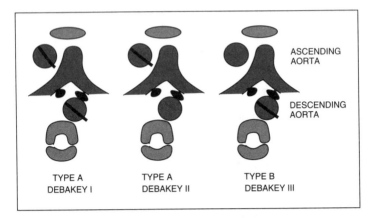

TYPE A
DEBAKEY I

TYPE A
DEBAKEY II

TYPE B
DEBAKEY III

ASCENDING
AORTA

DESCENDING
AORTA

1. **Stanford type A dissections**
   a. Begin several centimeters above the aortic valve.
   b. Usually treated surgically since the dissection may extend proximally to involve the pericardial sac (leading to tamponade), aortic valve, and/or coronary arteries (usually right coronary artery). Involvement of the great vessels is also important.
2. **Stanford type B dissections**
   a. Start distal to the ligamentum arteriosum.
   b. Usually treated medically with antihypertensive medications. Surgery is possible if there is acute ischemia.

C. CT findings
   1. **Unenhanced findings**
      a. **Dissection versus aneurysm.** Inward displacement of atherosclerotic calcifications is indicative of a dissection, while peripheral calcifications occur in an aneurysm.
      b. Mediastinal hemorrhage/pericardial effusion
   2. **Enhanced findings**
      a. Intimal flap separating the vessel into true and false lumina
      b. True lumen of a dissection is usually **smaller** than the false lumen.
      c. Aortic dilatation
      d. Aortic root thickening

D. Pitfalls
   1. An atelectatic lung adjacent to the aorta will enhance brightly after administration of contrast. Do not mistake this for extraluminal contrast from a leaking dissection.
   2. Streak artifact can occur with heart motion, but this usually extends beyond the wall of the vessel.
   3. Do not mistake normal structures for dissections.
      a. Left brachiocephalic vein: runs anterior to the ascending aorta
      b. Left superior intercostal vein: runs on the left aspect of the arch

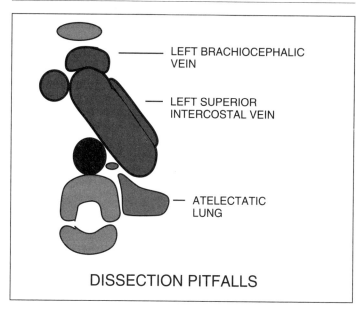

LEFT BRACHIOCEPHALIC VEIN

LEFT SUPERIOR INTERCOSTAL VEIN

ATELECTATIC LUNG

DISSECTION PITFALLS

**4.** A thrombosed false lumen can be mistaken for a mural thrombus in an aneurysm.

**5.** Atherosclerotic ulcers

# Nontraumatic Acute Abdomen

**I. Clinical history**

**A. Fever of unknown origin and abdominal pain. Rule out abscess.** In our institution, "rule out abscess" is often used as a catch-all phrase to justify an abdominal and pelvic CT examination. The overwhelming majority of these patients do not have an abscess but may have another intra-abdominal disease.

**B. Barium exams.** High-density barium used for most fluoroscopic studies must be cleared from the bowel before a CT exam can be performed.

**II. Checklist.** We use an "organ approach" and specifically look at each major abdominal organ for signs of common disease processes. The following is a list of common etiologies to consider in the diagnosis of the nontraumatic acute abdomen.

**A. Liver:** Abscess

**B. Gallbladder:** Cholecystitis

**C. Kidneys**
　　**1.** Pyelonephritis
　　**2.** Ureteral calculus

**D. Pancreas:** Pancreatitis

**E. Appendix:** Appendicitis

**F. Bowel**
　　**1.** Ischemia
　　**2.** Inflammatory bowel disease

       3. Obstruction
       4. Perforation
       5. Diverticulitis

  **G. Peritoneum:** Abscess

  **H. Vasculature**
       1. Thrombosis
       2. Aortic dissection
       3. Leaking abdominal aortic aneurysm
       4. Vascular access device thrombus

**III. Disease entities**

  **A. Hepatic abscess.** At our institution, hepatic abscesses most commonly occur in liver transplant patients. Other etiologies include cholangitis, infarction, trauma, and infection with *Entamoeba histolytica*.
     1. Unilocular or multilocular fluid collection
     2. Single or multiple
     3. Density: water to soft tissue (0–80 HU)
     4. Gas: specific for abscess
     5. Enhancing rim (rare)
     6. Pleural effusion
     7. Differential diagnosis: necrotic metastasis, lymphoma, biliary cystadenoma

  **B. Acute cholecystitis** is most commonly caused by a gallstone impacted in the cystic duct.
     1. Gallstones/sludge
     2. Gallbladder hydrops: diameter greater than 5 cm
     3. Wall thickening (>4 mm): nonspecific
     4. Pericholecystic fluid
     5. Intramural air (emphysematous cholecystitis)
     6. Intrahepatic bile duct dilatation (implies common duct obstruction) of one week's duration or more
     7. **Pitfall.** Pure cholesterol stones are isodense to bile and are therefore not detectable on CT.

  **C. Pyelonephritis** usually is caused by ascending infection from the bladder. A normal appearance on CT does **not** exclude infection.
     1. Cortical, wedge-shaped area of low density in an infused study
     2. Striated nephrogram
     3. Kidney enlargement
     4. Associated anatomic abnormality: kidney stone, obstructing mass

  **D. Ureteral calculus.** If suspicion is high, perform a helical scan with 5-mm thick sections and at a table speed of 5 mm/sec. All calculi (even "radiolucent" uric acid or cystine stones) appear radiopaque (200–600 HU) on CT.
     1. Hydronephrosis
     2. Hydroureter with intraluminal calculus (1- to 2-mm reconstructions may be helpful in suspicious areas)
     3. Perinephric fat stranding
     4. Unilateral increase in renal cortical thickness
     5. Perinephric fluid: perform delayed scans to check for contrast extravasation
     6. **Pitfall.** Phleboliths can be mistaken for calculi. Look for a lucent center on plain film and know the expected course of the ureter.

E. **Pancreatitis** is usually caused by gallstones, alcoholism, or trauma. The diagnosis rests on results of blood tests (i.e., amylase and lipase) and clinical criteria; a CT exam is usually done in unclear cases or to exclude complications. A normal appearance on CT does **not** exclude pancreatitis. A dedicated pancreatic protocol obtaining 3-mm slices scanning caudocephalad can be performed.

1. **Major findings**
   a. Pancreas: focal or diffuse enlargement, contour irregularities
   b. Pancreatic necrosis: nonenhancing, low-density area
   c. Peripancreatic fatty infiltration: thickening of left Gerota's fascia common
   d. Phlegmon/pseudocyst: commonly in lesser sac, transverse mesocolon, lower abdomen, mediastinum, peritoneal reflections (can be almost anywhere)

2. **Ancillary findings**
   a. Biliary obstruction
   b. Left pleural effusion
   c. Invasion of adjacent vasculature (e.g., pancreaticoduodenal, splenic, gastroduodenal artery) with pseudoaneurysm formation and possible hemorrhage
   d. Portal and splenic vein thrombosis

3. **Differential diagnosis:** neoplasm (invasion of superior mesenteric artery/superior mesenteric vein is usually **not** seen in pancreatitis)

F. **Appendicitis** is the most common cause of acute abdomen. Etiologies include fecalith, lymphoid hyperplasia, foreign body (e.g., chicken bone), and Crohn's disease. Always specifically check the appendix.

1. Peri-appendiceal fatty infiltration
2. Fluid collection/abscess
3. Appendicolith
4. Appendiceal wall thickening (>2 mm)
5. Appendix greater than 6 mm in diameter
6. **Differential diagnosis:** cecal diverticulitis, perforating cecal neoplasm

G. **Mesenteric ischemia and bowel infarction** have non-specific signs and symptoms. They are easily overlooked on imaging studies.

1. **Pneumatosis:** may be seen in benign processes. Look for gas on the **dependent** side of a fluid-filled bowel (i.e., intramural gas).
2. Portal venous or superior mesenteric vein air-blood level. Lung or bone windows (Window 2000–4000, Level 350–450) may be helpful to visualize air.
3. Bowel wall thickening or "featureless" bowel wall
4. Pneumoperitoneum
5. Thrombus in superior mesenteric artery/inferior mesenteric artery

Note that **linear air collections in the liver** are either in the bile ducts or portal vein. As a general rule, pneumobilia usually occurs centrally while portal venous gas is found peripherally (i.e., gas follows the flow of bile or blood).

H. **Inflammatory bowel disease:** Crohn's disease or ulcerative colitis

1. Bowel wall thickening
2. Mesenteric infiltration
3. Strictures
4. Fistulas: enterovesical (pneumobilia, bladder wall thickening)
5. Lymphadenopathy
6. Abscess
7. Fatty proliferation ("creeping fat")

**I. Small-bowel obstruction (SBO).** Often, an SBO can be diagnosed by plain films alone, rendering further studies unnecessary. In equivocal cases (e.g., SBO versus adynamic ileus), perform a CT examination **before** a barium study. The sensitivity and specificity of CT is greater than 90% in demonstrating an SBO. If a dedicated small-bowel exam is done first, a CT cannot be performed until the high-density barium used for fluoroscopic studies is cleared from the bowel.

1. Transition point: dilated proximal bowel (>2.5–3.0 cm in diameter) and nondilated distal bowel
2. Ischemia/strangulation
   a. Circumferential bowel wall thickening
   b. Pneumatosis intestinalis. In the proper clinical context, it indicates ischemia until proved otherwise.
   c. Increased density of adjacent mesenteric fat
3. **Types of SBO**
   a. **Intussusception**. Low-density mesenteric fat and vessels are seen within a dilated bowel loop (in adults, the majority are associated with a lead point such as a neoplasm)
   b. **Adhesion:** transition from dilated to nondilated bowel without visible cause (diagnosis of exclusion)
   c. **Closed loop (incarcerated) obstruction:** fluid-filled, U-shaped, dilated loop with nondistended proximal and distal bowel loops; prone to ischemia
   d. **Volvulus:** twisting of bowel and mesentery (whirl sign); bowel narrows to the shape of a beak (beak sign)
   e. **Hernia**
      (1) Inguinal
      (2) Internal
         i. Left paraduodenal: bowel loops herniating through peritoneal defect in the transverse mesocolon; small bowel loops between stomach and pancreas
         ii. Other types difficult to diagnose by CT

**J. Bowel perforation.** Common etiologies include peptic ulcer disease, obstruction, necrotic tumor, and appendicitis. If clinical suspicion is high, **gastrografin** should be used in the place of barium.

1. Pneumoperitoneum: collects under anterior abdominal wall, often anterior to liver (lung windows may be helpful to visualize air)
2. Extraluminal contrast extravasation
3. Free fluid/ascites
4. **Pitfalls:** postoperative air (should resolve in approximately 7 days but may persist for 2–4 weeks in very thin individuals)

**K. Diverticulitis.** Inspissated fecal material in a diverticulum leads to mucosal erosion and perforation of the diverticulum with a localized abscess. The sigmoid colon is most commonly affected.
1. Diverticula with adjacent fatty infiltration
2. Intramural abscess
3. Free intraperitoneal fluid or tiny air bubbles
4. Smoothly tapering symmetric bowel wall thickening (4–20 mm)
5. Fistula/sinus
6. Colonic or ureteral obstruction
7. **Differential diagnosis:** neoplasm (wall thickening >2 cm, shouldering, complete bowel obstruction, mucosal destruction); appendicitis
8. **Follow-up:** barium enema

**L. Abscess.** Nuclear medicine studies (gallium or indium WBC) may also be helpful to localize sites of inflammation. Make a conscious effort to follow all bowel loops to ensure contiguity; good bowel contrast is essential. An abscess can mimic a bowel loop but will appear isolated with respect to other bowel loops.
1. Fluid collection with thick enhancing rim
2. Internal gas (10–20%)
3. Variable density: water to soft-tissue density (0–80 HU)
4. **Pitfalls:** Abscess mimics (ascites, low-density neoplasm, bladder diverticulum, bowel loops)

**M. Venous thrombosis** (including deep venous, portal venous, inferior vena cava, and gonadal veins)
1. Low-density luminal clot in infused study
2. Vessel expansion
3. Central venous catheter
4. **Pitfall.** Early imaging on a helical scanner can simulate intraluminal thrombus.

**N. Abdominal aortic aneurysm.** Usually *infra*renal, fusiform, and the result of atherosclerotic disease. Typically enlarge at a rate of about 0.2 cm per year.
1. If an aneurysm is seen, document the following:
   a. Location and length
   b. Extent of mural thrombus and calcification
   c. Extension into iliac arteries (1 cm normal diameter) or proximal aorta
2. Size (>4–5 cm is indication for surgery)
3. Periaortic hemorrhage (indication for surgery)
   a. Posterior to kidneys adjacent to the psoas muscle
   b. May see focal wall interruption (especially if calcified)
   c. **Pitfalls**
      (1) May be confused with perianeurysmal fibrosis, masses, or lymph nodes (these should enhance)
      (2) May be confused with other retroperitoneal hemorrhage (e.g., renal neoplasm, pancreatitis)
4. Renal obstruction (indication for surgery)

**O. Aortic dissection.** See the discussion of aortic dissection in this chapter.

# Abdominal and Pelvic Trauma

I. **Clinical history**
   A. **Peritoneal lavage.** Free air and fluid on a CT exam is meaningless if the patient has undergone peritoneal lavage. Peritoneal lavage is an excellent, inexpensive manner to evaluate the peritoneal cavity; however, it is insensitive to retroperitoneal injuries (duodenum, pancreas, ascending and descending colon, kidneys), cannot localize the site of injury, and may not distinguish between significant and minor hemoperitoneum. The false-positive rate due to traumatic placement may be as high as 25%.
   B. **Cause of injury.** Both the manner in which the patient was injured (e.g., blunt versus penetrating) and the area are important considerations before attempting to analyze any scan. Essentially anyone with serious trauma should be evaluated by CT scan or taken directly to surgery if unstable.
   C. **Suspicion for aortic transection.** Although somewhat controversial, CT is generally **not** indicated for aortic transection in blunt or penetrating trauma. If the patient is stable without neurologic injury, he 'or she should be brought directly to the angiography suite for aortography.
II. **Imaging**
   A. Administer 500–750 ml of 3% Hypaque solution or dilute gastrografin (mix one capful full-strength gastrografin in a large cup of water) PO at least 15–30 minutes before starting the study if possible.
   B. If possible, give 20 ml of IV contrast 5 minutes before scanning (this will increase the likelihood of renal and bladder opacification). Alternatively, perform delayed scans through the areas of interest.
   C. Use a helical scanner and infuse 180 ml of nonionic contrast at 2 ml/sec with a 50- to 70-second scan delay.
   D. Always obtain bone windows (Window 4000, Level 350). They aid in the ability to detect unsuspected fractures and are valuable in detection of **free air** and **pneumothorax.**
   E. Third-trimester pregnancy is not a contraindication to CT scanning.
III. **Checklist**
   A. **Free air**
      1. Use bone or lung windows on the monitor and scan through the body to see a subtle pneumoperitoneum.
      2. Intraperitoneal air
         a. Usually collects under the anterior abdominal wall. Less common locations are the leaves of the mesentery, ligamentum venosum, and bowel wall.
         b. The most common etiology is a perforated hollow viscus. Less common etiologies are pneumothorax, pneumomediastinum, peritoneal lavage, and bladder perforation with Foley catheter placement.
      3. Retroperitoneal air: usually indicates duodenal perforation
   B. **Hemoperitoneum**
      1. May occur with injury to any abdominal organ
      2. Paracolic gutters, Morison's pouch, pelvic cul-de-sac

(rectovesical and rectouterine pouches) are the most dependent areas in a supine patient.

3. **Sentinel clot.** An area of increased density (clotted blood) in gross hemoperitoneum often indicates the site of initial hemorrhage. It may mimic an opacified bowel loop or ovary.

4. **Pitfalls.** Even acute blood may appear **low** in density due to the wide window settings used in body scanning. Blood is usually 50–60 HU, while the opacified liver and spleen are 70–80 HU. Note that this is different from the brain, when acute blood is nearly always **high** in density compared to brain parenchyma (40 HU) unless the patient is anemic.

## C. Spleen

1. Most commonly injured organ in major **blunt** abdominal trauma. Associated with left-sided rib injuries.

2. Look for lacerations, fractures, parenchymal hematomas, or vascular pedicle injuries.

3. **Pitfalls**

   a. The spleen can look very inhomogeneous if imaged early in the contrast bolus. Obtain delayed scans if equivocal.

   b. Congenital clefts, lobulations, and accessory spleens can mimic fractures. Clefts usually occur medially and have a smooth border, and blood is absent. Lacerations are jagged and frequently occur laterally.

   c. An unopacified bowel loop adjacent to the spleen can mimic a fracture.

   d. Infarct

   e. Ascites can mimic hemorrhage.

   f. A slow infusion can mask isoattenuating hematomas.

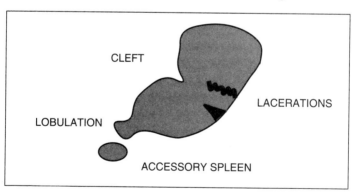

## D. Liver

1. Second most common injured organ. Up to 90% of hepatic injuries are associated with **other** visceral injuries.

2. Common injuries include contusions, hematomas, lacerations (usually occur parallel to hepatic veins), and fractures.

3. The right lobe (usually posterior segment) is more commonly affected than the left.

**4. Pitfalls**

    **a.** An air-fluid level in the stomach can create a linear artifact that mimics a laceration. Obtain repeat scans in the left lateral decubitus position if the findings are equivocal.

    **b.** Fatty liver may mask the laceration.

    **c.** Unopacified vessels can mimic a fracture.

**E. Kidneys and ureters**

  **1.** Commonly injured in either penetrating or blunt abdominal trauma

  **2.** Injuries include lacerations, fractures, parenchymal hematomas, or vascular pedicle injuries.

  **3.** Treatment is usually conservative unless complete loss of renal perfusion occurs (vascular pedicle transection).

  **4.** Delayed views at 30 minutes can be very helpful in equivocal cases.

  **5.** The absence of ureteral opacification caudal to the kidney suggests ureteral transection.

  **6. Pitfalls**

    **a.** Respiratory motion can create a low-density artifact around the kidney mimicking a subcapsular hematoma.

    **b.** Pseudofracture: smooth lobulation or invagination of the parenchyma without associated perirenal fluid

**F. Bladder**

  **1.** Intraperitoneal rupture

    **a.** Extravasated contrast outlines bowel loops.

    **b.** Treated surgically

  **2.** Extraperitoneal rupture

    **a.** Associated with pelvic fractures

    **b.** Extravasated contrast may enter perivesical fat, scrotum, anterior abdominal wall, thigh, or obturator foramen.

    **c.** Usually treated with suprapubic cystostomy

  **3.** Can perform CT cystogram by infusing 350 ml of 3% contrast (e.g., 3% Hypaque solution) into bladder

  **4. Pitfall.** Diverticulum may mimic extravasation.

**G. Adrenal glands**

  **1.** The right side is affected more than the left.

  **2.** Post-traumatic hemorrhage may occur.

**H. Pancreas**

  **1.** Longitudinal fracture line

  **2.** Diffuse swelling

  **3.** Retroperitoneal fluid (may be between splenic vein and pancreas)

  **4.** Thickening of Gerota's fascia

  **5. Pitfalls**

    **a.** A streak artifact can mimic a fracture.

    **b.** An adjacent unopacified bowel loop can mimic a fracture.

    **c.** An undulating pancreatic border can mimic a fracture.

**I. Inferior vena cava (IVC) thrombosis**

  **1.** Dark clot in bright vessel

  **2. Pitfall.** Vessels can appear very inhomogeneous early on helical scans. Obtain delayed images if the findings are equivocal.

**J. Bowel**
  1. Duodenal hematoma or perforation
     **a.** Pneumoperitoneum or pneumoretroperitoneum
     **b.** Peritoneal or retroperitoneal contrast extravasation
     **c.** Free fluid in anterior pararenal space
  2. Perforations
**K. Bones**
  1. Ribs
  2. Vertebral column: vertebrae, transverse processes, pedicles, lamina, spinous processes
  3. Pelvis: sacrum, ilium, ischium, pubic rami, acetabula
  4. Femora
**L. Hypoperfusion syndrome:** severe systemic hypotension usually manifesting in children
  1. Persistent, dense nephrograms
  2. Marked enhancement of bowel wall
  3. Decreased caliber of IVC and aorta

# Head

I. **Clinical history**
  A. **Suspicion of cancer, superior sagittal sinus thrombosis, or CNS infection.** In general, these are the only reasons to perform an infused scan. However, if you believe that contrast will help make a diagnosis, then by all means infuse. Do not infuse a patient with an acute stroke; it will not help in making the diagnosis and there is some (limited) evidence to suggest that contrast infusion will result in a worse prognosis in patients with acute stroke. If a stroke is manifest clinically with a normal CT appearance, the diagnosis is made.
II. **Imaging.** Typically, 5-mm contiguous axial slices are taken from the vertex to the skull base.
III. **Checklist.** Look for asymmetry, mass effect, air, and blood (may be isointense in anemics—8–10 g/dl—or if old). Wide window settings are helpful for demonstrating extra-axial hemorrhage (Window 220, Level 94). Specifically check the following:
  A. **Gyri and sulci**
  B. **Gray-white junction**
  C. **Cisterns**
    1. Perimesencephalic: ambient, interpeduncular
    2. Quadrigeminal
    3. Suprasellar
  D. **Ventricles**
    1. Lateral
    2. Third
    3. Fourth
  E. **Interhemispheric fissure**
  F. **Mass effect**
  G. **Extra-axial fluid**
  H. **Bones**
  I. **Sinuses**
    1. Mastoid
    2. Ethmoid
    3. Maxillary
    4. Frontal

**5.** Sphenoid

**J. Soft tissues**

**IV. Disease entities**

**A. Subarachnoid hemorrhage (SAH).** Aneurysms are the etiology in 80–90% (anterior communicating, posterior communicating, middle cerebral artery). Familiarize yourself with the appearance of subtle SAH because its detection is one of the more difficult "eye tests" in radiology. Always make a conscious effort to look for it.

  **1. Blood** (high-density if <1 week old—approximately 60 HU)

    **a.** Sulci

    **b.** Sylvian fissure

    **c.** Interhemispheric fissure: will appear thickened and "chunky"

    **d.** Cisterns: speck of blood in interpeduncular cistern

    **e.** Ventricles

      **(1)** Blood level in occipital horn of lateral ventricles

      **(2)** Communicating hydrocephalus: blood occludes pacchionian granulations interfering with CSF resorption

    **f. Pitfalls**

      **(1)** Subacute hemorrhage and anemia. Blood that is more than several days old or blood in anemic patients may be isodense to brain parenchyma. The only finding may be nonvisualization of one of the cisterns (i.e., cistern is filled with blood and is isodense to brain parenchyma).

      **(2)** Recent myelography: contrast in subarachnoid space may simulate blood.

      **(3)** Diffuse edema. Brain parenchyma may become very hypodense, causing arteries to appear dense and mimicking SAH.

      **(4)** Purulent meningitis may simulate SAH.

**B. Stroke** is a dynamic process of cerebral ischemia progressing to infarction. Greater than 75% of strokes occur in the area of the middle cerebral artery. In general, the purpose of imaging in suspected stroke is to exclude other intracranial processes such as hemorrhage, tumor, vascular malformation, and subdural hematoma, which can mimic stroke clinically. Clearly, the causes, treatment, and prognosis of these entities are different from those of nonhemorrhagic stroke. Specifically, gross hemorrhage is a contraindication to anticoagulation.

  **1. Hyperacute (<12 hours)**

    **a.** Normal (50%) appearance on CT

    **b.** Hyperdense artery containing thrombus

    **c.** Obscuration of lentiform nuclei (basal ganglia, insula, external/internal capsules)—associated with later intracranial hemorrhage

  **2. Acute (12–24 hours)**

    **a.** Low-density basal ganglia

    **b.** Effacement of sulci with mass effect

    **c.** Loss of gray-white junction (indicates edema)

  **3. Subacute (1–3 days)**

    **a.** Increased mass effect

**b.** Wedge-shaped low-density area involving both gray and white matter

**c.** Hemorrhage (basal ganglia, cortex)

4. **Hypertensive intracranial hemorrhage**

   **a.** External capsule/putamen

   **b.** Thalamus

   **c.** Pons

   **d.** Cerebellum

5. **Pitfalls**

   **a.** Stroke cannot be excluded in the first 12 hours.

   **b.** The sulci often appear less prominent in the region of the posterior parietal lobe. Check the gray-white junction in this area to exclude an early, subtle stroke.

   **c.** Cerebellar strokes are easily missed. Look for mass effect on the fourth ventricle and compare folia with sulci and gyri.

C. **Trauma**

1. **Subarachnoid hemorrhage.** The findings are the same as above.

2. **Subdural hematoma (SDH):** crescent-shaped collection of blood conforming to the outline of the skull. SDHs are usually caused by a sudden velocity change and subsequent injury to a "bridging cortical vein" as it crosses the subdural space to empty into the adjacent dural sinus. Most are found contra-coup to the site of injury. **SDHs are the most lethal of all head injuries, with a mortality rate of 70%.**

   **a.** Crosses **suture lines** but not dural attachments (will not extend across midline).

   **b.** Bilateral (15%). Ventricles assume a ")(" shape. Common in infants.

   **c.** Slight association with **linear** skull fractures

   **d.** Rebleeding (20%)

   **e.** Medial displacement of gray-white junction

   **f.** The surface sulci do not extend to the inner calvarial table. This may be the only finding in a subacute hematoma, as blood may be isodense to parenchyma.

   **g.** Significant mass effect

   **h. Pitfalls**

   (1) The transverse sinus posterior to the cerebellum often appears very dense and mimics extra-axial hemorrhage (especially in children). Make an effort not to "overcall" blood in this area. If this sinus appears too dense, consider the possibility of diffuse cerebral edema.

   (2) Subacute SDH may be isodense to brain parenchyma. Always follow the sulci to the inner table of the skull.

   (3) In some patients (especially children), the subarachnoid space anterior to the frontal lobes may appear prominent and simulate subacute or chronic SDHs. In these cases, it is helpful to obtain an infused scan to evaluate the bridging cortical vessels. In the absence of a fluid collection, these vessels course through the prominent subarachnoid space to the skull. If the vessels are

compressed against the brain, this is indicative of an extra-axial collection. Also look for mass effect on sulci and gyri, which indicates SDH.

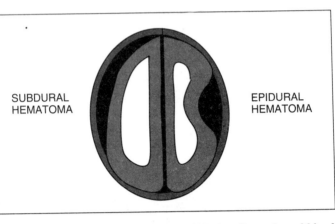

SUBDURAL
HEMATOMA

EPIDURAL
HEMATOMA

3. **Epidural hematoma (EDH):** lentiform-shaped blood collection between the cranial vault and the dura that is most commonly located in the temporal region (95%) and usually caused by injury to the middle meningeal artery (90%). Another less common etiology is superior sagittal sinus thrombosis. In the posterior fossa, most are caused by venous injury. EDHs are generally regarded as surgical emergencies!
   a. Crosses **dural attachments** but not suture lines (can extend across the midline)
   b. Bilateral 5%
   c. Associated with linear skull fractures (90%) and secondary herniation
   d. Rebleeding at 24–48 hours (20%)
   e. **Pitfall:** Because of partial volume averaging, an EDH adjacent to the base of the skull may protrude superiorly, mimicking an intraparenchymal contusion.
   A common clinical presentation is injury followed by a "lucid interval" followed by neurologic deterioration (50%).
4. **Intraparenchymal contusion.** Focal collection of blood is most common in the frontal and temporal lobes, caused by brain striking bone or the dural fold.
   a. Look for contra-coup injury opposite to the injury site.
   b. Associated with **depressed** skull fractures
   c. Delayed hemorrhage (20%)
5. **Fractures.** Usually, only skull fractures depressed one cortical width or greater are treated surgically.
   a. Air fluid levels in the sinuses, opacified sinuses, or clouded mastoids
   b. Intracranial air
   c. Coronal cuts may be helpful for suspected orbital **"blow out"** fractures, but always obtain axial cuts first. Look for inferior rectus muscle entrapment.
   d. Depressed skull fractures are usually associated with

intraparenchymal contusions while linear fractures are more often associated with EDH or SDH.

 **e.** Basilar skull fractures

  **(1)** Longitudinal (75%): associated with ossicular derangement and conductive hearing loss

  **(2)** Transverse (25%): associated with sensorineural hearing loss

**6. Diffuse axonal injury (DAI):** axonal shear strain injury usually located bilaterally at the gray-white junction, corpus callosum (especially splenium), and dorsolateral upper brain stem caused by acceleration, deceleration, and/or rotational forces. It is the most important cause of morbidity in patients with head trauma.

 **a.** Normal (70%) appearance on CT

 **b.** Optimally seen 3–7 days after injury

 **c.** Petechial hemorrhage at gray-white junction and/or corpus callosum

 **d.** Hemorrhage 5–15 mm (smaller than cortical contusion)

Loss of consciousness with DAI is common. These scans typically appear more innocuous than the clinical situation would suggest.

**D. Herniation**

 **1. Descending transtentorial.** The uncus (medial portion of the temporal lobe) and the parahippocampal gyrus of the temporal lobe are displaced medially over the free tentorial margin due to a **supratentorial** process. Descending herniation is more common than ascending herniation.

  **a.** Ipsilateral suprasellar cistern effaced (early), leading to obliteration of all basal cisterns (late)

  **b.** Ipsilateral cerebellar pontine angle widened due to brain stem displacement

  **c.** Ipsilateral posterior cerebral artery compression against tentorial incisura, leading to occipital infarct

  **d. Kernohan notch:** contralateral cerebral peduncle compressed against the tentorium, causing midbrain contusion (better seen on MRI)

TRANSTENTORIAL HERNIATION

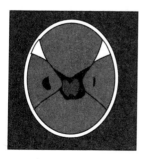
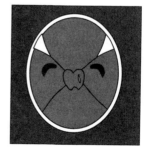

Early        Late

    **e. Duret hemorrhage:** midbrain hemorrhage (central tegmentum) due to compression of perforating vessels of the basilar artery in the interpeduncular cistern (better seen on MRI)

    **f.** Periaqueductal necrosis

    **g.** Tonsillar herniation (better seen on MRI)

2. **Ascending transtentorial:** upward herniation of the vermis and cerebellum through the tentorial incisura due to an **infratentorial** process

    **a.** The fourth ventricle is compressed and displaced anteriorly (early), leading to quadrigeminal cistern deformation and anterior displacement of the midbrain

    **b.** Aqueductal compression, leading to hydrocephalus

    **c.** Tonsillar herniation (better seen on MRI)

3. **Subfalcine (synonymous with midline shift)**

    **a.** Cingulate gyrus displaced across the midline under the margin of the falx cerebri

    **b.** Anterior cerebral artery (callosomarginal artery) compressed, leading to infarction (rare)

    **c.** Contralateral dilated ventricle due to foramen of Monro compression

4. **Transalar (transsphenoidal)**

    **a. Descending:** frontal lobe forced posteriorly over the greater sphenoid ala, causing backward displacement of sylvian fissure, middle cerebral artery (MCA), and temporal lobe

    **b. Ascending:** temporal lobe, sylvian fissure, and MCA displaced anteriorly over sphenoid ridge

**E. Cerebral edema.** Diffuse brain swelling due to increased intravascular blood volume and/or increased brain water content

1. Effacement of sulci and basal cisterns (suprasellar, quadrigeminal, perimesencephalic)

2. Small lateral ventricles

3. Homogenous decreased attenuation of supratentorial parenchyma with "white" cerebellum and brain stem (spared) 24–48 hours after injury

4. Herniation common

5. Mortality 50%

6. More common in children

**F. Ventriculoperitoneal shunts. Always compare the current study with the previous.** Even normal-appearing ventricles may represent hydrocephalus (i.e., shunt malfunction) if previously the ventricles were slitlike.

**G. Hydrocephalus:** occurs due to obstruction to CSF flow. The temporal horns are usually the first portions of the ventricles to dilate.

1. Communicating

    **a.** Ventricles appear large with respect to the sulci

    **b.** SAH, meningitis, normal-pressure hydrocephalus

2. Noncommunicating: obstruction at foramen of Monro, cerebral aqueduct, or fourth ventricle

# References

## General

Herts BR et al. Power injection of intravenous contrast material through central venous catheters for CT: In vitro evaluation. *Radiology* 200:731, 1996.

## Aortic Dissection

Fisher ER, Stein EJ, Godwin JD et al. Aortic dissection: typical and atypical imaging features. *Radiographics* 14:263, 1994.

Hartnell G. MRA of the aorta. Radiology Society of North America handout, October 21, 1995, Pp 1–11.

Lipton MJ. CT of thoracic aortic disease. American College of Radiology syllabus for the categorical course on cardiovascular imaging 1995, Pp 107–113.

Zegel HG, Chmielewski S, Freiman DB. The imaging evaluation of acute thoracic aortic dissection. *Applied Radiol* June 1995, Pp 15–25.

## Nontraumatic Acute Abdomen

Shirkhoda A. Diagnostic pitfalls in abdominal CT. *Radiographics* 11:969, 1991.

Taourel P, Pradel J, Fabre JM et al. Role of CT in the acute nontraumatic abdomen. *Semin Ultrasound CT MRI* 16:151, 1995.

## Abdominal and Pelvic Trauma

Federle MP, Brant-Zawadzki M. *Computed Tomography in the Evaluation of Trauma* (2nd ed). Baltimore: Williams & Wilkins, 1986.

Gay SB, Sisrom CL. Computed tomographic evaluation of blunt abdominal trauma. *Radiol Clin North Am* 30:367, 1992.

Pretorius ES, Fishman EK. Spiral computed tomography of upper abdominal trauma. *Emerg Radiol* 2:285, 1995.

Raptopoulos V. Abdominal trauma: Emphasis on computed tomography. *Radiol Clin North Am* 32:969, 1994.

Roberts JL, Dalen K, Bosanko CM, Jafir SZH. CT in abdominal and pelvic trauma. *Radiographics* 13:735, 1993.

Shirkhoda A. Diagnostic pitfalls in abdominal CT. *Radiographics* 11:969, 1991.

## Head

Laine FJ, Shedden AI, Dunn MM, Ghatak NR. Pictorial essay. Acquired intracranial herniations: MR imaging findings. *AJR Am J Roentgenol* 165:967, 1995.

Osborn AG. *Diagnostic Neuroradiology*. St. Louis: Mosby, 1994.

Provenzale J. Radiologic evaluation of intracranial trauma. *Appl Radiol* 23:11, 1994.

Ramsey RG. *Neuroradiology* (3rd ed). Philadelphia: Saunders, 1994.

Woodruff WW. *Fundamentals of Neuroimaging*. Philadelphia: Saunders, 1993.

# Magnetic Resonance Imaging

## General Considerations

I. **Clinical history**
   A. **Rule out cord compression or aortic dissection.** At the University of Chicago Hospital, cord compression and aortic dissection are the only routine indications for an emergent MRI. Other requests are handled on a case by case basis.
   B. **Patient's renal function.** If the creatinine level is higher than 2.0 mg/dl, dialysis should be performed after an infused scan.

II. **Common contraindications**
   A. Pacemakers
   B. Aneurysm clips (if a copy of the operative report documenting placement of a "safe" clip is provided, the requested scan is performed at our institution)
   C. Embolization coils less than 2 weeks old
   D. Inferior vena cava (IVC) filters less than 2 weeks old
   E. Thermodilution Swan-Ganz catheters
   F. Some ear implants (e.g., stapes prosthesis, drainage tubes, cochlear implants)
   G. Bullets in the brain
   H. Patient weight greater than 300 lb
   I. Halo vests or cervical fixation devices
   J. Carotid artery vascular clips (Poppen-Blalock clamp)
   K. Some dental implants
   L. Breast tissue expanders and implants
   M. Some penile implants
   N. Implantable venous access devices
   O. Diaphragms
   P. Muscle or nerve stimulators
   Q. Ventilators not specifically designed for use in an MRI scanner
   R. Chemotherapy pumps
   S. Metal fragments in the eye
   T. Holter monitors
   U. Transcutaneous electrical nerve stimulation (TENS) units
   V. IMED, IVAC, or morphine pumps

III. The following devices and situations are **not** contraindications for MRI:
   A. Heart valve prostheses
   B. Orthopedic devices
   C. Intravascular coils, filters, or stents 6 weeks after placement when positioned properly
   D. Status post–retinal surgery, lens implantation, or cataract surgery
   E. Dental implants attached to bone
   F. Joint prostheses, screws, plates, or suture wires
   G. Surgical clips
   H. Feeding or nasogastric tubes

**IV. Pregnant patients.** All pregnant patients should be aware that although MRI and MRI contrast agents pose no *known* hazards to mother or fetus, these procedures have not yet been *proved* safe. At our institution, breast-feeding is routinely stopped for 36 hours after gadolinium administration.

**V. Contrast reactions** are very rare with gadolinium administration but do occur. They should be treated in the same manner as other contrast reactions (see Ch. 1).

# Aortic Dissection

**I. Clinical history**

**A. Aortic dissection**

1. Twice as common as rupture of an abdominal aortic aneurysm
2. Usually occurs in men in their 60s and 70s
3. Classically, patients present with tearing chest pain radiating to the back.
4. Predisposing conditions include hypertension, bicuspid aortic valve, connective tissue disease, and pregnancy.

**B. Contraindications to CT.** At our institution, an emergent CT exam for aortic dissection can be performed more quickly than an MRI exam. Since the sensitivity and specificity are similar for both imaging modalities, at night, CT is usually our study of choice. However, if the patient has an allergy to iodinated contrast or will be followed with serial exams (e.g., Marfan's syndrome), an MRI exam should be considered. In a stable patient, MRI is considered by many to be the imaging modality of choice for evaluating suspected aortic dissection.

| Modality | Strengths | Weaknesses |
|---|---|---|
| Transthoracic echocardiography | Assesses aortic valve, hemopericardium, left ventricular function<br>Can be done portably | Cannot evaluate entire aorta |
| Transesophageal echocardiography | Assesses aortic valve, hemopericardium, left ventricular function<br>Can be done portably | Blind spots: behind the trachea, below the diaphragm |
| CT | Images the entire aorta and adjacent organs<br>Widely available | Cannot assess aortic valve or left ventricular function<br>Requires contrast |
| MRI | Assesses entire aorta, branch vessels, and valves | May not be tolerated by very ill patients<br>Other contraindications: |

| Modality | Strengths | Weaknesses |
|---|---|---|
| | | pacemakers, many patient monitoring devices |
| Aortography | Gold standard | Invasive Requires contrast |

II. **Imaging.** To achieve the best study, imaging parameters must be tailored to each patient. However, the general images we obtain are the following:

A. **Chest radiograph**
   1. Exclude other etiologies such as pneumothorax and rib fractures.
   2. Comparison films are extremely helpful.

B. **MRI of the thorax (with cardiac gating)**
   1. Scout view.
   2. T1 axial images from 2 cm above the arch to the diaphragm
   3. T1 sagittal oblique images (4-mm thickness)
   4. Cine GRASS axial images covering 6–12 images of the most suspicious area of aorta
   5. Cine two-dimensional (2D) phase contrast axial images (optional) to differentiate slow flow from thrombus (2–4 images)(venc 40 cm/sec)

C. **MRI of the abdomen (with cardiac gating)**
   1. T1 axial images from diaphragm to bifurcation
   2. Magnetic resonance angiography (MRA) 2D time of flight axial images (10-mm thickness) with breath hold of suspicious area
   3. Cine 2D phase contrast axial images (optional)—to differentiate slow flow from thrombus (venc 125 cm/sec) (2–4 images)

III. **Interpretation**

A. **Chest radiograph**
   1. Widened superior mediastinum (>8 cm)
   2. Superior extension of left mediastinal stripe above aortic arch, forming apical cap
   3. Right paratracheal widening
   4. Left pleural effusion
   5. Inward displacement of atherosclerotic calcifications (>6 mm)
   6. Tracheal (ET tube) or esophageal (NG tube) deviation to the right
   7. Inferior displacement of left main stem bronchus

B. **MRI general considerations**
   1. Flowing blood with velocity greater than 4 cm/sec will appear black on spin echo images.
   2. An intimal flap, thrombus, or slow-flowing blood will appear intermediate in signal on spin echo images, so gradient echo or phase contrast images should be obtained.

C. **Aortic dissection**
   1. Intimal flap separating vessel into true and false lumina (true lumen of a dissection is usually smaller than the false lumen)

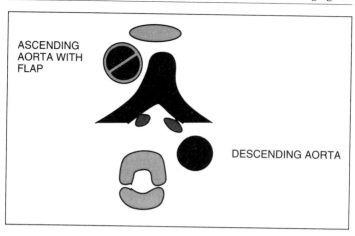

**ASCENDING
AORTA WITH
FLAP**

**DESCENDING AORTA**

**2.** Focal wall thickening with intramural hyperintense foci
(may represent blood) on T1-weighted images
**a.** No visible flap or compression of the true lumen
**b.** Must differentiate hyperintense foci (met-hemoglo-
bin) from normal fat in adventitial layer or thrombus
in an aneurysm

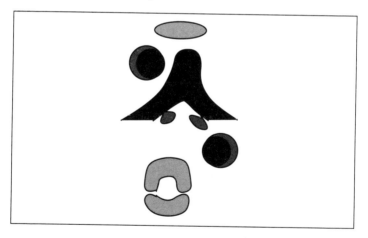

**3.** Mediastinal hemorrhage/pericardial effusion
**D. Classification.** MRI findings of aortic dissection are similar to CT findings:

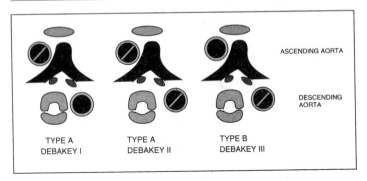

1. **Stanford type A dissections**
   a. Begin several centimeters above the aortic valve.
   b. Usually treated surgically since the dissection may extend proximally to involve the pericardial sac (leading to tamponade), aortic valve, and/or coronary arteries. Involvement of the great vessels is also important.
2. **Stanford type B dissections**
   a. Start distal to the ligamentum arteriosum.
   b. Usually treated medically with antihypertensive medications. Surgery is possible if acute ischemia exists.

IV. **Pitfalls**
   A. Normal structures that may be confused with dissections:
      1. Left brachiocephalic vein: runs anterior to the ascending aorta
      2. Left superior intercostal vein: runs on the left aspect of the arch

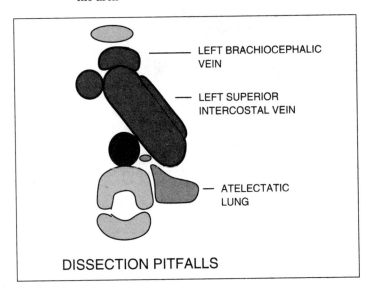

DISSECTION PITFALLS

**B.** Atrial and ventricular arrhythmias degrade image quality.
**C.** Motion artifact can be a serious problem, especially in critically ill patients.
**D.** An abdominal flap may be the only manifestation of dissection that does in fact extend into the thoracic aorta (occurs in approximately 5% of cases).
**E.** Mimics
   1. Aortitis: mural thickening with skip areas
   2. Atherosclerosis: may produce mural thickening but usually is diffuse rather than focal
   3. Thrombus in aneurysm: more common in the abdominal aorta than the thoracic aorta

# Spinal Cord

**I. Clinical history: rule out cord compression.** Most spinal cord MRIs performed emergently after-hours at our institution are performed on cancer patients who present with a focal neurologic exam or loss of bladder function. Always ask the location of the suspected lesion(s) since several types of scans can be performed based on the suspected area of cord compression and degree of suspicion. If the requesting service is quite certain of the level of compression (e.g., bone metastases are seen on a plain film), offer a dedicated exam (cervical, thoracic, or lumbar). If the service is uncertain, suggest a spine survey.

**II. Imaging.** Due to the physical size of the MRI coil used in spine surveys, only one-half the spine can be imaged in an acquisition. Therefore, the most suspicious half should be imaged *first*. We perform two general types of surveys based on the expected location of the lesion (extradural, intradural-extramedullary, or intramedullary).

   **A. Suspected extradural lesions** (e.g., suspected prostate cancer metastases)
   1. T1/T2/PD sagittal images
   2. T1 axial images
   3. T2/PD axial images (optional)—only if there is known thecal sac or cord compression

   **B. Suspected intradural or intramedullary lesions** (e.g., melanoma metastases)
   1. T1 axial images with and without **gadolinium**
   2. T1 sagittal images with and without **gadolinium**
   3. T2/PD sagittal images
   4. T2/PD axial images (optional)—only if there is known thecal sac or cord compression

   Suspected metastases are the indication for most spine surveys. In the majority of cases, IV contrast is unnecessary. In fact, osseous metastases are commonly **less conspicuous** on postinfused images. If the primary carcinoma is prostate or colon cancer, perform the first type of survey; IV contrast is unnecessary because these malignancies almost never metastasize to the spinal cord. For other primary lesions including lung, breast, melanoma or CNS that may cause leptomeningeal carcinomatosis, select the second type of survey that includes contrast infusion.

**III. Interpretation.** The T1 sagittal images (white cord surrounded by black CSF) give the best overall first impression of the cord. After detecting an anomaly on the sagittal images, proceed to axial views to confirm findings. Signs of cord compression include the inability to visualize CSF adjacent to cord and/or extension of a mass into the vertebral canal, narrowing the cord. Describe what is seen (e.g., "There is some flattening of the left side of the cord at T3–5").

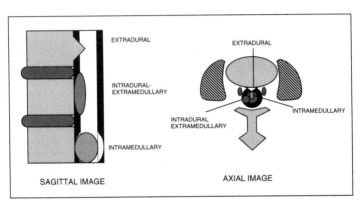

### A. Extradural
1. Tumor
    a. Colon
    b. Prostate
    c. Lung (may also be intradural)
    d. Breast (may also be intradural)
2. Trauma
    a. Hematoma
    b. Bone fragment
3. Disk: cervical spine, lumbar spine
4. Infection
    a. Bacterial
    b. Tuberculosis
    c. Abscess
5. Degenerative: Osteophyte
### B. Intradural extramedullary
1. Tumor
    a. Meningioma
    b. Lipoma
    c. Ependymoma
    d. Neurofibroma
    e. Metastasis
2. Abscess
### C. Intramedullary
1. Tumor
    a. Ependymoma
    b. Astrocytoma
    c. Hemangioblastoma
2. Trauma: Hematoma

   **3.** Syrinx
   **4.** Postradiation
IV. **Pitfalls**
   A. **Syrinx**
   1. On sagittal T1WI, a truncation artifact (Gibb's phenomenon) can occur, producing a dark band centrally in the cord that mimics the appearance of a syrinx. Always confirm findings on the axial and T2-weighted images. A true syrinx will appear on all images.
   2. Many primary spinal cord tumors may simulate the appearance of a syrinx. Administer gadolinium and check for an enhancing tumor nodule if a syrinx is identified.
   B. **Vertebral osteoporotic compression fractures and pathologic fractures** may be difficult or impossible to differentiate.
   1. Both may have hypointense areas that enhance with contrast.
   2. Benign compression fractures tend to have a straight horizontal or vertical demarcation between the hypointense and hyperintense regions.
   3. Pathologic fractures tend to exhibit a more irregular border between hypointense and hyperintense areas.

# References

### General

Shellock FG. *Pocket Guide to MR Procedures and Metallic Objects: Update 1994*. Hagerstown, MD: Lippincott-Raven, 1994.

### Aortic Dissection

Hartnell G. MRA of the aorta. Radiology Society of North America handout, October 21, 1995, Pp 1–11.
Wolff KA, Herold CJ, Tempany CM et al. Aortic dissection: Atypical patterns seen at MR imaging. *Radiology* 181:489, 1991.
Zegel HG, Chmielewski S, Freiman DB. The imaging evaluation of acute thoracic aortic dissection. *Applied Radiol* June 1995, Pp 15–25.

### Spinal Cord

Osborn AG. *Diagnostic Neuroradiology*. St. Louis: Mosby, 1994.
Ramsey RG. *Neuroradiology* (3rd ed). Philadelphia: Saunders, 1994.

# Gastrointestinal and Genitourinary Studies

## Bowel Obstruction

### I. Clinical history

**A. Rule out obstruction or free air.** One of the most common requests for an emergent abdominal radiograph is to exclude obstruction or free air. Further follow-up is based on the findings of this examination. The small bowel is the site of approximately 75% of obstructions and the colon is the site of the remaining 25%.

**B. Bowel sounds.** Auscultation is the easiest way to distinguish ileus from obstruction. However, the absence of bowel sounds does not rule out an obstruction; bowel sounds often vanish late in obstruction and may be absent in patients with fluid-filled bowel loops.

### II. Imaging

**A. Plain film.** Obtain upright and supine plain films.

    **1. Pneumoperitoneum.** Air in the peritoneal space is usually due to ruptured hollow viscus or recent abdominal surgery.

        **a. Findings**

            **(1) Rigler's sign:** both sides of the bowel wall are visualized. Need approximately 1 liter of intraperitoneal air

            **(2) Air** under right hemidiaphragm on **upright** chest radiograph (not portable)—both PA and lateral views should be obtained.

            **(3) Triangle sign:** gas between three bowel loops or two bowel loops and parietal peritoneum

            **(4) Hyperlucent liver**

            **(5) Hepatic edge sign:** air outlining the inferior portion of the liver

            **(6) Anterior superior oval:** oblong air collection anterior to the liver

            **(7) Ligamentum teres sign:** sharply defined vertical slit or oval at the porta hepatis

            **(8) Doge hat sign:** triangle-shaped air collection in Morison's (hepatorenal) pouch

        **b. Pitfalls**

            **(1) Postoperative air** usually resolves within **7–10 days** but may persist up to 2–4 weeks in very thin patients.

            **(2) Rigler's sign** may be mimicked by abundant air swallowing causing omental or mesenteric fat or meteorism (multiple dilated gas-filled loops apposing each other).

        **c. Follow-up: left lateral decubitus exam**

            **(1)** Perform a left side down decubitus plain film centering on the liver to achieve horizontal beam. Do **not** request "upright" portable film.

(2) Air usually collects between the right lateral liver margin and lateral hemidiaphragm. In patients with wide hips, it may collect in the right pelvis.

2. **Small bowel versus colon**

   **a.** Valvulae conniventes (plicae circulares, Kerckring's folds) of the small bowel completely encircle the bowel and appear finer and closer together than colonic haustra, which occupy only a portion of the transverse diameter of the bowel. Valvulae conniventes are the most prominent in the duodenum and jejunum; the ileum may appear featureless.

   **b.** Small-bowel loops are located in the central abdomen, while colonic-bowel loops are situated in the peripheral abdomen.

   **c.** Solid or semisolid material is present only in the colon; only gas or liquid is present in the small bowel.

3. **Small-bowel obstruction (SBO)**

   **a.** The diameter of the small-bowel loop is greater than 3 cm (the proximal bowel is usually more dilated than the distal bowel)

   **b.** Greater than two air fluid levels (AFLs) in the small bowel

   **c.** AFLs in the small bowel (not colon) at different heights

   **d.** "String of beads": most specific sign of obstruction on plain radiographs

   **e.** Decreased or absent colonic gas: nonspecific

   **f.** Gasless abdomen (fluid-filled loops): "nonspecific bowel gas pattern"

   **g.** Stacked coins

   **h.** **Pitfalls**

      (1) Remember that the level of the obstruction cannot be determined since several fluid-filled loops may be interposed between the dilated air-filled loops and the level of obstruction.

      (2) The "string of beads" sign is often subtle and easily overlooked. Do not confuse it with pneumatosis.

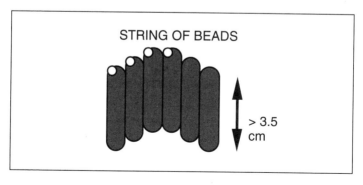

STRING OF BEADS

> 3.5 cm

4. **Colonic obstruction**

   **a.** The cecum is the most dilated segment of the colon.

   **b.** The colon is more than 7–8 cm in diameter.

**c.** The colon "cut-off sign" (abrupt end of gas-filled bowel loop) is present.

**d.** Small-bowel dilatation (25%) is due to an incompetent ileocecal valve.

**e.** AFLs in the colon are **not** significant.

If obstruction is suspected on upright and supine views, obtain a right lateral decubitus view and/or prone views to determine if air will move distal to the suspected obstruction into the left colon or rectum. This will exclude obstruction.

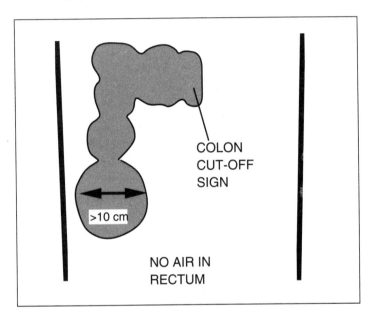

5. **Cecal volvulus**
   **a.** A dilated cecum extending to the left upper quadrant, displacing the stomach downward to the left, is present.
   **b.** Colonoscopy is the diagnostic and therapeutic procedure of choice.
6. **Sigmoid volvulus**
   **a.** "Coffee bean" or inverted U-shaped loop that migrates cephalad to the transverse colon and "points" to the right upper quadrant
   **b.** Absent haustra and plicae
   **c.** Proximal colonic dilatation (less severe than sigmoid loop)
7. **Ileus**
   **a.** Gas throughout small bowel and colon. This pattern is also present in a partial or "early" SBO (i.e., gas is not yet out of the bowel distal to the obstruction)
   **b.** Obtain serial examinations. In an obstruction, air will usually pass through the colon over several

hours, resulting in a more typical appearance of SBO. It may take 1–2 days for all the air to pass through the colon.

8. **Meteorism** (extensive air swallowing): AFLs absent
B. **Follow-up studies**
  1. **SBO:** see the section on Small-Bowel Obstruction.
  2. **Colonic obstruction:** see the section on Colonic Obstruction.

# Small-Bowel Obstruction

I. **Clinical history**
  A. **Patient with nausea, vomiting, and inability to pass gas.** In a patient with distended, air-filled bowel loops, the differential diagnosis is ileus versus obstruction. The small bowel is the site of 75% of intestinal obstructions. With very few exceptions, a mechanical SBO is an indication for urgent surgical relief. There is a 60% mortality for complete, untreated SBO. With treatment, the mortality drops to 5%.
  B. **Risk factors**
    1. **SBO etiologies**
      a. Adhesions (75%)
      b. Hernias (inguinal, femoral, umbilical, internal)
      c. Neoplasm
      d. Inflammatory disease
      e. Volvulus
    2. **Ileus etiologies**
      a. Postsurgical
      b. Medications (atropine, morphine, Lomotil, L-dopa)
      c. Electrolyte imbalance (especially hypokalemia)
      d. Any abdominal inflammatory process
II. **Imaging**
  A. **Plain films.** See the section on Bowel Obstruction.
  B. **CT.** Often, an SBO can be diagnosed by plain films alone, rendering further studies unnecessary. In equivocal cases, **perform a CT examination** before a barium study. The sensitivity and specificity of CT is greater than 90% in demonstrating an SBO. It also will give the best overall evaluation of the abdomen in most cases. If a dedicated small-bowel exam is done first, a CT **cannot** be performed until high-density barium used in the fluoroscopic study is cleared from the bowels. Administer two bottles of CT barium 1–2 hours before CT scanning, then one bottle immediately before scanning.
    1. Transition point: dilated proximal bowel (>2.5–3.0 cm in diameter) and nondilated distal bowel
    2. Ischemia/strangulation
      a. Circumferential bowel wall thickening
      b. Pneumatosis intestinalis: in the proper clinical context, it indicates ischemia until proved otherwise
      c. Increased density of adjacent mesenteric fat
  C. **Contrast study.** Avoid fluoroscopic studies in cases of suspected distal SBO. If the service insists on a **dedicated small bowel exam,** remember the following:

1. If there is any question of a proximal colonic obstruction rather than a distal SBO, **perform a barium enema first.** In a distal SBO, reflux through the ileocecal valve may delineate the level of obstruction. More important, if barium is given by mouth in a proximal colonic obstruction, it will solidify in the colon and exacerbate an already poor clinical situation.
2. Do **not** give metoclopramide (Reglan).
3. In a proximal SBO, use **barium** rather than gastrografin. Barium is denser than gastrografin and thus will allow better visualization of the small bowel (especially when mixed with bowel contents). More important, it is inert. Because gastrografin is hyperosmolar, fluid will be drawn into the bowel, diluting the contrast and possibly exacerbating an obstructive presentation.

III. **Types of SBO**
   A. **Intussusception:** low-density mesenteric fat and vessels are seen within a dilated bowel loop (in adults, the majority are associated with a lead point such as a neoplasm).
   B. **Adhesion:** transition from dilated to nondilated bowel without visible cause (diagnosis of exclusion)
   C. **Closed loop (incarcerated) obstruction:** fluid-filled, U-shaped dilated loop with nondistended proximal and distal bowel loops; prone to ischemia
   D. **Volvulus:** twisting of bowel and mesentery (whirl sign); bowel narrows to the shape of a beak (beak sign)
   E. **Hernia**
      1. Inguinal
      2. Internal
         a. Left paraduodenal: bowel loops herniating through the peritoneal defect in the transverse mesocolon; small-bowel loops between the stomach and pancreas
         b. Other types are difficult to diagnose by CT.

# Colonic Obstruction

I. **Clinical history**
   A. **Rule out distal obstruction.** Colonic obstruction represents 25% of intestinal obstructions.
   B. **Barium versus dilute gastrografin.** If the clinical service has any suspicion of perforation or the patient is taking steroids, use **gastrografin.** Barium peritonitis is a disastrous complication of barium enema (BE) and should be avoided. Also, some surgeons prefer not to operate on a colon containing barium if the patient should need emergent surgery. If gastrografin is chosen, remember that it is very hypertonic (and thus will draw a great deal of fluid into the colon); tell the clinical service to keep the patient **well hydrated** after the procedure. Warn the service that a CT exam cannot be performed until barium is cleared from the colon since the barium used in fluoroscopic exams is much more dense than that used in CT and will result in extensive streak artifact.

### C. Contraindications

1. Toxic megacolon: dilated colon (the transverse colon is the most dilated in the supine view) with effaced haustra and possibly pseudopolyps. It often occurs in patients with a history of ulcerative colitis.
2. Pneumatosis
3. Portal venous gas
4. Extraluminal gas ("free air")
5. Pseudomembranous colitis (severe cases)

## II. Imaging

### A. Abdominal plain film

1. Always obtain plain films before attempting a BE. Never perform a BE if there is "free air." Remember, an **upright** chest radiograph is the most sensitive plain film exam for detection of free air. If the patient is unable to stand, perform a left lateral (left side down) decubitus exam. If possible, keep the patient in the left side down position for 5–10 minutes before obtaining the radiograph.
2. See the section on Bowel Obstruction.

### B. Barium enema.
If the cecum is larger than 10 cm in diameter or impending bowel perforation is suspected, use **gastrografin** or other water-soluble contrast rather than barium.

Barium ultra–low density (15–20% w/v)

KVP—120 KeV

1. Take the powder-containing bag and add 2 liters of warm (**not hot**) water, then shake vigorously.
2. Attach tip.
3. Attach a clamp to control flow.
4. In some kits, before the barium will flow out of the bag, a sponge "plug" that prevents barium from entering the tube during shaking must be removed. This is done by squeezing the tube just distal to the plug to force it backwards into the barium bag.
5. Administer 1 ml of glucagon IV or IM.
6. Place the patient in the left lateral decubitus position and perform a digital rectal exam. If a mass or stricture is palpated, do **not** inflate the retention balloon.
7. Lubricate, then insert, the tip. A common error is to continue to direct the tip anteriorly after it has passed the anus. Remember that the normal course of the rectum is **posterior** once it has passed the anus. Directing the tip anteriorly after it has passed the anus can result in rectal perforation.
8. Begin the flow of barium. The bag should be approximately 2–3 feet above the level of the table.
9. If the patient is unable to hold the barium in the rectum, inflate the retention balloon with fluoroscopic monitoring. Air is put into the balloon until it displaces nearly all of the barium between itself and the rectal wall. Do not overinflate the balloon! Rectal perforation is a well-documented complication of BE. The balloon should not substantially contact or expand the rectal wall.

10. Take images of the sigmoid and rectum while slowly turning the patient supine.
11. Image the entire colon to the ileocecal valve or level of obstruction.
12. Obtain postevacuation films.

### C. Gastrografin enema

Gastrografin 800 ml 1:1 dilution

KVP—80–85 KeV

1. Add gastrografin to the empty bag and proceed as above.
2. Remember that gastrografin is very hypertonic and will draw fluid into the colon; it is an effective therapeutic enema in constipated patients.

### D. Ostomy study

1. Discuss the postsurgical anatomy and expected findings with the clinical service.
2. Cut a small hole in the tip of an infant feeding nipple and 4 × 4 gauze.
3. Insert a 26–30 French soft, rubber catheter with multiple side holes through the gauze pad and nipple tip.
4. Attach the contrast bag to the catheter.
5. If air contrast is desired, insert an 18-gauge needle attached to an insufflation bulb into the proximal portion of the catheter.

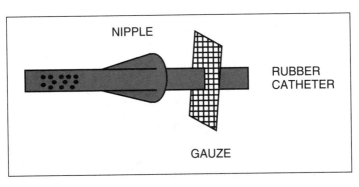

6. Lubricate the tip of the rubber catheter and insert approximately 15–20 cm into the stoma with the patient supine.
7. Occlude stoma by firmly holding the nipple and gauze at the skin opening (the patient may be able to perform this function) and begin contrast flow.

Occasionally, it is necessary to put a balloon within the colostomy. This should only be done if all other attempts fail and the procedure is a true emergency.

1. Insert the smallest catheter that will fit into the ostomy (usually 8–10 French).
2. Insert the balloon beyond the abdominal wall and slowly inflate it while monitoring with fluoroscopy while jiggling the catheter back and forth.

3. Once the balloon will occlude the ostomy (but remain movable inside the bowel), gently pull back on the catheter and use the balloon as a ball valve to prevent contrast from coming out of the ostomy.
4. If the patient complains of any discomfort while you are inflating the balloon, stop inflating it!

### III. Interpretation

**A. Cancer versus diverticulitis.** In many cases, it is impossible to differentiate the two diseases, and both occur simultaneously in up to 30% of patients.

1. **Diverticulitis**
   a. There is a gradual transition zone into an area of thickened but intact mucosa, often in the region of the sigmoid colon.
   b. Fixation and spiculation of bowel loops
   c. Filling of an abscess cavity or fistula tract (best seen on postevacuation films)
   d. Other diverticula

2. **Neoplastic process**
   a. Abrupt transition zone ("shouldering")
   b. Nodularity of the affected segment with mucosal destruction
   c. More commonly results in complete obstruction

**B. Perforation.** Small perforations can be difficult to detect.

1. **Follow-up abdominal plain film.** After 2–4 hours, gastrografin will be secreted by the kidneys if a perforation exists.

**C. Ostomy study**

1. Fistula
2. Stenosis
3. Recurrence

**D. Sigmoid volvulus**

1. "Bird's beak": contrast extends to the point of rotation of the bowel
2. BE may be diagnostic and therapeutic.

### IV. Pitfalls

**A. Retention balloons** should not be inflated in any patient who has rectal disease, such as known stricture or tumor. They also should not be inflated in patients who are status post–recent anorectal surgery or pelvic radiation therapy.

**B. Ostomy studies.** Foley catheters inflated in ostomies can perforate bowel and should be avoided if possible.

**C. Pseudo-obstruction (Ogilvie's syndrome).** Right lateral decubitus or prone views will usually confirm that a true obstruction is absent.

# Esophagram

### I. Clinical history: rule out esophageal perforation.

Early diagnosis of esophageal perforation is critical. Untreated perforations of the thoracic esophagus have a mortality of 100% (70% if treated within 24 hours). Cervical esophageal perforations, while less serious, still have a 15% overall mortality. Most perforations (75–80%) occur as a result of endoscopy, foreign-body ingestion, or intubation.

## II. Imaging
### A. Plain films
1. **Cervical perforation**
   a. Subcutaneous emphysema after 1 hour progressing to pneumomediastinum
   b. Prevertebral air or abscess
2. **Thoracic perforation**
   a. Pleural effusion (left greater than right)
   b. Hydropneumothorax (75% on left)
   c. Pneumomediastinum (usually develops later than effusion)
   d. If perforation is distal, air may dissect into the lesser sac or retroperitoneum
   e. Usually **no pneumoperitoneum**
   f. Spontaneous perforation (Boerhaave's syndrome) usually occurs immediately above the gastroesophageal junction on the anterior left side of the esophagus.
3. **Foreign body**
   a. Perform lateral view with patient phonating, "Eeee" to distend the pharynx.
   b. Frontal view to confirm location
### B. Contrast study: barium versus gastrografin. Each type of contrast has particular advantages and disadvantages. The figure below should dictate the choice of contrast. Ask the clinical service the approximate location of the suspected tear. If the service is unsure of the location of the suspected perforation, begin with gastrografin and if a tear is not seen, proceed to barium.
1. **Proximal tears**
   a. Use barium (e.g., high-density 220–240% w/v E-Z-HD)
   b. Advantages: barium is far superior to gastrografin for demonstrating esophageal tears due to its higher density.
   c. Disadvantages
      (1) Barium extravasation into the mediastinum is associated with fibrosing mediastinitis.
      (2) Barium peritonitis is a possible complication if the patient has a distal tear.
2. **Distal tears**
   a. Use gastrografin.
   b. Advantages: no risk of fibrosing mediastinitis or peritonitis
   c. Disadvantages
      (1) Since it is hyperosmolar (6 times normal serum), if aspirated into the lungs, gastrografin will cause pulmonary edema (i.e., it will draw water into the lungs), which may be fatal.
      (2) Tears are more difficult to visualize with gastrografin because of the contrast's low density.

If perforation into the mediastinum is suspected (symptoms of chest pain, fever, subcutaneous emphysema, especially after endoscopy), gastrografin should be the initial contrast agent, followed by barium if no leak is seen. If rupture into the airway is suspected (paroxysmal coughing or choking after ingestion of liquids, especially with a history of esophageal cancer) or severe vomiting is present, barium should be chosen.

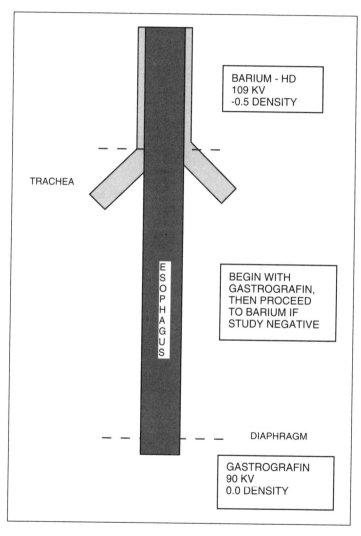

### 3. Procedure
**a.** Begin by administering one-half dose of gas granules and approximately 25 ml of contrast in a small cup. Remember to **always** begin with small boluses and control the size of the bolus given to the patient.

**b.** Position the patient left posterior oblique and administer bolus under fluoroscopic monitoring. (If a tracheoesophageal fistula is suspected, place the patient in the lateral position.)

**c.** If extravasation is not seen, proceed to larger boluses and place the patient in multiple recumbent positions (if possible).

**d.** If extravasation is not seen with gastrografin, proceed to barium, repeating the above steps. Decrease KVP from 109 KV to 90 KV.

**e.** If extravasation is seen, instruct the patient to stop drinking and take spot films of the area in several projections.

**f.** Sometimes CT can be helpful if extravasation is not seen and clinical suspicion remains high.

# Excretory Urogram

**I. Clinical history**

**A. Choice of CT, ultrasound, or intravenous excretory urogram (IVU).** There is no general consensus on the imaging evaluation of choice in suspected renal colic. The three popular modalities—IVU, noninfused helical CT, and ultrasound (with or without abdominal radiograph)—have comparable sensitivities and specificities for renal obstruction. Traditionally, the IVU was the study of choice and still provides the best overall anatomic evaluation of the urinary tract if intervention is planned. Ultrasound is generally the study of choice for pregnant women and children since exposure to ionizing radiation is eliminated. Noninfused helical CT has been used and may provide the most rapid information with the added benefit of visualization of other abdominal and pelvic structures.

**B. Patient allergies.** If the patient has any allergies, perform a noninfused helical CT examination or ultrasound instead of the IVU.

**C. BUN and creatinine levels.** Elevation of either is not an absolute contraindication to IVU; however, a creatinine above 1.5 is associated with higher risk of atubular necrosis. Again, suggest a noninfused helical CT or ultrasound examination instead.

**II. Imaging.** Tell the clinical service to stop hydrating the patient and to make sure the patient has a functional IV.

**A. Equipment**

1. Two 60-ml syringes
2. Butterfly needle or IV with connecting tubing
3. Tourniquet
4. Contrast (we recommend liberal use of nonionic contrast, such as 75 cc of Omnipaque 300 at night). Specific indications for nonionic contrast are listed in Ch. 1.

**B. Emergency medications and equipment**

1. Oxygen
2. Bag-ventilation device

      **3.** Stethoscope and blood pressure cuff
      **4.** Crash cart
      **5.** IV fluids
      **6.** Do **not** inject contrast and leave the patient unmonitored! Always be aware of the possibility of a contrast reaction.

  **C. Procedure for intravenous excretory urogram**
      **1.** Check the scout film (should include adrenals to 1–2 cm below the symphysis pubis)
      **2.** Inject 75–100 ml of contrast at approximately 1–2 ml/sec. A faster injection will give a better nephrogram but is associated with more minor reactions, such as nausea and vomiting.
      **3.** After the infusion, raise the arm and flush with saline.
      **4.** Image at 1, 5, 15, and 30 minutes after injection if the study appears normal (in a child, images at 1 and 15 minutes will usually suffice). Tailor the exam depending on the findings. Standing, supine, or oblique views are frequently helpful to better demonstrate the course of the ureters. If the study is abnormal, obtain images at 2, 4, 8, and 24 hours or until the level of the obstruction is visualized.
      **5. Pre- and postvoid image of the bladder.** Sometimes, a postvoid image will decompress the ureter and distinguish "pseudo-obstruction" from true obstruction.

**III. Checklist**
  **A. Scout film**
      **1.** Calcification: aortic aneurysm, renal stones
      **2.** Splinting
      **3.** Ileus
  **B. Nephrogram**
      **1.** Delay on one side suggests acute renal obstruction
      **2.** Delay bilaterally may be due to hypotension! **Assess the patient!**
  **C. Collecting systems and ureters**
      **1.** Unilateral hydronephrosis can occur with acute renal obstruction or a recently passed calculus or bladder lesion at the ureterovesical junction.
      **2.** The study should be performed until the level of obstruction is determined.
  **D. Bladder**
      **1.** Diverticula
      **2.** Calculi
      **3.** Postvoid residual
  **E. Perinephric fluid:** Ruptured calyx

**IV. Disease entities**
  **A. Nephrolithiasis**
      **1.** Calculi are usually radiopaque (>90%)
      **2.** Cystine and uric acid stones are radiolucent
      **3.** The size of the stone has important therapeutic implications: stones greater than 5 mm are generally removed with intervention. Stones less than 5 mm are managed expectantly and usually pass spontaneously.
  **B. Acute obstruction**
      **1.** Faint nephrogram that gradually intensifies over hours
      **2.** Delayed appearance of collecting system enhancement
      **3.** Poor opacification of collecting system

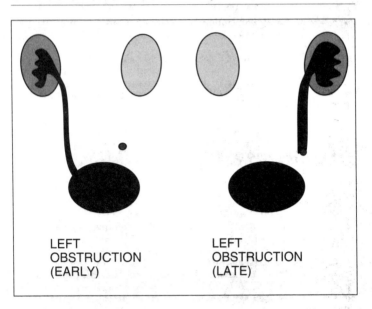

LEFT
OBSTRUCTION
(EARLY)

LEFT
OBSTRUCTION
(LATE)

C. **Hypotensive nephrogram.** Initially, good nephrograms are seen and contrast is excreted from the collecting systems. Contrast stops being excreted as blood pressure drops, and only nephrograms are seen as the kidney is less well perfused. **Assess the patient!**

D. **Hydronephrosis/hydroureter**
  1. Often, after passing a calculus, a reflex hydronephrosis and hydroureter are seen on the affected side.
  2. Obstruction

V. **Pitfalls**
  A. **Contrast extravasation.** One hopes that only a small amount of contrast will have been extravasated since the infusion is being monitored (See Ch. 1).
  B. **Allergic reactions**
    1. See Ch. 1.
    2. We prefer using an IV rather than a butterfly needle. If the patient has a contrast reaction, we already have IV access and can rapidly administer medications or fluids as needed.

# Retrograde Urethrogram/Cystogram

I. **Clinical history**
  A. **Trauma patient with blood at urethral meatus, a "high-riding" prostate, and inability to void spontaneously.** Urethral injury occurs in 5–10% of males and 5% of females with pelvic fractures. Associated bladder injury is present in 10–20% of patients with posterior urethral trauma. In the absence of pelvic fractures, posterior urethral injury is rare. A urethrogram should be per-

formed before urethral catheterization in any male patient with an anterior pelvic arch fracture, straddle-type injury, or penetrating injury of the buttocks or perineum.

B. **Placement of Foley catheter.** Although a Foley catheter should never be placed in patients with suspected urethral trauma, placement does occasionally occur. If a Foley catheter has been successfully placed, complete urethral transection is doubtful. Do **not** remove the catheter to perform the study; instead, defer the study until the catheter is no longer required. Alternatively, an 8 French pediatric feeding tube can be placed adjacent to the catheter to perform a contrast study.

C. **Angiography.** Do not perform a urethrogram until angiography has been completed. Extravasated contrast material may interfere with interpretation of the vascular study.

D. **Contrast allergy.** Retrograde urethrography is associated with contrast reactions in patients with contrast allergies.

II. **Imaging. Never attempt to pass a Foley catheter into the bladder in someone with urethral trauma!**

A. Attach an 8 or 10 French Foley catheter to a syringe filled with contrast (e.g., Conray 30). Make sure that all air bubbles are out of the catheter.

B. Pass the catheter into the navicular fossa (1-cm-long bulbus dilatation of the distal anterior urethra) and inflate **gently** with 2–3 ml of water until secure. The navicular fossa is wider than the external meatus so the urethra is sealed for contrast infusion.

C. Place the patient supine in a left or right posterior oblique position. Flex the dependent leg, tape the catheter to the thigh, and extend the superior leg.

D. **Slowly** infuse contrast (approximately 25–30 ml) and take spot films. Steady pressure will overcome the initial resistance due to the external sphincter. Injecting too quickly in a urethral injury will result in flooding the field with contrast.

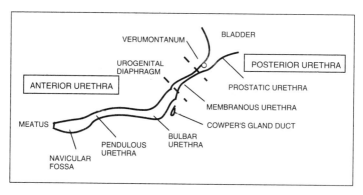

E. If there is no evidence of extravasation, deflate the Foley balloon and gently pass the catheter into the bladder to perform a cystogram.

F. After infusing approximately 100 ml, check for extravasation and obtain frontal and oblique spot films.

G. Fill the bladder until the patient has the urge to void (usually a total of approximately 300–350 ml). Document any extravasation.

H. Always take a postvoid bladder image. Occasionally, this will be the only film showing extravasation.

### III. Interpretation

A. **Posterior urethral injuries.** In patients with pelvic fractures, classically the prostatomembranous urethra is injured above the urogenital diaphragm. Urine does not escape the bladder unless it is also injured. Posterior urethral injuries are classified as follows:

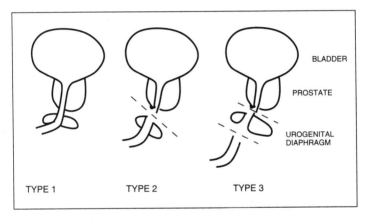

BLADDER

PROSTATE

UROGENITAL DIAPHRAGM

TYPE 1            TYPE 2            TYPE 3

1. **Type 1.** Stretched, intact posterior urethra with torn puboprostatic ligaments. The urethra may appear narrowed by proximal displacement of the prostate or hematoma, elevating the bladder.

2. **Type 2 (rare).** Urethral rupture at the membranoprostatic junction above the intact urogenital diaphragm. There is contrast extravasation into the pelvic extraperitoneal space. There is no contrast extravasation into the perineum.

3. **Type 3 (most common).** Urethral rupture with extension into the bulbar urethra and/or urogenital diaphragm. Contrast extravasation is above and below the urogenital diaphragm into the perineum. Contrast may extend into the scrotum and outline the testicle. The prostate is dislocated proximally.

B. **Anterior urethral injuries** occur most commonly with **straddle-type accidents** (e.g., falling on a bicycle bar).

1. Injuries usually occur at the bulbar urethra.

2. Associated fractures are uncommon.

3. Extravasation will occur between Buck's fascia and the tunica albuginea if Buck's fascia is intact. If Buck's fascia is lacerated, contrast will extend into Colles' fascia.

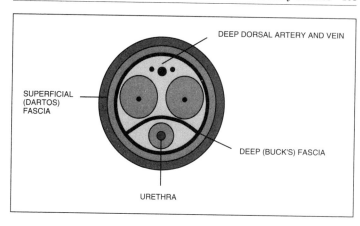

DEEP DORSAL ARTERY AND VEIN

SUPERFICIAL (DARTOS) FASCIA

DEEP (BUCK'S) FASCIA

URETHRA

## C. Bladder injuries

### 1. Intraperitoneal rupture

**a.** Usually occurs at the dome (weakest portion)

**b.** Contrast outlines bowel and flows into paracolic gutters

**c.** Associated with pelvic fractures in approximately 25% of cases

**d.** Occurs more commonly when the bladder is full

### 2. Extraperitoneal rupture

**a.** Usually caused by anterior pelvic arch fracture (lacerates the bladder)

**b.** Approximately twice as common as intraperitoneal rupture

## IV. Pitfalls

**A. Cowper's glands** are located in the urogenital membrane adjacent to the membranous urethra. The ducts from the gland extend distally to empty into the anterior urethra. Reflux into these ducts should not be confused with extravasation.

# References

**Bowel Obstruction**

Shaffer HA Jr. Perforation and obstruction of the gastrointestinal tract: Assessment by conventional radiology. *Radiol Clin North Am* 30:403, 1992.

**Small-Bowel Obstruction**

Frager DH, Baer JW. Role of CT in evaluating patients with small bowel obstruction. *Semin Ultrasound CT MRI* 16:127, 1995.

Gelfand DW. Complications of gastrointestinal radiologic procedures. I. Complications of routine fluoroscopic studies. *Gastrointestinal Radiol* 5:99, 1980.

Megibow AJ. Bowel obstruction. Evaluation with CT. *Radiol Clin North Am* 32:861, 1994.

Taourel PG, Fabre JM, Pradel JA, et al. Value of computed tomography in the diagnosis and management of patients with suspected acute small bowel obstruction. *AJR Am J Roentgenol* 165:1187, 1995.

## Colonic Obstruction

Burhenne, HJ. Technique of colostomy examination. *Radiology* 97:183, 1970.

Gelfand DW. Complications of gastrointestinal radiologic procedures. I. Complications of routine fluoroscopic studies. *Gastrointestinal Radiol* 5:99, 1980.

Goldstein HM, Miller MH. Air contrast colon examination in patients with colostomies. *AJR Am J Roentgenol* 127:607, 1976.

Shaffer HA Jr. Perforation and obstruction of the gastrointestinal tract: Assessment by conventional radiology. *Radiol Clin North Am* 30:403, 1992.

## Esophagram

Gelfand DW. Complications of gastrointestinal radiologic procedures. I. Complications of routine fluoroscopic studies. *Gastrointestinal Radiol* 5:99, 1980.

Ghahremani GG. Radiologic evaluation of suspected gastrointestinal perforations. *Radiol Clin North Am* 31:1219, 1993.

Levine MS. Questions and answers. *AJR Am J Roentgenol* 162:1243, 1994.

White CS, Templeton PA, Attar S. Esophageal perforation: CT findings. *AJR Am J Roentgenol* 160:767, 1993.

## Excretory Urogram

Choyke PL. The urogram: Are rumors of its death premature? *Radiology* 184:33, 1992.

## Retrograde Urethrogram/Cystogram

Amis ES. The urethra. Radiology Society of North America Categorical Course in Genitourinary Radiology 1994, Pp 147–157.

# Nuclear Medicine

## Gastrointestinal Bleeding Study

I. **Clinical history**
   A. **Bleeding bright red blood per rectum.** Endoscopy is the study of choice for the evaluation of upper GI hemorrhage, while either nuclear medicine scanning or angiography is best for lower GI bleeding. As a rule, the darker the blood, the more proximal the source. If no blood is aspirated via nasogastric tube, there is a 90% chance that bleeding is from a lower GI source.
   B. **Angiogram versus nuclear medicine bleeding study.** In general, perform the nuclear medicine study first because its sensitivity is greater than angiography. The rate of bleeding must be **at least 0.5–1.0 ml/min for angiographic detection.** This is approximately 2–3 units per 24 hours or a 10% drop in hematocrit. A **nuclear medicine scan may be positive with bleeding rates of 0.1–0.2 ml/minute.** Also, if positive, the nuclear medicine scan can be helpful in guiding the angiogram. Arterial bleeding usually occurs intermittently, followed by vessel spasm and temporary cessation of bleeding. Often, by the time the patient begins to pass blood per rectum, bleeding will have stopped. If a technetium-99m (Tc-99m)–labeled RBC study has been initiated, the patient can be reimaged at a latter time (up to approximately 24 hours). Under certain circumstances (i.e., if the patient is bleeding actively from the rectum in large amounts), proceed directly to an angiogram.
   C. **Tc-99m RBC versus Tc-99m sulfur colloid.** Sulfur colloid has a better target to background ratio early; however, its disadvantages are that its vascular half life is only 2.5–3.5 minutes (preventing acquisition of delayed images), and normal uptake by the liver and spleen can obscure an upper GI tract hemorrhage. Tc-99m–labeled RBCs remain in the intravascular space and thus can be imaged at any time up to 24 hours after injection in a patient with intermittent bleeding. At our institution we almost always use Tc-99m–labeled RBCs.
   D. **Recent barium studies.** Retained barium in the bowel can interfere with the nuclear medicine study by attenuating signal from a bleeding source.
   E. **Recent nuclear medicine scans.** The half-life and activity of certain isotopes (e.g., gallium-67, indium-111) preclude further scanning within several days.

II. **Imaging**
   A. Tc-99m RBCs: 25 mCi
   B. Tc-99m sulfur colloid: 10 mCi
   C. Children and infants:
      1. (Age in years +1)/(Age in years + 7) × Adult dose
      2. Mimimal dose: 2 mCi for either sulfur colloid or labeled RBCs

    **D. Potassium perchlorate:** 400 mg PO (two 200-mg tablets). (This prevents thyroid uptake of radiotracer in case of a poor tag. It can be given after the scan is started if forgotten initially.)

    **E. Image acquisition.** The angiographic phase is performed by acquiring images every 4 seconds for 60 seconds, followed by the blood pool phase, which consists of images every 2 minutes for 2 hours or until the study becomes positive. A computerized cine loop should be done in addition to hard copies. If Tc-99–labeled RBCs are used and the scan is negative, the patient can be brought back for further blood pool images at any time in the next 24 hours if further bleeding occurs.

**III. Interpretation**

  **A. GI bleeding**

    1. A lower GI bleeding site will initially appear as a focal area of increased uptake that should both intensify and expand over time.

    2. The tracer should move distally in the bowel, but occasionally it will move proximally as well.

    3. The cine loop should be visualized to exclude rapidly moving extravasated blood or transient bleeding. It also may be helpful in cases of confusing anatomy. *"If it don't move, it ain't blood."*

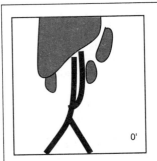
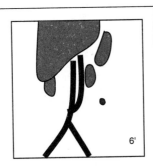
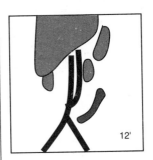
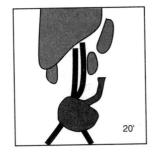

DISTAL COLONIC BLEEDING

B. **False-positive findings.** Always consider false-positive findings when interpreting bleeding studies.
1. Cavernous hemangioma
2. Vascular: aneurysm, varices, arteriovenous malformation, left gonadal vein, graft, portal and splenic veins (may mimic transverse colon, duodenum, or stomach)
3. Horseshoe kidney
4. Penis: have technician tape the penis to the opposite side and reimage.
5. Excretion of free pertechnetate due to poor tag: visualize stomach, kidney, and bladder
6. Menstruation
7. Abscess
8. Gallbladder
C. **Poor labeling.** Certain drugs can cause decreased labeling efficiency. Gastric uptake of pertechnetate can mimic bleeding (should not move with time).
1. Heparin
2. Methyldopa
3. Hydralazine
4. Quinidine
5. Digoxin
6. Propranolol
7. Doxorubicin
D. See the section on the Mesenteric Angiogram in Ch. 8.

# Hepatobiliary Scan

I. **Clinical history**
A. **Ultrasound versus hepatobiliary scan.** In general, because ultrasound provides rapid evaluation of the gallbladder and other abdominal structures, it should be the first study performed on call. If stones and other manifestations of acute cholecystitis are identified (e.g., wall thickening, common bile duct [CBD] dilatation, ultrasonic Murphy's sign), many surgeons will take the patient immediately to the operating room. However, others may prefer to first perform a hepatobiliary scan to assess the patency of the cystic and common bile ducts. A hepatobiliary scan is also helpful if the ultrasound findings are equivocal.
B. **Recent barium studies.** Retained barium in the bowel can "mask" isotope activity.
C. **Recent nuclear medicine scans.** The half-life and activity of certain isotopes (e.g., gallium-67, indium-111) preclude further scanning within several days.
D. **Time of patient's last meal.** Fasting for at least 2–4 hours is required.
II. **Imaging**
A. **Tc-99m Mebrofenin (DISIDA):** 5–10 mCi IV
1. Rapid hepatic excretion
2. Bilirubin <25 mg/dl
B. **Sincalide (CCK):** 0.02–0.04 mg/kg IV slowly (over 5 minutes)
1. Causes the gallbladder to contract
2. Used if bowel is not seen with gallbladder visualization

or if the patient has been fasting for more than 24–48 hours before the test

C. **Morphine:** 0.04 mg/kg IV slow push
1. Causes spasm of the sphincter of Oddi, forcing the tracer into the cystic duct
2. Used if the gallbladder is not seen by 60 minutes
3. Contraindicated in pancreatitis

D. **Children and infants**
1. (Age in years + 1)/(Age in years + 7) × Adult dose
2. Mimimal dose: 1 mCi

E. **Image acquisition.** Anterior images are taken at 2 minutes, 4 minutes, and then every 3 minutes for 1 hour or until both bowel and gallbladder are seen. Right lateral views are obtained at 30 minutes and 1 hour. Delayed views can be done at 3–4 hours if the gallbladder is not visualized.

## III. Interpretation

A. **Normal scan**
1. Liver, heart, and vasculature enhance early with progressive concentration in the liver.
2. Gallbladder and CBD visualized by 30–60 minutes
3. Gallbladder should be seen **before** bowel.
4. Minimal renal uptake occurs unless bilirubin is elevated.
5. Oblique or right lateral views with administration of water are helpful in unclear cases.

B. **Acute cholecystitis**
1. Nonvisualization of the cystic duct or gallbladder after 90 minutes with morphine augmentation or 4 hours without morphine
2. Delayed visualization of the gallbladder after bowel in 3.5% (indistinguishable from chronic cholecystitis or normal variant)
3. **"Rim sign":** increased uptake in hepatocytes at the right inferior liver edge above the gallbladder fossa without visualization of the gallbladder; may indicate perforation with gangrene

C. **Chronic cholecystitis**
1. Delayed visualization of gallbladder (bowel seen before gallbladder and cystic duct)
2. Differential diagnosis: bile stasis due to hyperalimentation, alcoholism, or other severe intercurrent disease. Delayed visualization of the gallbladder can be a **normal variant.**

D. **Common bile duct obstruction**
1. No opacification of bowel
2. May see spectrum of findings from hepatic uptake only without excretion into the hepatic ducts to visualization of liver, bile ducts, gallbladder, and proximal CBD without bowel activity
3. The size of CBD **cannot** be determined on nuclear medicine studies. The intensity of signal is **not** directly related to the diameter of the CBD.

E. **Pitfalls**
1. The gallbladder can reside in multiple locations.
2. The radiotracer may reflux into the stomach, giving a confusing picture (administer a glass of water to wash the tracer distally).

3. If the bladder is visualized, assess the kidneys. Occasionally, a horseshoe kidney or ectopic kidney can simulate bowel.
4. Cystic duct remnant visualized distal to the obstruction can simulate the gallbladder in approximately 5% (compare with the size of gallbladder on ultrasound if that has been performed).
5. Radiotracer in the duodenum or in a duodenal diverticulum can occasionally simulate the gallbladder (administer a glass of water to wash the tracer distally).
6. A hepatic adenoma can mimic the gallbladder.
7. **False-positive**
   a. Cancer
   b. Inadequate fasting
   c. Hyperalimentation
   d. Chronic cholecystitis
8. **False-negative**
   a. Acalculous cholecystitis
   b. Accessory or dilated cystic duct

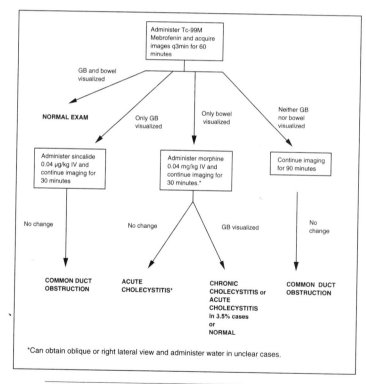

*Can obtain oblique or right lateral view and administer water in unclear cases.

# Osteomyelitis Scan

## I. Clinical history
   **A. Age of the patient.** Due to different patterns of blood

supply, hematogeneous osteomyelitis generally involves the metaphysis and epiphysis in infants, the metaphysis in children, and the epiphysis in adults. The sensitivity of a triple-phase bone scan in neonates is decreased in comparison to children and adults.

B. **Plain films** are generally normal early in acute osteomyelitis but should always be done before bone scanning or MRI since they rule out other sources of pathology (such as fractures and tumors) and aid in choosing the next appropriate study.

C. **MRI versus nuclear medicine study.** At our institution, MRI is reserved for complicated cases (e.g., diabetic foot with suspected superimposed osteomyelitis) or for evaluating the extent of infection.

D. **Triple-phase bone scan, indium-labeled leukocyte, or gallium study.** For acute osteomyelitis, a triple-phase Tc-99m HDP bone scan is generally the best choice (except in spinal osteomyelitis). Most on-call studies are done with Tc-99m HDP. In neonates, a combination of triple-phase bone scan and gallium can be helpful in equivocal cases. In general, we do not perform indium studies in children due to the high radiation dose to the spleen. In patients with underlying bone abnormalities (e.g., chronic osteomyelitis), we do an MRI exam. Many institutions are beginning to perform Tc-99m HMPAO–labeled leukocyte studies in place of indium studies since a higher dose of radionuclide can be given (without the large splenic dose), which improves image quality. Unlike indium studies, delayed scans cannot be obtained since the half-life of Tc-99m is 6 hours.

E. **Recent nuclear medicine scans.** The half-life and activity of certain isotopes (e.g., gallium-67) preclude further scanning within several days.

II. **Imaging**
  A. **Plain films**
  B. **Triple-phase bone scan**
    1. **Tc-99m HDP:** 25 mCi (pinhole collimator)
    2. **Image acquisition.** The angiographic phase is performed by acquiring images every 3 seconds for 45 seconds followed by a blood pool image at 3–5 minutes and static images at 3 hours. **Delayed** images at 24 hours may be helpful in equivocal cases.
    3. **Children and infants**
      a. (Age in years $+1$)/(Age in years $+ 7$) × Adult dose
      b. Mimimal dose: 2 mCi
    4. Insensitive to spinal osteomyelitis
  C. **Gallium scan**
    1. **Gallium 67:** 5 mCi
    2. **Image acquisition.** Images are obtained 48–72 hours after injection
    3. **Children and infants**
      a. (Age in years $+1$)/(Age in years $+ 7$) × Adult dose
      b. Mimimal dose: 0.25 mCi
  D. **MRI**
    1. T1-weighted images
    2. T2-weighted images
    3. Postinfused images with fat saturation

## III. Interpretation
### A. Plain films
1. Fat planes obliterated in 2–5 days
2. Osteopenia in 7–10 days (indicates at least 30% of bone matrix is destroyed)
3. Periostitis in 14 days
4. Sclerosis in chronic osteomyelitis

### B. Triple-phase bone scan
1. **Cellulitis**
   a. Diffuse soft-tissue uptake on angiographic images
   b. **Decreased** activity on delayed views
2. **Osteomyelitis**
   a. Increased activity on angiographic images. If angiographic images are normal, osteomyelitis is extremely **unlikely**
   b. Continued focal accumulation
3. **Pitfalls**
   a. **False-negatives:** subperiosteal abscess
   b. **False-positives:** diabetic neuropathic osteoarthropathy, fractures

|                          | Angio-graphic | Blood pool | Delayed |
|--------------------------|---------------|------------|---------|
| Osteomyelitis/ fracture  | +++           | +++        | +++     |
| Cellulitis               | +++           | ++         | Normal  |
| Noninflam- matory        | Normal        | Normal     | +++     |

+++ = very increased uptake; ++ = increased uptake.

### C. Gallium scan
1. Usually combined with bone scan
2. If the intensity of gallium uptake is equal to or greater than Tc-99m HDP uptake, osteomyelitis is **likely**; if it is less than Tc-99m HDP uptake, osteomyelitis is **unlikely.**

### D. MRI
1. **Osteomyelitis**
   a. T1-weighted images: marrow dark (fat is replaced), bony cortex interrupted
   b. T2-weighted images: marrow and surrounding soft tissues bright due to edema
   c. Fat suppressed postinfused images: enhancement of area of infection
2. **Strengths.** Excellent for determining marrow involvement of infection and distinguishing cellulitis from osteomyelitis
3. **Weaknesses**
   a. **False-positives:** other processes that involve the marrow such as infarction, healing fractures, and tumors
   b. **Artifacts:** Joint implants and other metal prostheses

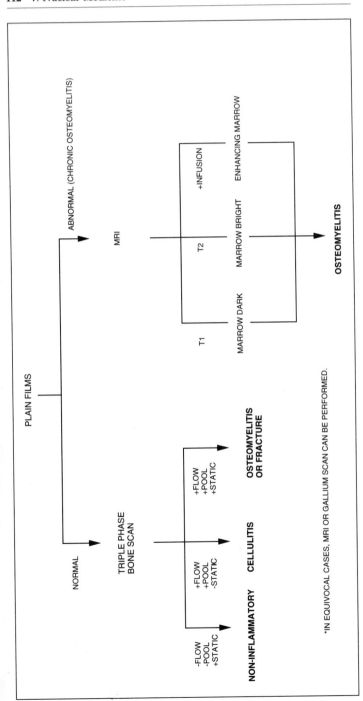

# Renal Scan

## I. Clinical history

**A. Time of transplant.** Acute tubular necrosis (ATN) and cyclosporine toxicity may appear identical. ATN typically occurs 4 days to 1 month post-transplantation. After this time, cyclosporine toxicity should be considered.

**B. Prior nuclear medicine studies.** In many cases a combination of abnormalities may be found; a single study will not differentiate between the various abnormalities, and serial scans need to be performed.

## II. Imaging.
At our institution, we use Tc-99m DTPA for evaluation of obstruction versus ATN. DTPA will wash out of the kidney in ATN and slowly accumulate in obstruction. If Tc-99m MAG3 is used, slow accumulation will occur with both entities. If rejection versus ATN is considered, many institutions prefer Tc-99m MAG3 since it is a tubular agent.

**A. Tc-99m-MAG3:** 10 mCi

**B. Tc-99m DTPA:** 15 mCi

**C. Children and infants**
1. (Age in years +1)/(Age in years + 7) × Adult dose
2. Mimimal dose: 2 mCi

**D. Renal blood flow:** Angiographic images are obtained every second for 60 sec.

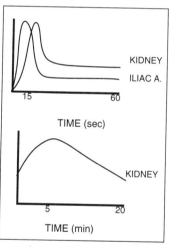

1. Opacification of iliac arteries at 15–20 sec with opacification of kidney 2–4 sec later
2. Maximal parenchymal opacification at 2–4 minutes
3. Bladder opacification at 4–5 minutes
4. Ureter may be visualized for up to 2 weeks (due to edema at ureterovesical junction) after transplantation

**E. Excretion.** Serial images are then obtained every 15 sec for 30 minutes.
1. Maximal uptake at 5 minutes
2. Cleared from kidney within 30 minutes

## III. Interpretation

**A. Rejection**
1. **Hyperacute:** occurs within 24 hours—no perfusion to kidney transplant

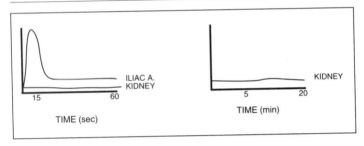

2. **Acute:** occurs within 1–3 weeks—decreased perfusion, cortical retention, and decreased excretion

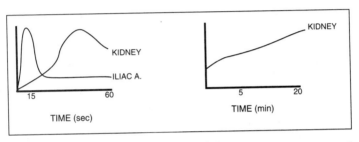

3. **Chronic:** occurs within months to years—decreased perfusion with normal excretion

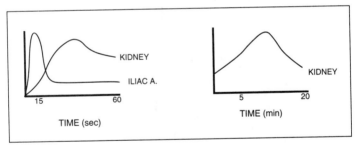

B. **Acute tubular necrosis**
   1. **Tc-99m MAG3**
      a. Four days to 1 month after transplantation
      b. Normal perfusion
      c. Decreased excretion

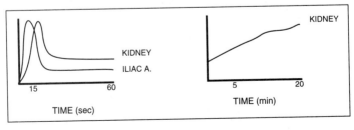

**2. Tc-99m DTPA**
    **a.** Four days to 1 month after transplantation
    **b.** Normal perfusion
    **c.** Slow wash out of tracer from the kidney

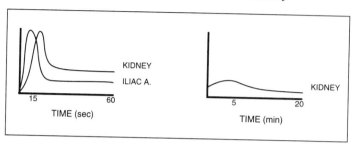

## C. Cyclosporine toxicity
    **1.** More than 1 month after transplantation
    **2.** Normal perfusion
    **3.** Decreased excretion
    **4.** Indistinguishable from ATN and rejection on renal study

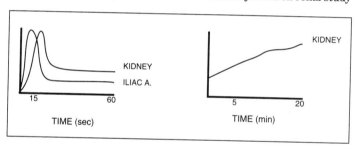

## D. Obstruction
    **1.** Any time after transplantation
    **2.** Normal or slightly decreased or delayed perfusion
    **3.** Decreased or absent excretion
    **4.** Radionuclide generally does not wash out of the kidney (as in ATN).

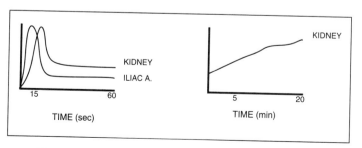

## E. Pitfalls
    **1.** The above curves are generalizations.

**2.** Both cyclosporine toxicity and rejection can cause decreased glomerular filtration rate and perfusion and frequently are indistinguishable.

**3.** An avascular graft may be due to arterial or venous thrombosis or rejection.

# Testicular Scan

**I. Clinical history**
   **A. Onset of pain and swelling.** In acute torsion, the testicle is salvageable for approximately 6–8 hours after the event.
   **B. History of trauma**
   **C. Most recent sexual intercourse.** In the acute nontraumatic painful testicle, the differential diagnosis is torsion versus infection.
   **D. Doppler ultrasound versus nuclear medicine scan.** Ultrasound has generally replaced the nuclear medicine scan as the study of choice because it is faster and equally or more sensitive than the nuclear medicine study. However, be aware that some attending physicians still prefer nuclear medicine studies, especially in prepubertal patients who have abnormal color Doppler evaluations.

**II. Imaging**
   **A. Tc-99m pertechnetate:** 15 mCi
   **B. Potassium perchlorate:** 400 mg PO (two 200-mg tablets). (This prevents thyroid uptake of radiotracer—can be given after the scan is started if forgotten.)
   **C. Children and infants**
      **1.** (Age in years +1)/(Age in years + 7) × Adult dose
      **2.** Mimimal dose: 2 mCi
   **D. Image acquisition.** Angiographic images are obtained every 2.5 seconds for 60 seconds; then delayed images are performed over 5 minutes for 20 minutes.

**III. Interpretation.** In a normal scan, the iliac arteries and scrotum will be visualized. The uptake in the thigh and scrotum should be approximately equal in intensity.
   **A. Increased testicular flow**
      **1.** Epididymo-orchitis
      **2.** Spontaneous detorsion
   **B. Decreased flow**
      **1.** Torsion
      **2.** Abscess
      **3.** Hydrocele
      **4.** Hematocele
      **5.** Hematoma
   **C. Photopenic area**
      **1.** Missed torsion
      **2.** Abscess
      **3.** Hydrocele
      **4.** Hematocele
      **5.** Hematoma
   **D.** See the section on Testicular Ultrasound in Ch. 2.

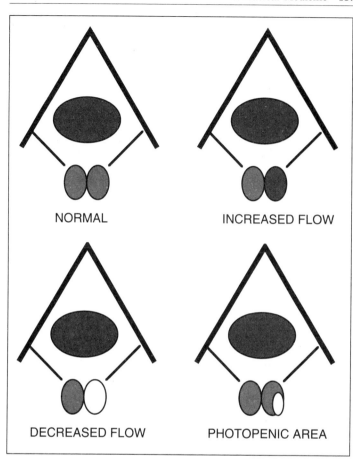

NORMAL  INCREASED FLOW

DECREASED FLOW  PHOTOPENIC AREA

# Ventilation-Perfusion Study

I. **Clinical history**
   A. **History of pulmonary embolism (PE).** Always check the prior scans! A common cause of a perfusion defect on a ventilation-perfusion ($\dot{V}/\dot{Q}$) scan is a prior embolism.
   B. **Use of results by clinical service.** Discuss the treatment algorithm with the clinical service requesting the study. If the patient is already being anticoagulated, an emergent scan is unnecessary. If there is contraindication to anticoagulation and an IVC filter will be desired in the event of a "high probability" scan, the interventional team can be alerted without delay.
   C. **Clinical symptoms.** Physical findings, ECG changes, and blood gas values are suggestive but not specific for PE. In general, if a patient does not have shortness of breath, chest pain, or tachypnea, PE is unlikely.

D. **Chest x-ray (CXR).** Entities such as pneumonia, congestive heart failure, pneumothorax, effusion, or rib fracture can cause symptoms similar to an acute PE. Also, some studies quote the probability of PE in a completely normal CXR as less than 10% (although it is unlikely that a normal CXR will dissuade the clinical service from ordering a $\dot{V}/\dot{Q}$ scan).

E. **Recent nuclear medicine studies.** The half-life and activity of certain isotopes (e.g., gallium-67) preclude further scanning within several days.

F. **Pregnancy** is **not** a contraindication to scanning. In fact, lower extremity venous ultrasound may be difficult in women in the third trimester and will often not detect pelvic vein thrombosis. Thus, $\dot{V}/\dot{Q}$ scan is the study of choice.

## II. Imaging

A. **CXR:** frequently abnormal in the setting of PE but rarely specific
   1. Small pleural effusion
   2. Hampton's hump: pleural-based wedge density seen with infarction
   3. Westermark's sign: focal oligemia distal to embolus
   4. Peripheral pruning of vessels
   5. Atelectasis

B. **Ventilation-perfusion scan.** In an ideal world, perfusion imaging would be performed before ventilation imaging. If the perfusion study was normal, ventilation imaging would then be unnecessary. This cannot be done with the most commonly used ventilation agent, xenon-133 (Xe-133). If the perfusion scan is done before ventilation imaging, the higher energy of Tc-99m (140 KeV) used in the perfusion study will cause downscatter into the Xe-133 (80 KeV) window used in the ventilation study and interfere with scan interpretation. Therefore, ventilation with Xe-133 is done before the perfusion study.
   1. **Ventilation:** 20 mCi of Xe-133
      a. Single breath, equilibrium, and washout views are performed imaging posteriorly.
      b. Other agents include:
         (1) **Krypton 81M:** short half-life (13 sec) does not allow equilibrium scanning; however, higher energy does allow ventilation images to be done after perfusion imaging.
         (2) **Tc-99m DTPA aerosols:** cannot obtain wash in or wash out views and may be difficult to achieve peripheral distribution. However, it can be given at the bedside if necessary, and ventilation images can be done after perfusion images.
         (3) **Xe-127:** very expensive with long half-life, so not widely used. Higher energy allows ventilation imaging after perfusion images.
   2. **Perfusion:** 4 mCi of Tc-99m MAA
      a. Approximately 300,000–500,000 particles of MAA are injected, which occlude one of every 1000 pulmonary capillaries in adults.
         (1) The number of particles should be decreased in patients with pulmonary arterial hypertension

or right-to-left shunts, in children, and in pregnant patients to 100,000 particles.

(2) A minimum of 60,000 particles (neonate) should be used to ensure an adequate study.

b. Evaluate for segmental or subsegmental defects, which should be seen on more than one of the eight views.

c. When a perfusion defect is seen, it may be helpful to get a reventilation in the projection best showing the perfusion defect.

3. Children and infants
   a. (Age in years +1)/(Age in years + 7) × Adult dose
   b. Mimimal dose: 5 mCi Xe-133, 0.2 mCi Tc-99m MAA
   c. PE is very rare in children.

## III. Interpretation

### A. Ventilation

1. An abnormality in either the single breath **or** washout phase of the ventilation study is considered a ventilation **defect.**

2. Abnormalities corresponding to noninfiltrate CXR abnormalities (e.g., fluid, mass, etc.) are disregarded.

3. **Pitfalls**
   a. Hepatic uptake may be caused by fatty infiltration of the liver.
   b. Stomach uptake may be caused by swallowed xenon.
   c. The heart does not cause significant defect on posterior images due to the low energy of xenon.

### B. Perfusion

1. A perfusion **deficit** (i.e., decreased, but not absent perfusion) should be treated the same as a perfusion **defect.**

2. Abnormalities corresponding to noninfiltrate CXR abnormalities (e.g., fluid, mass, etc.) are disregarded.

3. A large perfusion abnormality should be seen on more than one view if it is not artifactual. Artifacts can easily affect only one projection whereas true defects are seen whenever that section of the lung is imaged.
   a. Breasts in women decrease activity at the lung bases.
   b. Hila may cause circular defects on lateral views.
   c. The shoulders may cause decreased activity in the upper lungs.

4. If a perfusion defect is nonsegmental (even if it is large), it should be disregarded (as far as considering PE).

5. **Stripe sign.** If a rim of activity is seen peripheral to the perfusion defect, PE can be **excluded** in more than 90% of patients since emboli should cause perfusion defects that extend to the pleural surface.

6. Cardiomegaly. An enlarged heart can cause apparent left lower lobe perfusion defects.

7. Pleural effusion: can cause defects at the bases and in the fissures

8. **Pitfalls**
   a. Sharp nonsegmental defects: metal jewelry or a pacemaker
   b. Bright spots in both lung fields: clotted MAA
   c. Kidney visualization: right-to-left cardiac shunts or pulmonary arteriovenous malformations

    **d.** Thyroid, gastric mucosa, and/or choroid plexus visualization: poor tag with free pertechnetate

    **e.** Nonembolic causes of $\dot{V}/\dot{Q}$ mismatch include neoplasm, vasculitis, sarcoidosis, and radiation.

    **f.** Whole lung mismatch: hilar tumor

    **g.** Decreased ventilation and perfusion to one lung: mucus plugging, endobronchial tumor, or foreign body

**9. Pulmonary embolism**

    **a.** The average patient with PE has 11 vessels occluded (smaller occluded vessels are not detectable on $\dot{V}/\dot{Q}$ scan).

    **b.** Emboli more commonly go to the lower lobes due to increased blood supply.

**C. Special considerations**

  **1. Chronic obstructive pulmonary disease (COPD).** With extensive COPD, scattered xenon retention occurs throughout both lungs.

    **a.** If the amount of retention occupies more than one-half to two-thirds of the lungs, and the perfusion outside the regions of retention is normal, then the scan cannot be adequately evaluated and it is considered **indeterminate.**

    **b.** If the amount of retention occupies more than one-half to two-thirds of the lungs, and there are $\dot{V}/\dot{Q}$ mismatches in a nonretaining portion of the lung that would qualify the scan as high probability, the scan can be interpreted.

    **c.** Perfusion defects are usually nonsegmental.

  **2. Asthma.** Asthma and mucus plugging can cause "embolic-like" perfusion defects; however, these are usually accompanied by matching ventilation defects

  **3. Prior pulmonary embolism**

    **a.** Up to 60% of patients on anticoagulants develop new perfusion defects (may be due to fragmentation).

    **b.** In young otherwise healthy adults, the majority of resolution of PE occurs within 10 days. Approximately 50% of perfusion defects resolve within 3–4 months. In older patients, resolution is slower and less complete. In most patients older than 60 years, defects commonly persist for life.

**IV. Classification schemes.** There is no consensus as to which is the best classification scheme for categorizing PE on nuclear scintigraphy. Recent literature suggests that in experienced readers, "gestalt" is as accurate as any scheme. Both the Biello criteria and PIOPED criteria are included here. We favor the Biello criteria for several reasons. We believe that it is the most straightforward scheme that results in the least number of intermediate interpretations. (In our institution, most patients with intermediate scans undergo pulmonary angiography. On call at 3 A.M., if given a choice, we would rather do fewer than more pulmonary angiograms.) Furthermore, the PIOPED criteria seem to be revised almost weekly and become increasingly confusing (e.g., a "triple-match" is low probability for PE except in lower lung zones when it is intermediate probability for PE; a "small" effusion favors PE whereas a "large" effusion does not). You should be familiar with at least one scheme and use the one accepted at your institution.

**A. Biello criteria** are adapted in the algorithm on p. 32.
**B. "Modified" revised PIOPED V̇/Q̇ scan criteria**
   **1. High** probability (≥ 80%): two or more large mismatched segmental perfusion defects or the arithmetic equivalent in moderate or large to moderate defects*
   **2. Intermediate** probability (≥ 79%)
      **a.** One moderate to two large mismatched segmental perfusion defects or the arithmetic equivalent in moderate or large to moderate defects
      **b.** Single matched ventilation-perfusion defect with clear chest radiograph†
      **c.** Difficuft to categorize as low or high, or not described as low or high
      **d.** Corresponding ventilation and perfusion defects and chest radiograph opacity ("triple match") in lower lung zone
      **e.** Corresponding ventilation and perfusion defects and **small** pleural effusion
   **3. Low** probability (≥ 19%)
      **a.** Nonsegmental perfusion defects (e.g., cardiomegaly, enlarged aorta, enlarged hila, elevated diaphragm)
      **b.** Any perfusion defect with a substantially larger chest radiographic abnormality
      **c.** Perfusion defects matched by ventilation abnormality provided that there are:
         **(1)** Clear CXR and
         **(2)** Some areas of normal perfusion in the lungs
      **d.** Any number of small perfusion defects with a normal CXR
      **e.** Corresponding ventilation and perfusion defects and chest radiograph opacity ("triple match") in upper or middle lung zone
      **f.** Corresponding ventilation and perfusion defects and **large** pleural effusion
      **g.** "Stripe sign"
   **4. Normal**
      **a.** No perfusion defects or perfusion outlines exactly the shape of the lungs seen on the CXR (note that hilar and aortic impression may be seen and the chest radiograph and/or ventilation study may be abnormal)
   **5. Comment**
      **a.** The sensitivity of a high probability scan is 41%; the specificity is 97%.
      **b.** Follow-up and angiography suggest that PE occured in 12% of patients with low-probablility scans.
See the sections on inferior vena cava filter placement and pulmonary angiogram in Ch. 8.

---

*Two large mismatched perfusion defects are borderline for "high probability." Individual readers may correctly interpret individual scans with this pattern as "high probability." In general, it is recommended that more than this degree of mismatch be present for the "high probability" category.
†Very extensive matched defects can be categorized as "low probability." Single V̇/Q̇ matches are borderline for "low probability" and thus should be categorized as "intermediate" in most circumstances by most readers, although individual readers may correctly interpret individual scans with this pattern as "low probability."

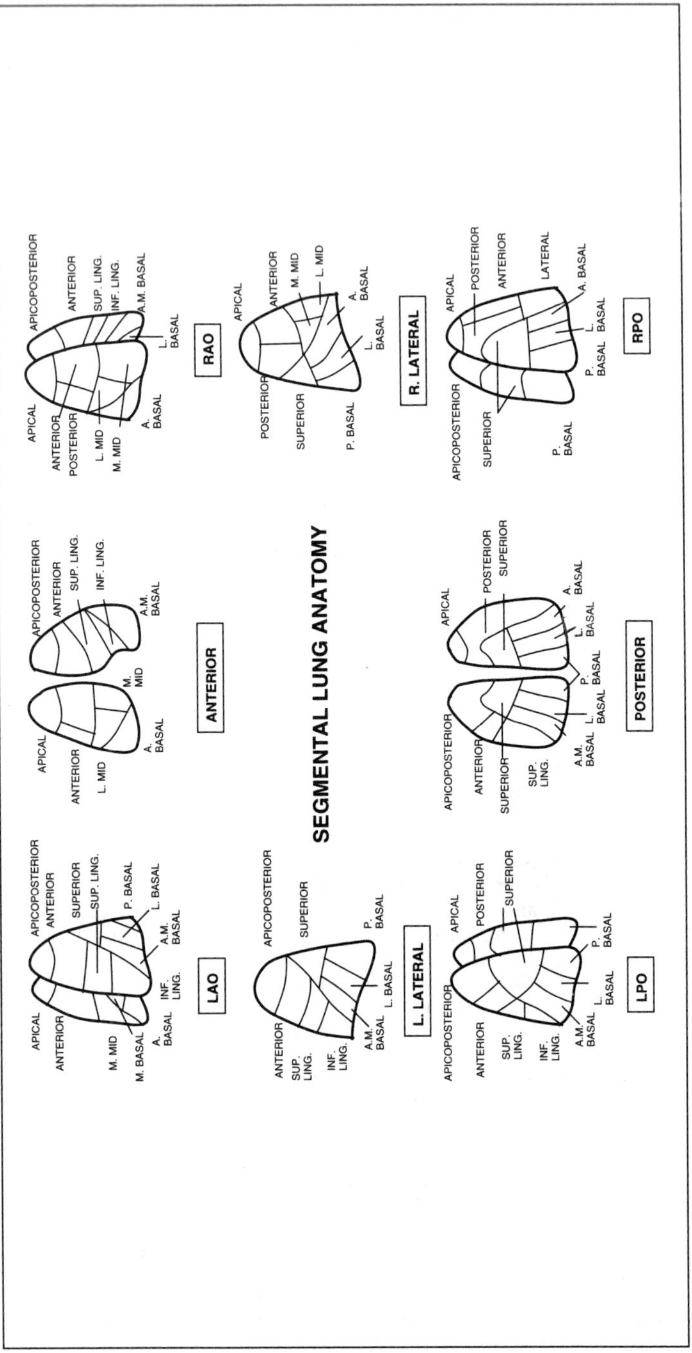

**SEGMENTAL LUNG ANATOMY**

RAO

R. LATERAL

RPO

ANTERIOR

POSTERIOR

LAO

L. LATERAL

LPO

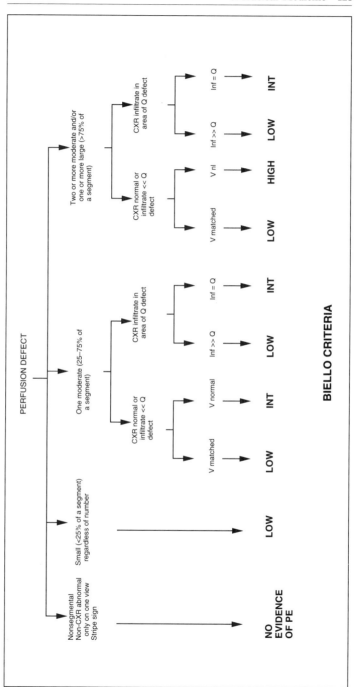

**BIELLO CRITERIA**

# References

### Gastrointestinal Bleeding Study

Datz FL, Patch GG, Arias JM, Morton KA. *Nuclear Medicine: A Teaching File*. St. Louis: Mosby, 1992.

Mettler FA, Guiberteau MJ. *Essentials of Nuclear Medicine* (3rd ed). Philadelphia: Saunders, 1991.

Prasad UR, Tisnado J, Jolles PR. Pitfalls in the scintigraphic evaluation of GI bleeding: Angiographic-clinical correlation. Presented at the meeting of the Radiological Society of North America, 1995.

Zuckerman DA, Bocchini TP, Birnbaum EH. Massive hemorrhage in the lower gastrointestinal tract in adults: Diagnostic imaging and intervention. *AJR Am J Roetgenol* 161:703, 1993.

### Hepatobiliary Scan

Datz FL, Patch GG, Arias JM, Morton KA. *Nuclear Medicine: A Teaching File*. St. Louis: Mosby, 1992.

Mettler FA, Guiberteau MJ. *Essentials of Nuclear Medicine* (3rd ed). Philadelphia: Saunders, 1991.

### Osteomyelitis Scan

Jaramillo D, Treves ST, Kasser JR, et al. Osteomyelitis and septic arthritis in children: Appropriate use of imaging to guide treatment. *AJR Am J Roetgenol* 165:399, 1995.

Schauwecker DS. The scintigraphic diagnosis of osteomyelitis. *AJR Am J Roetgenol* 158:9, 1992.

### Renal Scan

Datz FL, Patch GG, Arias JM, Morton KA. *Nuclear Medicine: A Teaching File*. St. Louis: Mosby, 1992.

Mettler FA, Guiberteau MJ. *Essentials of Nuclear Medicine* (3rd ed). Philadelphia: Saunders, 1991.

### Testicular Scan

Datz FL, Patch GG, Arias JM, Morton KA. *Nuclear Medicine: A Teaching File*. St. Louis: Mosby, 1992.

Mettler FA, Guiberteau MJ. *Essentials of Nuclear Medicine* (3rd ed). Philadelphia: Saunders, 1991.

### Ventilation-Perfusion Study

Biello DR, Mattar AG, McKnight RC, Siegel BA. Ventilation-perfusion studies in suspected pulmonary embolism. *AJR Am J Roentgenol* 133:1033, 1979.

Gottschalk A, Sostman HD, Coleman RE, et. al. Ventilation-perfusion scintigraphy in the PIOPED study. Part II. Evaluations of the scintigraphic criteria and interpretations. *J Nucl Med* 34:1119, 1993.

Sostman HD, Coleman RE, DeLong DM, et al. Evaluation of revised criteria for ventilation-perfusion scintigraphy in patients with suspected pulmonary embolism. *Radiology* 193:103, 1994.

Value of the ventilation/perfusion scan in acute pulmonary embolism. Results of the prospective investigation of pulmonary embolism diagnosis (PIOPED). *JAMA* 263:2753, 1990.

Webber MM, Gomes AS, Roe D, et al. Comparison of Biello, McNeil, and PIOPED criteria for the diagnosis of pulmonary emboli on lung scans. *AJR Am J Roentgenol* 154:975, 1990.

Worsley DF, Alavi A, Palevsky HI. Role of radionuclide imaging in patients with suspected pulmonary embolism. *Radiol Clin North Am* 31:849, 1993.

# Interventional Procedures

Although interventional procedures at most institutions are performed with an attending physician or fellow, the resident should be familiar with the examination and general sequence of the procedure. Before calling in the interventional team, always make sure that the patient will **consent** to the procedure. Call the attending or fellow on-call to discuss the case. At our institution, the service accompanies the patient to the interventional radiology suite and monitors the patient during all on-call emergency procedures. If there is no contraindication (e.g., urethral trauma), make sure the patient has a Foley catheter in place.

I. **Laboratory tests**
   A. **Prothrombin time (PT)**
      1. Less than 15 sec for arterial puncture
      2. Less than 18 sec for venous puncture
      3. If the patient is on warfarin (Coumadin), ideally the medication should be stopped for several days before the procedure. Clearly, this does not occur in emergent procedures.
      4. The patient can be given fresh frozen plasma (FFP) before the procedure; the procedure must be performed **30 minutes to 6 hours** after administration.
   B. **Partial thromboplastin time (PTT)**
      1. In general, should be less than 50 secs. Isolated elevation usually occurs only with heparin use.
      2. Stop heparin 2 hours or more before the study and restart immediately after the procedure.
      3. Can give protamine sulfate (rarely necessary)
   C. **Creatinine**
      1. More than 1.5 mg/dl is a relative contraindication (since most cases performed on call are emergencies, they will be done regardless of the creatinine level)
      2. Can hydrate (75 ml/hour normal saline for 24 hours) before and after the procedure
   D. **Platelets:** Greater than 75,000/$\mu$l for most procedures
II. **Medications**
   A. **Midazolam (Versed)**
      1. Contraindications: allergy, acute narrow-angle glaucoma
      2. Dosing: 1.0–2.0 mg loading dose with incremental 0.5-mg doses after 2 minutes not to exceed more than 5–6 mg (endpoint is slurred speech)
      3. Reversal: flumazenil (Reversed, Mazicon, Romazicon), 0.2 mg over 15 seconds with repeat 0.2-mg doses at 1-minute intervals to a maximum dose of 1 mg if no response
   B. **Fentanyl**
      1. Contraindications: monamine oxidase inhibitors, respiratory disorders
      2. Dosing: 50-$\mu$g slow push (over 1–2 minutes) loading, then 50 $\mu$g q30min maintenance. Total dose not to exceed more than 200 $\mu$g/hour.
      3. Reversal: naloxone (Narcan), 0.2 mg over 2–3 minutes

**III. Injuries.** Always take the proper precautions when in the angiography suite. Most of the following injuries can be prevented with proper precautions. If possible, do not rush when performing procedures; injuries commonly occur when you try to do too many things at the same time. Common injuries include:

**A.** Flipping a wire or catheter in the eye or mouth
**B.** Needle-stick injuries
    **1.** Recapping needles
    **2.** Reaching back to a tray without looking
    **3.** Reaching for a needle that someone else is holding
**C.** Sprayed in face with body fluids
    **1.** Removing catheters. It is helpful to insert a wire into a pigtail catheter before removal to straighten the loop.
    **2.** Performing arterial punctures
    **3.** Injecting forcefully into an obstructed catheter (syringe detaches at the hub connection)

If you do injure yourself during a procedure, report the injury **immediately** to the proper personnel in your hospital.

| Examination | Wire size | Catheter | Cut film Rate[a] | Cut film Dose[b] | Digital Rate[a] | Digital Dose[b] | Filming rate |
|---|---|---|---|---|---|---|---|
| Aortic arch | 0.038 | 6F pigtail | 35 | 70 | 35 | 40 | 3 f/sec for 7 sec biplane |
| Internal carotid artery | 0.035 | 5F WB, HI, S3 | 6 | 8 | 6 | 8 | 2–3 f/sec for 5 sec |
| External carotid artery | 0.035 | 5F WB, HI, S3 | 4 | 6 | 4 | 6 | 2–3 f/sec for 5 sec |
| Common carotid artery | 0.035 | 5F WB, HI, S3 | 7 | 9 | 7 | 9 | 2–3 f/sec for 5 sec |
| Vertebral artery | 0.035 | 5F WB, HI, S3 | 5–6 | 8–9 | 5–6 | 8–9 | 2–3 f/sec for 5 sec |
| Subclavian artery | 0.035 | 5F WB, HI, S3 | 6–8 | 20 | 6–8 | 15 | 2–3 f/sec for 5 sec |
| Thoracic aorta | 0.038 | 6F pigtail | 35 | 70 | 35 | 35 | 3 f/sec for 7 sec biplane |
| Abdominal aorta | 0.035 | 5F pigtail | 18 | 50 | 18 | 25 | 3 f/sec for 7 sec biplane |
| Celiac axis | 0.035 | 5F RC-1 | 6–8 | 60 | 6–8 | 30 | 1f/sec for 10 sec— 1 f/2 sec out |
| Superior mesenteric artery | 0.035 | 5F RC-1 | 6–8 | 60 | 6–8 | 30 | 1f/sec for 10 sec— 1 f/2 sec out |
| Inferior mesenteric artery | 0.035 | 5F Sos | 3 | 15–20 | 3 | 15–20 | 2–3 f/sec for 5 sec |

| Exami-nation | Wire size | Catheter | Cut film Rate[a] | Cut film Dose[b] | Digital Rate[a] | Digital Dose[b] | Filming rate |
|---|---|---|---|---|---|---|---|
| Renal artery | 0.035 | 5F RC-1 | 6 | 12 | 6 | 12 | 4 f/sec for 3 sec—2 f/sec out |
| Femoral artery | 0.035 | 5F pigtail | 6 | 30 | 6 | 15 | 3 f/sec for 4 sec |
| Pulmonary artery | 0.038 | 7F Van Aman | 20 | 50 | 20 | 25 | 4–7 f/sec for 5 sec |
| Inferior vena cava | 0.035 | 5F pigtail | 20 | 50 | 20 | 20 | 4 f/sec for 5 sec |

HI = Headhunter 1; WB = Weinberg 1; S3 = Simmonds 3.
[a]Rate: ml/sec.
[b]Dose: ml.

# Abscess Drainage

**I. Clinical history**
   **A. Abdominal abscess that needs drainage.** An abscess is a thick-walled, well-defined, infected cavity that exhibits mass effect and may contain gas. The mortality of untreated abdominal abscesses approaches 80%.
   **B. Contraindications**
      **1.** PT greater than 15 sec
      **2.** PTT greater than 45 sec
   **C. Relative contraindications**
      **1.** Fungal abscesses
      **2.** Extensively loculated abscesses
      **3.** Fistulas

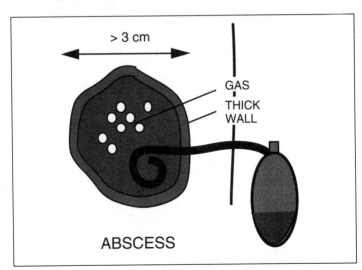

**II. Procedure**
  **A.** Choose a guidance modality (CT versus ultrasound) if necessary and plan the path.
    **1.** Avoid bowel loops and other organs.
    **2.** Measure depth to abscess.
  **B.** Mark the skin with indelible ink at the planned puncture site and clean the area with povidone-iodine solution.
  **C.** Anesthetize skin with 1% lidocaine and nick the skin with a scalpel.
  **D.** Puncture the expected site of the abscess with an 18-gauge Teflon sheath–needle combination.
  **E.** Remove the needle and aspirate 5–10 ml of fluid for the following:
    **1.** Gram's stain
    **2.** Aerobic
    **3.** Anaerobic
    **4.** Fungal
    **5.** Mycobacterial cultures
  **F.** Inject a 1:1 mixture of contrast and saline to confirm the position in the abscess.
  **G.** Insert a 0.018-inch large J wire and coil as much as possible into the cavity.
  **H.** Advance the sheath over the wire as far as possible.
  **I.** Exchange the 0.018-inch wire for a 0.038-inch Amplatz wire (again, coiling as much wire as possible into cavity).
  **J.** Remove the Teflon sheath and dilate the tract with sequential (e.g., 7, 9, 11 French) dilators.
  **K.** Insert and deploy a drainage catheter (e.g., Cope 10 French locking loop catheter).
  **L.** Suture to the skin and attach bulb suction.

| Catheter size (French) | Abscess |
| --- | --- |
| 8 | Low-viscosity fluid |
| 10 | Average-viscosity fluid |
| 12 | High-viscosity fluid |
| 16 | Infected hematomas, necrotic tissue |

**III. Pitfalls**
  **A. Abscess mimics**
    **1.** Necrotic tumor
    **2.** Bladder diverticula
    **3.** Ovary
    **4.** Leiomyoma
    **5.** Ascitic fluid (no wall)
  **B. Hepatic abscesses.** Remember that the pleura extends below the apparent costophrenic angle. Therefore, in general, approach hepatic abscesses from **below the ribs** to avoid the pleural space.
  **C. Pancreatic abscesses:** best to avoid if possible
  **D. Small abscesses.** If the diameter is less than 3 cm, aspirate the cavity without placing a drainage catheter.

# Aortogram

## I. Clinical history

**A. Patient in motor vehicle accident: rule out transection.** Although somewhat controversial, in a case of suspected transection, angiography—not CT or MRI—is generally considered the study of choice. Some institutions perform CT as a screening test before angiography.

**B. Suspected dissection: evaluate.** Despite widespread use of CT, MRI, and transesophageal echocardiography, angiography remains the gold standard for the diagnosis of aortic dissection.

## II. Plain films

**A. Radiographic findings of aortic laceration**
1. Widened superior mediastinum (>8 cm)
2. Superior extension of left mediastinal stripe above the aortic arch, forming the apical cap
3. Right paratracheal stripe widening
4. Hemothorax
5. Rib fractures
6. Tracheal or esophageal deviation to the right of the T4 vertebral body
7. Inferior displacement of the left mainstem bronchus more than 40 degrees below horizontal

## III. Procedure

**A.** Puncture the femoral artery (preferably the right) and exchange a Seldinger needle for a 6 French pigtail catheter over a large J wire.

**B.** Do not allow the pigtail to reform. Advance the catheter and J wire together into the aortic arch until the tip is approximately 3 cm above the aortic valve. If resistance is encountered, perform a small test injection to confirm the position of the catheter (it may be in the false lumen of a dissection).

**C.** Perform an angiogram in the anteroposterior, lateral, and 45-degree left anterior oblique planes (steep right anterior oblique may also be helpful).
1. Inject
   **a.** 70 ml at 35 ml/sec with a 0-sec delay: **cut film**
   **b.** 40 ml at 35 ml/sec with a 0-sec delay: **digital**
2. Film at 3/sec for 7 sec in each plane
3. Pull the catheter back to the descending aorta and perform aortography of the descending aorta since a **small percentage of transections occur at the esophageal hiatus.**

## IV. Interpretation

**A. Laceration (transection)**
1. The vast majority (approximately 90%) of aortic transections occur immediately distal to the origin of the left subclavian artery.
2. Angiographic findings include spasm, dissection, pseudoaneurysm, coarctation, extravasation, and an intimal flap in either or both projections.

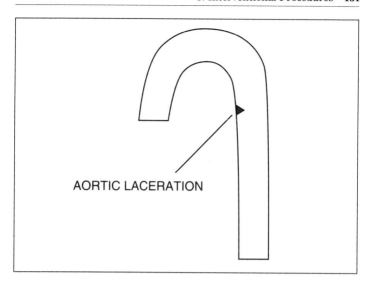

AORTIC LACERATION

## B. Dissection

1. The false lumen is usually located **anteriorly and to the right** in the ascending aorta and **posteriorly and to the left** in the arch and descending aorta.
2. Commonly, the false lumen is larger than the true lumen and generally opacifies and clears after the true lumen.

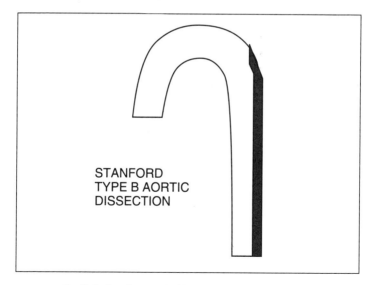

STANFORD
TYPE B AORTIC
DISSECTION

3. **Stanford type A dissections**
   **a.** Start several centimeters above the aortic valve.
   **b.** Usually treated surgically since the dissection may

extend proximally to involve the pericardial sac (leading to tamponade), aortic valve, and/or coronary arteries (usually right coronary artery). Involvement of the great vessels is also important.

**4. Stanford type B dissections**
  **a.** Start distal to the ligamentum arteriosum.
  **b.** Usually treated medically with antihypertensive medications. Surgery possible if acute ischemia exists

## V. Pitfalls

**A. Ductus diverticulum versus aortic laceration.** These entities can be easily confused. Obtain multiple views in different projections if findings are equivocal.

  **1. Aortic lacerations** tend to have jagged, linear margins and irregular outlines. An overlap of densities with acute angles is usually visible.

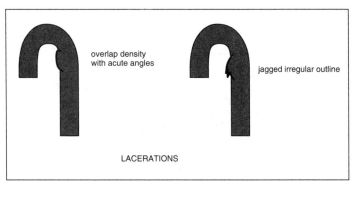

overlap density with acute angles

jagged irregular outline

LACERATIONS

  **2. Ductus diverticuli** have smooth outlines with obtuse angles and no overlap density. Occasionally, vessels will be visible arising from the apex of the diverticulum.

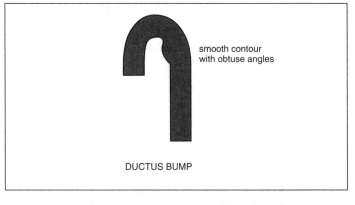

smooth contour with obtuse angles

DUCTUS BUMP

  **3.** Both lacerations and ductus bumps may exhibit delayed washout.

# Extremity Angiogram

I. **Clinical history**
   A. **Assess vessels in a patient with a gunshot or stab wound.** The indications for an emergency extremity angiogram are somewhat controversial. In general angiograms are obtained for patients with:
      1. Hemodynamic instability
      2. Expanding hematoma
      3. Loss of distal pulse
      4. Neurologic deficits
      5. Bruit or thrill at injury
      6. Extensive fracture or dislocation
      7. Ischemia (pallor, cold)
      The evaluation of a "proximity injury" (i.e., injury near a vascular structure) is also controversial. Some surgeons want an angiogram, whereas others will do nothing unless vascular symptoms manifest. A vascular surgery consult should be obtained if an angiogram is contemplated.
   B. **Consent.** Because the vertebral artery arises from the subclavian artery, there is a small risk of stroke when performing upper extremity angiography.

II. **Procedure**
   A. **Upper extremity**
      1. Catheterize the femoral artery and exchange a Seldinger needle for a Headhunter 1 (H1) catheter over a large J wire.
      2. Manipulate the catheter into the subclavian artery of interest. A glide wire may be helpful in difficult cases.
      3. Administer a test dose to determine delay, then perform run.
         a. Inject
            (1) 20 ml at 6–8 ml/sec: **cut film**
            (2) Manual injection of 1:1 contrast to heparinized saline: **digital**
         b. Film at 2 films/sec through the venous phase
   B. **Lower extremity**
      1. Catheterize the femoral artery on the contralateral side of the injury and exchange a Seldinger needle for a 5 French sheath.
      2. Advance a Chung catheter over the aortic bifurcation to the area proximal to injury.
      3. Administer a test dose to determine delay (usually 3–8 sec), then perform run.
         a. Inject
            (1) 30 ml at 10 ml/sec: **cut film**
            (2) 12 ml at 10 ml/sec (alternatively do hand injection): **digital**
         b. Film at two films/sec for 5 sec, then one film/sec through the venous phase.

III. **Interpretation**
   A. **Vascular injury**
      1. Transection
      2. Pseudoaneurysm
      3. Arteriovenous fistula

**4.** Intimal injury: may be difficult to differentiate from spasm or adjacent hematoma

**B. Pitfall: projectile migration.** Bullets and pellets can gain entrance to the vascular system and travel far from the initial site of injury. Fluoroscopy is helpful in locating "lost" fragments.

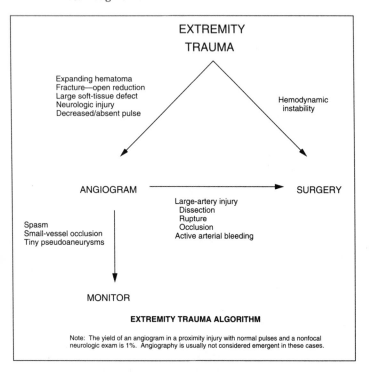

EXTREMITY TRAUMA

Expanding hematoma
Fracture—open reduction
Large soft-tissue defect
Neurologic injury
Decreased/absent pulse

Hemodynamic instability

ANGIOGRAM → SURGERY

Large-artery injury
Dissection
Rupture
Occlusion
Active arterial bleeding

Spasm
Small-vessel occlusion
Tiny pseudoaneurysms

MONITOR

**EXTREMITY TRAUMA ALGORITHM**

Note: The yield of an angiogram in a proximity injury with normal pulses and a nonfocal neurologic exam is 1%. Angiography is usually not considered emergent in these cases.

# Inferior Vena Cava Filter Placement

**I. Clinical history**

**A. Documentation of pulmonary embolism (PE).** Indications for emergent inferior vena cava (IVC) filter placement are:

**1. Documented** recurrent PE despite anticoagulation

**2.** High-probability ventilation-perfusion scan or documented deep venous thrombosis (DVT) with contraindication to anticoagulation

**3.** Documented iliofemoral thrombus ("floating thrombus")

**4.** Septic emboli or phlebitis

**B. Contraindications to short-term anticoagulation.** Ideally, patients are anticoagulated overnight for filter placement in the morning. The **only absolute** contraindications to short-term (8–16 hours) heparin therapy are:

**1.** Subacute or acute bacterial endocarditis

2. Recent neurologic surgery or CNS disease known to increase the risk of bleeding
3. Heparin-induced thrombocytopenia **with** documented heparin antibodies
4. Septic emboli or phlebitis

**Relative** contraindications are:
1. Major injury to viscera or long bones
2. Recent abdominal or thoracic surgery
3. Active bleeding (**not** heme-positive stools or microscopic hematuria)

C. **Laboratory values**
1. PT ≤ 15 sec
2. Platelets ≥ 100,000/$\mu$l
3. PTT ≤ 42 sec
4. Activated clotting time ≤ 200 sec

II. **Contraindications to IVC filter placement**
A. Ongoing bacteremia
B. Uncontrollable coagulopathy
C. Pediatric patient (the risk of caval thrombosis over the child's life span is unacceptably high)

III. **Complications**
A. IVC thrombosis (10–20%): probably the most significant common complication
B. Recurrent PE (5%)
C. Misplacement
D. Air embolism
E. Pneumothorax—via internal jugular approach

IV. **Procedure**
A. Perform right femoral vein puncture (1 cm medial to artery) at the level of the midfemoral head, then exchange a Seldinger needle for a pigtail catheter over a large J wire. If access cannot be obtained in either of the femoral veins, puncture either the right antecubital vein or internal jugular vein.
B. Bolus test dose of contrast to confirm position in IVC
C. Insert metal ruler below patient/IVC
D. Perform IVC-gram with pigtail tip at confluence of iliac veins:
1. Inject
a. 30 ml at 15 ml/sec: **digital**
b. 50 ml at 18 ml/sec: **cut film**
2. Film
a. Four films/sec with 0-sec delay: **digital**
b. Four films/sec with 1-sec delay: **cut film**

| | |
|---|---|
| If the IVC is less than 28 mm in diameter, any filter can be deployed | (9–14 French sheath) |
| If the IVC is 28–40 mm in diameter, use bird's nest filter | (14 French sheath) |
| If the IVC is more than 40 mm in diameter, deploy bilateral iliac vein filters | (9–14 French sheath) |
| If using the antecubital approach, use the Simon-Nitinol filter | (9 French sheath) |

E. Determine the level of the renal veins (approximately at

the level of the L2 pedicle). In general, the filter is placed **below** the level of the renal veins. In pregnant women, young patients, patients with renal transplants, and patients with renal vein thrombosis, it is usually placed **above** the renal veins

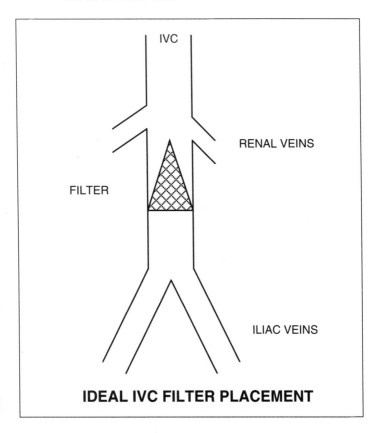

**IDEAL IVC FILTER PLACEMENT**

  **F.** Always make sure that the filter being used is appropriate for your route of access (so the filter will not be deployed upside down).
    **1. Vena Tech filter**
      **a.** Exchange pigtail catheter for Vena Tech sheath and dilator over 0.038 Amplatz wire.
      **b.** Advance sheath and dilator **together.**
      **c.** Remove the wire/dilator together, then insert filter into sheath.
      **d.** Use plastic trocar to push the filter to the tip of the sheath under fluoroscopic monitoring.
      **e.** Ensure that the tip of the sheath is immediately **below** the renal veins (as determined by cavagram). A filter placed too high could result in thrombosis of renal veins.

**f.** Pull the **sheath** caudally to release the filter (rather than pushing the filter out of the sheath). If the filter is pushed out of the sheath, it will be placed too far cephalad—possibly in one of the renal veins.

2. **Simon-Nitinol filter**

**a.** Make sure the filter is correct for the route of access (in the femoral approach, the filter is oriented so that the top portion emerges first, whereas in the antecubital approach, the bottom portion exits the sheath first).

**b.** Exchange the pigtail catheter for a sheath/dilator over a 0.038 Amplatz wire.

**c.** Attach saline-filled syringe to filter apparatus.

**d.** Remove the wire and dilator, then attach the filter apparatus to the sheath.

**e.** Use the pusher to advance the filter to the end of the sheath.

**f.** Make sure the tip of the sheath is immediately below the level of the renal veins (as determined by cavagram). If the antecubital approach is used, the tip must be slightly lower (since this position marks the bottom of the filter rather than the top). A filter placed too high can result in thrombosis of the renal veins.

**g.** Slowly pull the **sheath** caudally holding the pusher steady to release the filter. Allow the top portion to expand, then reposition the tip if necessary by manipulating the entire sheath/filter assembly to the desired level. (The top portion usually drops 1–2 cm caudally when it forms.) Then continue to pull the sheath caudally to release the bottom portion (legs) of the filter.

3. **Giantureo-Roehm bird's nest filter:**

**a.** Exchange the pigtail catheter for the sheath/dilator over a guide wire.

**b.** Align the tip of the sheath immediately below the level of the renal veins and insert the filter-catheter.

**c.** Flush the filter catheter with heparinized saline.

**d.** Pull back on the catheter/sheath while holding the inner pusher wire steady to release the top portion of the filter. Push the entire apparatus cephalad once approximately 1–3 mm to secure the legs of the filter into the IVC wall.

**e.** Push the inner wire cephalad while holding the sheath steady and align the cranial tip of the bottom portion of the filter so that it overlaps the top portion by approximately 5 mm.

**f.** Again, pull back on the sheath while holding the inner wire steady to release the bottom portion of the filter. Secure the legs into the wall of the IVC by pulling back slightly or using a to-and-fro motion on the inner wire.

**g.** Tear off the peel-away shrink tubing and push the innermost wire cranially while holding the outer wire steady (this releases the last leg of the bottom portion of the filter).

**Note that** the bird's nest filter is the longest filter, measuring 6–7 cm in length; make sure the infrarenal IVC is long enough for filter deployment.

## V. Pitfalls
  A. Anomalous venous anatomy
   1. Circumaortic left renal vein
    a. Occurs in 5–10% of patients
    b. Filter placement between the two left renal veins may allow recurrent embolization through the renal vein ring.
    c. Place the filter below the renal veins or place one filter in each common iliac vein.
   2. Double IVC
    a. Rare anomaly (<1%)
    b. Placement of filter in one IVC allows embolization through duplicated IVC
    c. Place filter in each IVC
  B. Deployment upside down. All filters can be deployed from either the jugular/axillary or femoral approach. Make sure you have the correct deployment system.
  C. Deployment in or adjacent to the IVC thrombus. Place a second filter above the first.
  D. Insertion via the left femoral vein approach. The sheath may kink due to tortuous anatomy. Vena Tech filters have thick-walled, reinforced sheaths.
  E. Incomplete opening or severe tilting. Place the second filter above the first.
  F. Embolization to right heart: may leave filter in place
  See the section on the Pulmonary Angiogram in this chapter and the section on the Ventilation-Perfusion Scan in Ch. 7.

---

# Lower Extremity Venogram

## I. Clinical history
  A. **Questionable DVT on lower extremity Doppler ultrasound study.** Always perform lower extremity ultrasound before attempting a venogram. Rarely, the ultrasound study will be equivocal.
## II. Procedure
  A. Cannulate dorsal foot vein.
  B. Place a tourniquet tightly at the level of the ankle. This maneuver forces contrast into the deep venous system.
  C. The patient stands on the block with the affected leg unsupported, dependent, and relaxed. In other words, if a clot is suspected in the left leg, the patient stands on the block with the right leg letting the left leg dangle free.
  D. Angle the table 45–60 degrees from vertical.
  E. Drip a 150-ml bottle of contrast through an IV line in the foot. Alternatively, attach a three-way stopcock to the IV line and inject 120 ml of contrast as fast as possible through two 60-ml syringes.
  F. Take anteroposterior and lateral spot films of the ankle, knee, femur, and hip following the course of the contrast using fluoroscopy. If the injection method is performed, most of the spot films of the lower leg will be taken before all of the contrast is injected.
  G. Fill the common iliac vein by turning the table horizontal. This maneuver "dumps" contrast into the pelvis. Monitor

the area with fluoroscopy and be prepared to take the spot film. The vein fills and empties **rapidly.**
H. "Wash out" contrast at the end of the study with heparinized saline.
III. **Interpretation**
   A. **DVT**
      1. Filling defect
      2. Nonvisualization of expected vessel
      3. Chronic DVT: collateral vessels or lumen smaller than expected
See the section on Lower Extremity Ultrasound in Ch. 3.

# Mesenteric Angiogram

I. **Clinical history**
   A. **Bleeding bright red blood per rectum.** Endoscopy is the study of choice for the evaluation of upper GI hemorrhage, while either nuclear medicine scanning or angiography is best for lower GI bleeding. Angiography may be requested in upper GI bleeding if embolization is desired.
   B. **Angiogram versus nuclear medicine bleeding study.** In general, perform the nuclear medicine study first because its sensitivity is greater than that of angiography. The rate of bleeding must be **at least 0.5–1.0 ml/minute for angiographic detection.** This is approximately 2–3 units per 24 hours or a 10% drop in hematocrit. A **nuclear medicine scan may be positive with bleeding rates of 0.1–0.2 ml/minute.** Also, if positive, the nuclear medicine scan can be helpful in guiding the angiogram. Arterial bleeding usually occurs intermittently followed by vessel spasm and temporary cessation of bleeding. Often, by the time the patient begins to pass blood per rectum, bleeding will have stopped. If a technetium-99m–labeled red blood cell study has been initiated, the patient can be reimaged at a latter time (up to approximately 24 hours). Under certain circumstances (e.g., if the patient is bleeding actively from the rectum in large amounts), proceed directly to an angiogram.
   C. **Recent barium studies.** Retained barium in the bowel can interfere with both the nuclear medicine study and the angiogram.
II. **Procedure**
   A. If there is no contraindication, make sure that the patient has a Foley catheter placed. Contrast pooling in the bladder can obscure rectal bleeding sites.
   B. Puncture the femoral artery (preferably the right) and exchange a Seldinger needle for a 5 French pigtail catheter over a large J wire.
   C. Perform an aortogram with a catheter tip at T11–12 (optional).
      1. Inject
         a. 50 ml at 20 ml/sec: **cut film**
         b. 25 ml at 20 ml/sec: **digital**
      2. Film at three films/sec with 1-sec delay.
   In cases of abdominal aortic aneurysms, perform a biplane aortogram to exclude aortoenteric fistula.

**D.** Exchange pigtail catheter for either:
  1. RC-1 catheter
  2. RC-2 catheter
  3. Simmonds 1 catheter
  4. Sidewinder catheter
  5. Chung catheter
**E.** Selectively catheterize the artery of interest based on findings of the nuclear medicine study:
  1. Celiac axis: supplies stomach and duodenum to ligament of Treitz
  2. Superior mesenteric artery (SMA): supplies ligament of Treitz to splenic flexure
  3. Inferior mesenteric artery (IMA): supplies splenic flexure to rectum

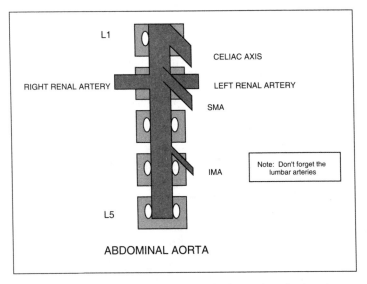

Note: Don't forget the lumbar arteries

**ABDOMINAL AORTA**

**F.** If the nuclear medicine study is equivocal or not performed, begin with the SMA (usually 1 cm below the celiac artery at approximately the L1–2 disk space).
  1. Inject
     **a.** 60 ml at 6–8 ml/sec: **cut film**
     **b.** 30 ml at 6–8 ml/sec: **digital**
  2. Film at one film/sec for 10 sec with 0.5-sec delay, then one-half film/sec out
**G.** Selectively catheterize the IMA. This artery is more difficult to catheterize. An Sos catheter, RIM catheter, or IMA catheter may be helpful in difficult cases.
  1. Inject
     **a.** 15 ml at 3 ml/sec: **cut film**
     **b.** 15 ml at 3 ml/sec: **digital**
     **c.** May also perform hand injection.
  2. Film at 2–3 films/sec for 5 sec
**H.** If no bleeding source is identified, proceed to the celiac artery (usually at the right L1 pedicle or T12–L1 disk level

approximately 1 cm above the SMA). Perform angiogram imaging the arterial and portal venous phases (same injection and filming rate as SMA injection).

III. **Interpretation.** A bleeding source will appear as pooling of contrast beginning in the arterial phase and persisting throughout the venous phase of the study.

IV. **Treatment**

A. **Vasopressin** infusion may be performed to treat bleeding distal to the ligament of Treitz (a more proximal bleeding source is usually embolized).

1. **Contraindications:** coronary artery disease, severe peripheral vascular disease, congestive cardiomyopathy, renal failure, severe hypertension, prior GI surgery (relative)

2. **Technique**

a. Mix 100 units of vasopressin in 500 ml of normal saline for a concentration of 0.2 units/ml.

b. Position the catheter selectively near the vessel of interest.

c. Infuse 0.2 units/minute for 20 minutes.

d. Repeat angiogram.

e. If the bleeding stops, admit the patient to the ICU and infuse at the same rate for 12–24 hours. Then cut the rate to 0.1 units/minute for 12–24 hours. Then infuse heparinized D5W at 20 ml/hour for 4–6 hours with removal of the catheter if bleeding has stopped.

f. If the bleeding continues after the first 20-minute infusion, increase the dose to 0.4 units/ml for 20 minutes.

g. Repeat the angiogram.

h. If the bleeding stops, taper the rate by 0.1 units/minute q6–12h. Then infuse heparinized D5W at 20 ml/hour for 4–6 hours.

i. If the bleeding continues at the infusion rate of 0.4 units/ml, consider embolization or surgery. Increasing the dose further is not indicated.

3. **Pitfalls**

a. Stop the infusion if any of the following occur: myocardial infarction or other cardiovascular event, mesenteric ischemia (severe abdominal pain >30 minutes after initiation of treatment), peripheral vascular ischemia (pain and extremity mottling), cerebral edema (rare), or sepsis.

b. Decreased urine output: treat with furosemide (Lasix).

c. Electrolyte imbalance: replace as needed.

B. **Embolization** may be performed to control bleeding proximal to the ligament of Treitz. The dual blood supply of the upper GI tract protects against bowel infarction.

1. **Contraindications:** before GI surgery, immediately after vasopressin infusion (wait at least 30 minutes), severe flow-limiting stenosis at the origin of the main mesenteric artery

2. **Technique**

a. Use digital road-mapping to guide the catheter to the vessel of interest. Occasionally, a coaxial system may be necessary to select the vessel of interest.

b. Super-selective embolization is desired, but either

the left gastric artery or gastroduodenal artery may be embolized safely.

   c. Agents include:

     (1) **Gelfoam pledgets:** 1- to 2-mm pledgets soaked in contrast and delivered through a small syringe

     (2) **Coils**

  **3. Pitfalls.** Fever after the procedure is common; strict adherence to sterile technique is essential.

## Nephrostomy Tube Placement

**I. Clinical history**

  **A. Confirmation of hydronephrosis and infection.** The only indication for an emergent nephrostomy placement is an **infected,** obstructed kidney.

**II. Procedure**

  **A.** Consider sedation.

  **B.** Use ultrasound from a posterolateral approach to localize a midpole calyx, and measure the distance from the skin to the target.

  **C.** Anesthetize the skin and puncture with a Teflon needle.

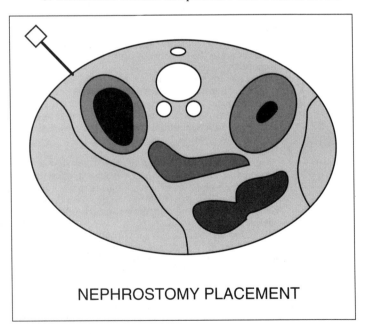

NEPHROSTOMY PLACEMENT

  **D.** With urine return, inject 1:1 saline to contrast mixture to opacify the collecting system and obtain spot film.

  **E.** Insert a large J wire and attempt to feed it down the ureter. This maneuver secures the wire for subsequent dilation and eventual nephrostomy tube placement. If this is not successful, coil the wire multiple times in the renal pelvis. This step is critical. If access is lost after decompressing the collecting system, it is extremely difficult to re-enter the septum.

**F.** Exchange the Teflon sheath for a multipurpose catheter. Again, attempt to pass it down the ureter if possible (may also try angled glide wire).

**G.** Exchange MPA catheter for 0.38 Amplatz wire, then use dilators (1 French larger than nephrostomy) to expand the tract.

**H.** Place a nephrostomy tube over the Amplatz wire, coiling the tip in the pelvis, and secure.

### III. Pitfalls

**A. Obstructed or leaking nephrostomy tube.**
Remember that unless the tube is infected, an "emergency" tube change is unnecessary.

**1.** Obtain an abdominal x-ray to assess the position of the tube. If it is in good position, bring several 5-ml syringes (remember that more pressure can be generated from a smaller syringe) and tape up to the floor.

**2.** Aspirate from the tube; if there is no fluid return, slowly inject 5 ml of saline into the tube. If the saline flows freely, then it is unlikely that the tube is obstructed. It may be in a poor location or the kidney may be functioning poorly. If you cannot inject fluid, instruct the nurse to keep the skin dry and plan for a tube change in the morning.

# Pulmonary Angiogram

### I. Clinical history

**A. Use of results by clinical service. Always** get a ventilation-perfusion scan before calling the interventional team. Discuss treatment options with the clinical service. If the patient has already been placed on heparin, the study can be done in the morning because an emergent study is unnecessary. If there is a contraindication to anticoagulation and an **IVC filter** will be desired in the event of a positive study, it can be done without delay or repuncture.

**B. Request for the study.** An emergent pulmonary angiogram should be performed only on a patient with a low or intermediate probability ventilation-perfusion scan and high clinical suspicion.

**C. Relative contraindications to angiography**

**1.** Left bundle branch block: place transvenous pacemaker to break complete heart block in the event that the catheter induces right bundle branch block

**2.** Pulmonary arterial hypertension greater than 50 mm Hg: perform subselective injections. A recent study concluded that elevated pulmonary artery pressure does not increase the risk of angiography when nonionic contrast is administered. In the most recent study with nonionic contrast, no deaths occurred.

**3.** Patient unable to lie supine

**4.** Patient weight greater 300 lb

**D. The mortality rate is 1 in 250 with ionic contrast (risk highest in patients with pulmonary hypertension).**

## II. Procedure
  **A.** Institute continuous cardiac monitoring.
  **B.** Perform femoral venous puncture, then exchange a Seldinger needle for a 7 French Van Aman or Grollman catheter.
  **C.** Advance the catheter through the right heart using a J or Rosen wire, if needed, into the main pulmonary artery. Pay particular attention to the cardiac monitor; withdraw the catheter if a run of three or more premature ventricular contractions (PVCs) or ventricular tachycardia occurs! In the event of continued PVCs, give a bolus of 50 mg lidocaine into the right atrium.
  **D.** Measure right heart pressures, perform a test injection, then inject the left or right pulmonary artery.
    **1.** Inject
      **a.** 50 ml at 20 ml/sec: **cut film**
      **b.** 20 ml at 25 ml/sec: **digital**
    **2.** Film
      **a.** Four films/sec out with a 0.5-sec delay: **cut film**
      **b.** Seven films/sec with a 0-sec delay: **digital**
  **E.** Film at maximal inspiration if possible and take oblique views as necessary.
  **F.** If a PE is seen, stop the exam—the diagnosis is made.

## III. Interpretation
  **A.** Acute pulmonary embolism
    **1.** Abrupt arterial cut-off
    **2.** Intraluminal filling defect
  **B.** Chronic pulmonary embolism
    **1.** Luminal narrowing and occlusion
    **2.** Webs
    **3.** Pouching defects
    **4.** Mural irregularities
See the section on Inferior Vena Cava Placement in this chapter and the section on the Ventilation-Perfusion Scan in Ch. 7.

# Thrombolysis

## I. Clinical history. Intra-arterial thrombolysis is successful in about two-thirds of cases of acute extremity arterial or bypass graft occlusion.
  **A. Laboratory tests**
    **1.** Hematocrit
    **2.** WBC count
    **3.** PT/PTT
    **4.** Bleeding time
    **5.** Thrombin time
  **B. Medications.** Discontinue aspirin, dextran, blood transfusions, and monobactam antibiotics.
  **C. Absolute contraindications**
    **1.** Irreversible ischemia or tissue loss (no motor or sensory function)
    **2.** Acute bleeding
    **3.** CNS abnormality within 3 months (hemorrhage, trauma, cerebrovascular accident, primary or metastatic neoplasm)

**D. Relative contraindications**
   1. Surgery within 10 days
   2. Recent obstetric delivery
   3. Left ventricular thrombus
   4. Severe hypertension
   5. Ulcerative colitis or GI bleeding
   6. Recent intra-arterial procedure
   7. Central venous line

**II. Complications.** Both remote and local complications increase as the time of infusion increases (8 hours: 5%; 40 hours: 35%).

   **A.** Major hemorrhage (remote or local)
   **B.** Distal embolization
   **C.** Thrombosis (decreased incidence with simultaneous heparin infusion)
   **D. Reperfusion syndrome:** sensory and motor deficits
   **E. Compartment syndrome**
      1. Edema and fluid retention in ischemic muscle cause the tissue pressure to rise (since this is a "closed space"). Increased tissue pressure can decrease blood flow further, which is manifested by decreased function and increased pain.
      2. Anterior tibial muscle is most vulnerable. Compromise is demonstrated by inability to dorsiflex the foot.
      3. Treatment: fasciotomy

**III. Procedure**

   **A.** Perform a femoral artery puncture using a single-wall puncture technique if possible and place a 5 French sheath. (If a clot is suspected in the lower extremity, puncture the contralateral femoral artery.)
   **B.** Perform an angiogram in the vessel of interest to visualize the presence and extent of the thrombus as well as the distal vasculature.
   **C.** Slowly advance a 0.035-inch Bentson guide wire or angled glide wire into the thrombus. Fresh clot is usually "soft" and feels like pushing a wire into butter.
   **D.** Advance Mewissen (multiple side holes with end-hole) or similar catheter into thrombus; some of the side holes should be within the thrombus while others should be proximal to it. (This ensures that the most proximal extent of the thrombus will be exposed to urokinase.)
   **E.** Confirm the position with a small injection of contrast.
   **F.** Attach a Tuohy-Borst side arm to the catheter and insert an end-hole occlusion wire.

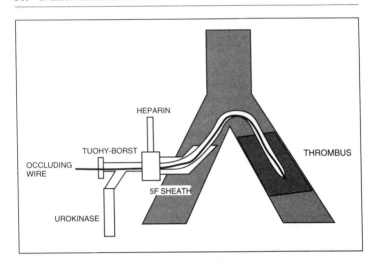

**G.** Prepare urokinase.
   **1.** Dissolve four 250K IU vials of urokinase in 20 ml of sterile water (5 ml for each vial).
   **2.** Add a total dose of 1,000,000 IU to 500 ml of 0.9% NaCl in water, yielding a concentration of 2000 IU/ml.
**H.** Administer urokinase through the Mewissen catheter.
   **1. McNamara** (high dose)
      **a.** Infuse at 250K IU/hour (125 ml/hour) using an infusion pump for 4 hours or until patent.
      **b.** Slow infusion if blood pressure drops more than 25 mm Hg or the patient has asthmatic symptoms.
      **c.** Repeat angiograms q4–12h.
   **2. Katzen** (low dose)
      **a.** Infuse 100K U/hour (50 ml/hour) overnight.
      **b.** Slow infusion if blood pressure drops more than 25 mm Hg or the patient has asthmatic symptoms.
      **c.** Repeat angiogram in the morning.
**I.** Infuse heparinized saline (1000 U in 500 ml) at 100 U/hour (50 ml/hour) through the sheath.
**J.** Administer 3000–5000 U heparin bolus IV with peripheral infusion of 1000 U/hour IV (1000 U in 500 ml at 20 ml/hour).
**K.** Transfer to ICU and monitor. Patients may have increased pain during thrombolysis.
   **1. PTT** 2–5 times normal
   **2. Fibrinogen** stop and redose if <100 mg/ml
   **3. Hematocrit**
   **4. No needle-sticks.** If absolutely necessary, venous sticks can be performed with a 23-gauge needle. Arterial puncture for air-blood gas assessment is done with physician monitoring and placing pressure for 30 minutes after the stick.
   **5. Measure vital signs** q4h
**L.** Stop infusion if:
   **1.** Resolution of thrombus with reperfusion
   **2.** Low-dose infusion: no response overnight

3. High-dose infusion: no response in 4–6 hours
4. Irreversible ischemia
5. Compartment syndrome

**M.** Assess for the etiology of the thrombus with repeat angiogram (e.g., underlying stenosis) and consider angioplasty.

**IV. Pitfalls**

**A. Bleeding** at catheter site
  1. Apply manual compression with fingertips and 4 × 4 sponges for 20 minutes.
  2. If bleeding continues, reduce the heparin and urokinase dose by 50% and apply manual pressure for an additional 15 minutes.
  3. If bleeding continues, stop heparin and apply pressure for an additional 15 minutes.
  4. If bleeding continues, decrease the urokinase dose by an additional 50%, give 3 units of cryoprecipitate, and apply pressure for an additional 15 minutes.
  5. If bleeding continues, decrease the urokinase dose by an additional 50% and apply pressure for an additional 15 minutes.
  6. If bleeding continues, stop urokinase and apply pressure until bleeding stops.

**B. Pain**
  1. Morphine, 5 mg IV; then, after 5 minutes, diazepam, 2.5 mg IV
  2. If pain persists, additional 2.5 mg diazepam IV
  3. Repeat 1–2 hours prn

**C. Nausea:** trimethobenzamide (Tigan), 200 mg IM q4–6h prn

# References

### General

Kandarpa K. *Handbook of Cardiovascular and Interventional Radiologic Procedures*. Boston: Little, Brown, 1989.

### Extremity Angiogram

Phillips CD. Emergent radiologic evaluation of the gunshot wound victim. *Radiol Clin N Am* 30:307, 1992.

### Inferior Vena Cava Filter Placement

Kaufman JA, Geller SC, Rivitz SM, Waltman AC. Operator errors during percutaneous placement of vena cava filters. *AJR Am J Roentgenol* 165:1281, 1995.

### Pulmonary Angiogram

Hudson ER et al. Pulmonary angiography performed with iopamidol: Complications in 1,434 patients. *Radiology* 198:61, 1996.

# Neurointerventional Procedures

## Cerebral Angiogram

### I. Clinical history

**A. Assess cerebral blood flow.** Emergencies will come from neurosurgery or vascular surgery. Most are either for trauma or for suspected aneurysms in patients with subarachnoid hemorrhage. Find out if the study needs to be done emergently. In general, these studies are never refused.

**B. Complications**
1. Bleeding
2. Infection
3. Stroke (1 in 1000 cases)

### II. Procedure

**A.** Catheterize femoral artery and exchange a Seldinger needle for a Weinberg 1 or Headhunter type catheter over a large J wire.

**B.** Advance the Weinberg 1 catheter into the ascending aorta with the wire in front of the catheter tip.

**C.** Pull wire back into catheter and then pull back on catheter with the tip facing the great vessels. Often slightly rotating the catheter counter-clockwise while retracting the catheter helps it to enter a vessel.

**D.** When the catheter "pops" into one of the great vessels, remove the wire and double flush with heparinized saline. Inject a test dose to confirm the location. Do not advance a catheter or guide wire past the origin of the vertebral or internal carotid artery without first performing a test injection to check for stenoses, plaques, and so forth. Always advance both the guide wire and catheter together with the guide wire leading.

**E.** Common carotid injection
1. Catheter tip should be below the bifurcation (approximately C4 level).
2. Inject 7 ml/sec for 9 ml.
3. Film at 2–3 films/sec for 5 sec.

**F.** Internal carotid injection
1. Catheter tip above the bifurcation at approximately C2 level
2. Inject 6 ml/sec for 8 ml.
3. Film at 2–3 films/sec for 5 sec.

**G.** External carotid injection
1. Catheter tip above bifurcation at approximately C2 level
2. Inject 4 ml/sec for 6 ml.
3. Film at 2–3 films/sec for 5 sec.

**H.** Vertebral artery injection
1. Catheter tip approximately 1 cm above the bifurcation
2. Inject 4 ml/sec for 6 ml.
3. Film at 2–3 films/sec for 5 sec.
4. Prone to spasm!

**I. Pitfalls**
1. If the vessel cannot be catheterized with the Weinberg 1 catheter, try a sidewinder catheter (remember to form a loop in the left subclavian artery).
2. At times, the internal carotid artery can be confused with the vertebral artery. If the patient turns his or her neck and the catheter remains superimposed over the spine, it is in the vertebral artery.
3. In patients with slow intracranial flow, prolonged filming may be necessary (e.g., subarachnoid hemorrhage).
4. **Bovine arch.** The left common carotid artery originates from the right brachiocephalic artery.

**III. Interpretation**
  **A. Aneurysms**
1. Usually involve the anterior communicating artery, posterior communicating artery, middle cerebral artery bifurcation, or basilar tip
2. Bleeding aneurysm
   **a.** Largest (90%)
   **b.** Anterior communicating artery
   **c.** May not be visualized due to spasm
  **B. Neck trauma.** Unstable patients are taken directly to surgery for exploration whereas angiography is performed for stable patients with low-velocity injuries. In high-velocity injuries (e.g., hunting or assault rifles), surgical exploration is usually performed.
1. Zone 1 (high)
   **a.** Above mandibular angle to skull base
   **b.** Angiogram in stable patient
2. Zone 2 (middle)
   **a.** Between mandibular angle and cricoid cartilage (approximately 1 cm above heads of clavicles)
   **b.** Controversial—angiography may **not** be indicated in the absence of physical signs of vessel injury (hematoma, hemorrhage, bruit)
3. Zone 3 (low)
   **a.** Below cricoid cartilage to sternoclavicular notch
   **b.** Angiogram in stable patient
4. Angiogram
   **a.** An aortic arch and four-vessel angiogram in multiple projections should be performed with *inclusion* of the venous phase.
   **b.** Cover the entire path of the bullet with generous margins.
   **c.** Oblique views are necessary if fragments are superimposed over the vessel.
   **d.** Check for pseudoaneurysms, arteriovenous fistula, intimal flaps, and transections.

# Myelography

**I. Clinical history**
  **A. Contraindications to MRI.** MRI is the exam of choice for most spine imaging. In general, emergent CT myelog-

raphy is reserved for patients who have spinal fixation rods that will result in significant metal artifact or in whom MRI is contraindicated (e.g., those with pacemakers, aneurysm clips).

**B. Rule out cord compression.** Most cases done emergently after-hours at our institution are performed on cancer patients who present with a focal neurologic exam or loss of bladder function. Always ask the location of the suspected lesion(s) because this will dictate the location of the puncture and area of the spine to be examined.

**C. Relative contraindications**
   1. Coagulopathy
   2. Previous myelogram within 1 week
   3. Sepsis
   4. Pregnancy
   5. Seizure history (may be premedicated)
   6. Allergy to contrast media
   7. Intracranial process with significant mass effect or impending herniation

**II. Procedure.** Always explain the procedure and risks to the patient and then obtain informed consent. **Possible complications include meningitis, CSF leak, arachnoiditis, headache, seizures, nausea, and vomiting.** If a complete block to contrast flow is present, progression occurs in up to approximately 25% of patients.

**A. Lumbar spine**
   1. Prepare the table before bringing the patient into the room. Load the syringe and connecting tubing with contrast, making sure that all air bubbles are out of the system. **Always make sure the contrast is labeled "approved for intrathecal use."** The dose of injected contrast is as follows:

   Omnipaque 180   10–17 ml
   Omnipaque 240   7.0–12.5 ml
   (Total dose not to exceed 3060 mg iodine)

   Isovue 200   8–17 ml
   Isovue 300   7–13 ml
   (Total dose not to exceed 4500 mg iodine)

   In children, we use Omnipaque 180 as follows:

   | 0–3 months | 2–4 ml |
   |---|---|
   | 3–36 months | 4–8 ml |
   | 3–7 years | 5–10 ml |
   | 7–13 years | 5–12 ml |
   | 13–18 years | 6–15 ml |

   2. Place the patient prone (the normal spinal lordosis will allow injected contrast to collect in the lumbosacral spine) with a pillow under the stomach. The pillow will help to "open up" the spinous processes, allowing better access to the cord. Alternatively, elevate one hip approximately 10–20 degrees with a pillow. This maneuver facilitates access to the cord since the spinous process is moved off the midline.

**3.** Use fluoroscopy to locate the L2–3 interspace and mark the skin with a pen. (Choose another interspace if this is the suspected location of pathology.)

**4.** Sterilize the skin with Betadine, then place a drape.

**5.** Anesthetize the planned tract liberally with lidocaine, using a 25-gauge needle followed by a 20-gauge needle. Leave the needle in the skin, remove the syringe, and, using fluoroscopy, confirm the needle position.

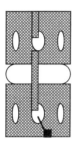
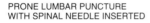
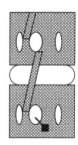

PRONE LUMBAR PUNCTURE
WITH SPINAL NEEDLE INSERTED

10- to 20-DEGREE OBLIQUE
WITH SPINAL NEEDLE INSERTED

**6.** Remove the lidocaine needle and puncture the skin with a 22-gauge spinal needle. Advance the needle in short 3- to 4-mm jabs. Periodically check the needle position with fluoroscopy and remove the inner cannula to check for backflow of CSF. Often you will feel a slight "pop" as the ligamentum flavum is crossed. Advance the needle another 3–5 mm and if CSF is desired for laboratory analysis, remove 6–10 ml before injecting contrast. (If a complete block is suspected, remove as little CSF as possible.)

**7.** Always inject contrast very **slowly**; the entire dose of contrast should be given over 3–4 minutes, keeping the patient flat or slightly head up with the neck extended and chin on a pillow. Contrast should flow freely away from the needle if it is in the subarachnoid space. If contrast "pools" around the tip, it is probably in the subdural or epidural space. The **pitfalls** are:

**a.** Do **not** allow contrast to run up into the brain, which could result in a seizure.

**b.** Be aware of warning signs of improper needle position, including Lhermitte's sign (electric shocks running down the arms or legs), which suggest the needle is pushing on a nerve, or complaints of pain or paresthesia.

**c.** If a complete block to contrast flow is encountered, do not inject the entire dose. Save at least 3 ml for cervical puncture.

**8.** At our institution, the following spot films are obtained:

**a.** PA views of the LS spine. Make sure to visualize the conus.

   **b.** Cross table lateral views of the LS spine. Make sure to visualize the conus.
   **c.** Shallow and steep left and right oblique views of the LS spine
   **d.** Flexion and extension lateral views if requested
   (If a block is identified, mark the skin at the level of the block with an indelible ink pen. Then proceed with a cervical tap.)
9. Bring the patient directly to the CT scanner and proceed with the scan.
10. After the scan the patient should be placed supine with the head slightly above the feet and watched for at least 6 hours. The incidence of postprocedural headache is approximately 40%.

**B. Thoracic spine**
1. Prepare the table before bringing the patient into the room. Load the syringe and connecting tubing with contrast, making sure that all air bubbles are out of the system. The dose of injected contrast is as follows:

   Omnipaque 240   7.0–12.5 ml
   (Total dose not to exceed 3060 mg iodine)

   Isovue 300        7.0–13 ml
   (Total dose not to exceed 4500 mg iodine)

2. Place the patient prone (the normal spinal lordosis will allow injected contrast to collect in the LS spine) with a pillow under the stomach. The pillow will help to "open up" the spinous processes, allowing better access to the cord. Alternatively, elevate one hip approximately 10–20 degrees with a pillow. This maneuver facilitates access to the cord since the spinous process is moved off the midline.
3. Use fluoroscopy to locate the L2–3 interspace and mark the skin with a pen.
4. Sterilize the skin with Betadine, then place a drape.
5. Anesthetize the planned tract liberally with lidocaine, using a 25-gauge needle followed by a 20-gauge needle. Leave the needle in the skin, remove the syringe, and, using fluoroscopy, confirm the needle position.
6. Remove the lidocaine needle and puncture the skin with a 22-gauge spinal needle. Advance the needle in short 3-to 4-mm jabs. Periodically check the needle position with fluoroscopy and remove the inner cannula to check for backflow of CSF. Often you will feel a slight "pop" as the ligamentum flavum is crossed. Advance the needle another 3–5 mm and if CSF is desired for laboratory analysis, remove 6–10 ml before injecting contrast. (If a block is suspected, remove as little CSF as possible.)
7. Always inject very **slowly**; the entire dose of contrast should be given over 3–4 minutes. Contrast should flow freely away from the needle if it is in the subarachnoid space. If contrast "pools" around the tip, it is probably in the subdural or epidural space.

**8. Pitfalls:**

  **a.** Do **not** allow contrast to run up into the brain, which could result in a seizure.

  **b.** Be aware of warning signs of improper needle position, including Lhermitte's sign (electric shocks running down the arms or legs), which suggest the needle is pushing on a nerve, or complaints of pain or paresthesia.

  **c.** If a complete block to contrast flow is encountered, do not inject the entire dose. Save at least 3 ml for cervical puncture.

**9.** After injecting contrast, turn the patient supine. The normal thoracic kyphosis will allow contrast to collect in the region of the thoracic spine. It is often useful to have the patient flex the neck, hips, and knees (i.e., curl up in the fetal position) while supine to exaggerate the kyphosis.

**10.** At our institution, the anteroposterior and lateral spot views of thoracic spine are obtained.
(If a block is identified, mark the skin at the level of the block with an indelible ink pen. Then proceed with a cervical tap.)

**11.** Bring the patient directly to the CT scanner and proceed with the scan.

**12.** After the scan the patient should be placed supine with the head slightly above the feet and watched for at least 6 hours. The incidence of postprocedural headache is approximately 40%.

**C. Cervical spine**

  **1.** Prepare the table before bringing the patient into the room. Load the syringe and connecting tubing with contrast, making sure that all air bubbles are out of the system. The dose of injected contrast for a cervical puncture is as follows:

Omnipaque 180   10–14 ml
(Total dose not to exceed 3060 mg I)

Isovue 200        10–14 ml
(Total dose not to exceed 4500 mg I)

Alternatively, a puncture can be performed in the lumbar area (see the section on the Lumbar Spine) with the head placed below the level of the feet. In that instance, the dose of injected contrast is as follows:

Omnipaque 240   7.0–12.5 ml
(Total dose not to exceed 3060 mg iodine)

Isovue 300        8–13 ml
(Total dose not to exceed 4500 mg iodine)

After injecting contrast, place the patient in a left lateral decubitus position and slowly run contrast up to the cervical spine.

  **2.** For a cervical puncture, place the patient prone with the head slightly extended and use lateral fluoroscopy to find the C1–2 interspace. Localize the posterior third of the spinal canal and mark the skin with a pen. The puncture should be made dorsal to the junction of the middle and posterior third of the spinal canal approximately 5 mm caudal to the posterior arch of the C1. (A cervical puncture can also be performed with the patient supine or in the left lateral decubitus position.)

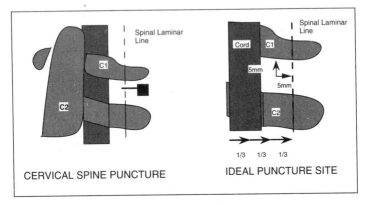

CERVICAL SPINE PUNCTURE          IDEAL PUNCTURE SITE

3. Sterilize the area with Betadine, then place a drape.
4. Anesthetize the planned tract liberally with lidocaine using a 25-gauge needle followed by a 20-gauge needle. Leave the needle in the skin, remove the syringe, and, using fluoroscopy, confirm the needle position.
5. Remove the lidocaine needle and puncture the skin with a 22-gauge spinal needle. Advance the needle in short 3- to 4-mm jabs. Periodically check the needle position with fluoroscopy and remove the inner cannula to check for backflow of CSF. Often you will feel a slight "pop" as the ligamentum flavum is crossed. Advance the needle another 3–5 mm and if CSF is desired for laboratory analysis, remove 6–10 ml before injecting contrast. (If a block is suspected, remove as little CSF as possible.) Do not advance the needle past the projected edge of the dens (on anteroposterior fluoroscopy).
6. Begin by injecting a tiny amount of contrast. It should flow freely away from the needle if it is in the subarachnoid space. If contrast "pools" around the tip or assumes a linear configuration, the needle tip is probably in the cord or subdural or epidural space. If the patient is supine, contrast will layer in the dependent portion of the canal; this looks almost exactly like a subdural injection. Inject contrast very **slowly**; the entire dose should be administered over a 3- to 4-minute period. **Do not** allow contrast to run up into the brain, which could result in a seizure. Be aware of warning signs, including Lhermitte's sign (electric shocks running down the arms or legs), which suggests the needle is pushing on a nerve, complaints of pain or paresthesia, or arterial blood flow from the needle.

7. If a complete block to contrast flow is encountered, do not inject the entire dose. Save at least 3 ml for cervical puncture.

8. At our institution, the following spot films are obtained:
   **a.** Anteroposterior view of the cervical spine—extension
   **b.** Anteroposterior view of the craniocervical junction—flexion
   **c.** Shallow and steep right and left obliques of the cervical spine
   **d.** Lateral view of the cervical spine
   (If a block is identified, mark the skin at the level of the block with an indelible ink pen. Then proceed with a cervical or lumbar tap.)

9. Bring the patient directly to the CT scanner and proceed with the scan.

10. After the scan the patient should be placed supine with the head slightly above the feet and watched for at least 6 hours. The incidence of postprocedural headache is approximately 40%.

## III. Pitfalls

**A. Contrast.** Always use only nonionic water-soluble contrast labeled **"approved for intrathecal use."** Administration of ionic contrast can result in **paralysis or death.**

**B. Complications of cervical puncture**

1. The most common complications of C1–2 puncture are hyperextension injuries of the spine. Death, paralysis, and worsening of pre-existing neurologic deficits have been reported. Patients at particular risk are those with spinal canal stenosis or severe spondylosis.

2. Rare cases of vascular injury have occurred with anomalous vessels. The posterior inferior cerebellar artery can extend to the C1–2 level. Aberrant vertebral arteries have also been punctured.

3. Paralysis and death have been reported with intraspinal injections. This risk is minimized if the amount of contrast injected is less than 0.5 ml.

**C.** Avoid using anything longer than a 3.5-inch spinal needle. Longer needles are more difficult to manipulate and usually unnecessary even in extremely obese patients.

## IV. Interpretation

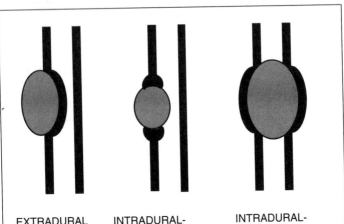

EXTRADURAL

INTRADURAL-
EXTRAMEDULLARY

INTRADURAL-
INTRAMEDULLARY

### A. Extradural
    1. Tumor
        **a.** Colon
        **b.** Prostate
        **c.** Lung
        **d.** Breast
    2. Trauma
        **a.** Hematoma
        **b.** Bone fragment
    3. Disk: C-spine, L-spine
    4. Infection
        **a.** Bacterial
        **b.** Tuberculosis
        **c.** Abscess
    5. Degenerative: osteophyte
### B. Intradural extramedullary
    1. Tumor
        **a.** Meningioma
        **b.** Lipoma
        **c.** Ependymoma
        **d.** Neurofibroma
        **e.** Metastasis
    2. Abscess
### C. Intradural intramedullary
    1. Tumor
        **a.** Ependymoma
        **b.** Astrocytoma
        **c.** Hemangioblastoma
    2. Trauma: hematoma
    3. Syrinx
    4. Postradiation

# References

## Cerebral Angiogram

Phillips CD. Emergent radiologic evaluation of the gunshot wound victim. *Radiol Clin N Am* 30:307, 1992.

## Myelography

Ramsey RG. *Neuroradiology* (3rd ed). Philadelphia: Saunders, 1994.

Robertson HJ, Smith RD. Cervical myelography: Survey of modes of practice and major complications. *Radiology* 174:79, 1990.

# Pediatrics

## Acute Abdomen

### I. Clinical history
  **A. Age of the patient.** The various etiologies of an acute abdomen in a child tend to be age dependent.
  1. Newborn: necrotizing enterocolitis (NEC), Hirschsprung's disease, meconium plug/small left colon, meconium ileus, midgut volvulus
  2. First 3 months: inguinal hernia (#1), Hirschsprung's disease, midgut volvulus
  3. 6 months to 2 years: ileocolic intussusception
  4. Older than 2 years: appendicitis
  **B. Bilious vomiting.** Any distal small-bowel or colonic obstruction can produce bilious vomiting. Hypertrophic pyloric stenosis will present with nonbilious vomiting.

### II. Imaging
  **A.** In any suspected acute abdomen, always obtain at least three abdomen views: supine, upright, and **prone.** The prone view is not done routinely but allows better differentiation of colon from small bowel (since gas will preferentially fill the rectum, ascending colon, and descending colon) as well as confirming or disproving fixation of bowel loops.
  **B.** Air should be in the stomach at birth, in the small bowel by 6 hours, and in the rectum by 24 hours. The appearances of the small bowel and the colon are indistinguishable in the newborn (i.e., the haustra and valvulae conniventes are not visible). Differentiation is usually made based on the position and location of bowel loops.

### III. Interpretation
  **A. Free air**
  1. Gastric perforation in the newborn
  2. NEC
  3. Obstruction (Hirschsprung's disease, meconium ileus)
  4. Dissection from pneumomediastinum
  5. Perforated ulcers, Meckel's diverticulum, appendicitis
  **B. GI hemorrhage**
  1. Neonates: NEC, infectious colitis
  2. Infant: Stress ulcer, Meckel's diverticulum, intussusception
  3. Child: polyp, inflammatory bowel disease
  **C. Necrotizing enterocolitis.** NEC is an ischemic bowel disease usually involving the distal ileum and ascending colon that occurs predominantly in premature infants (<2500 g, 37 weeks) 3 days or older. **Barium enema is contraindicated.**
  1. **Clinical history**
    **a.** Bloody diarrhea
    **b.** Abdominal distention
  2. **Abdominal radiograph**
    **a.** Bowel distention

**b.** Pneumatosis (80%): may appear linear or bubbly and should be seen on multiple views; supine cross table lateral view is frequently helpful

**c.** Portal venous air

**d.** Fixed bowel: arranged in concentric coils on various views (>50% perforation within 24–48 hours)

**e.** Thumb printing

**f.** Free air: usually indicates ileocecal perforation—surgery is mandatory

**3. Treatment**

**a.** Bowel rest

**b.** Antibiotics

**D. Midgut volvulus:** torsion of entire GI tract around the axis of the superior mesenteric artery. It is usually associated with malrotation and/or duodenal (Ladd) bands.

**1. Clinical history**

**a.** Bilious vomiting in a previously asymptomatic infant developing several days to weeks after birth

**b.** Normal girth and inguinal canal

**c.** Usually in children less than 1 month of age although it can present later in life

**2. Abdominal radiograph**

**a.** Four basic plain film patterns

    **(1)** Gastric obstruction ("single bubble")

    **(2)** Duodenal obstruction ("double bubble sign")

    **(3)** Small-bowel obstruction: air-fluid levels are usually not seen because the obstruction is at the level of the duodenum. In children with midgut volvulus, this is an ominous pattern with a high incidence of ischemia and infarction.

    **(4)** Normal

**b.** Perform a left side down decubitus.

    **(1)** Obstruction at the gastric outlet suggests pyloric stenosis.

    **(2)** Obstruction at the duodenum suggests midgut volvulus.

**c.** Free air

**d.** Often paucity of gas distally

**e.** Midgut volvulus **cannot be excluded** by plain films alone. In the proper context, an upper GI exam must be performed emergently.

**3. Upper GI exam**

**a.** Place a nasogastric tube (NGT) and aspirate the gastric contents. Put the child in a left side down decubitus position and administer barium through the NGT.

**b.** When the fundus of the stomach is well distended, place the child in a right anterior oblique position (nearly prone with the right side in contact with the table) and watch for filling of the duodenal bulb.

**c.** As contrast is seen passing through the bulb, quickly turn the child supine and follow the contrast to the ligament of Treitz.

    **(1)** In normal children, the ligament of Treitz should be seen on the left side of the spine slightly above the level of the fourth portion of the duodenum (at the level of the pylorus). It may be as medial as the left pedicle or as inferior as the greater curvature of the stomach.

  (2) In midgut volvulus, the ligament of Treitz most commonly will be lower and to the right of the spine.

  **d.** Obtain frontal, supine, oblique, and lateral projections as necessary.

  **e.** Interpretation

    (1) Obstruction of duodenum ("beak sign")

    (2) Thumb printing of the duodenum

    (3) Corkscrew or spiral appearance of the second and third portion of the duodenum

    (4) Jejunum in the right upper quadrant

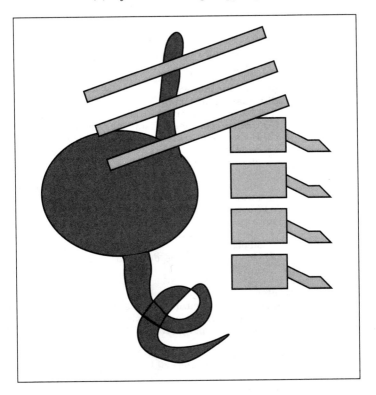

  **f.** Pitfalls

    (1) Bowel distention may displace the duodenal-jejunal junction inferiorly, mimicking malrotation

    (2) A single loop in the duodenum or jejunum in the right upper quadrant may be normal if the ligament of Treitz is in normal position.

  **4.** Treatment: surgical emergency

**E. Hirschsprung's disease.** Absence of parasympathetic ganglia in the muscle and submucosal layers of the colon due to an arrest of migration of neural crest cells

1. **Clinical history:** no passage of meconium in the first 24 hours of life
2. **Abdominal radiograph:** obtain a supine and prone cross table lateral view, centering on the rectum to look for the transition zone.
3. **Barium enema**
   a. Use a straight-tipped nonbulbous catheter (not balloon tip) and do not perform a cleansing enema.
   b. Findings
      (1) Aganglionic segment (normal size) with proximal dilatation
      (2) Retention of barium on 24-hour delayed views
      (3) Transition zone may be gradual or abrupt
      (4) Normal in one-third of patients
4. **Treatment:** surgery

F. **Hypertrophic pyloric stenosis (HPS)**
   1. **Clinical history:** usually presents in male infants 3–6 weeks of age as nonbilious projectile vomiting. If an "olive" is palpated, the child is usually taken directly to surgery.
   2. **Ultrasound**
      a. Aspirate gastric contents through NGT
      b. Look for a "pseudokidney" in the right upper quadrant
      c. Muscle (serosa to mucosa) greater than 3 mm
      d. Length of pylorus greater than 12 mm

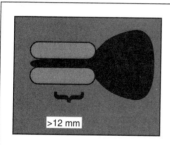
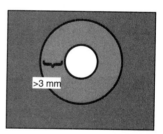

LONGITUDINAL               TRANSVERSE

   e. **Pitfalls**
      (1) Nonuniform muscle echogenicity at 6 and 12 o'clock positions can render the muscle isoechoic to surroundings and difficult to measure (worse on longitudinal images).
      (2) If the pylorus is imaged tangentially rather than in cross section, it may appear artifactually enlarged.
      (3) Pylorospasm: usually no muscle hypertrophy
      (4) Posteriorly directed antrum. Occasionally, administering a small amount of water may help to distend the stomach and bring the pylorus into better position for visualization.
   3. **Upper GI exam**
      a. Aspirate gastric contents with NGT.

**b.** Place the child in right anterior oblique position and administer 20–25 ml barium through NGT (may also give 15 cc of air if desired).

**c.** Turn the child left anterior oblique and compress the fundus with a leaded glove.

**d.** Look for hypertrophied pyloric muscle mass and narrowing plus elongation of the pylorus.

**e.** If contrast flows unobstructed into the duodenum, HPS is unlikely.

# Child Abuse

## I. Clinical history

**A. Suspected abuse.** Most children with radiographic evidence of child abuse are less than 2 years old and almost all are less than 6 years of age. The mechanism of injury is often violent shaking. In the absence of physical signs of abuse, radiographic findings are rarely present. In cases of suspected abuse, telephone the physician responsible for the patient and document the call in the report.

## II. Imaging

**A.** Screening examination should include:

1. Anteroposterior (AP) and lateral skull
2. AP thorax, abdomen, and pelvis
3. Lateral spine
4. AP extremities

**B.** If plain films are negative and clinical suspicion remains high, a nuclear medicine bone scan can be performed. In most institutions, a bone scan is not the screening examination of choice since the growth plates are difficult to assess (i.e., increased uptake occurs in normal and pathologic conditions).

**C.** If neurologic signs are present, obtain a head CT.

**D.** If blunt abdominal trauma is suspected, obtain a CT examination of the abdomen and pelvis.

## III. Interpretation

**A. Plain films**

1. **The hallmark of radiographically detectable child abuse is the presence of multiple fractures in various stages of healing with marked callus formation and subperiosteal hemorrhage.**

2. Although many abused children present with nonspecific soft-tissue injuries and fractures, other fractures are considered specific for child abuse:

   **a.** Metaphyseal-epiphyseal fractures ("corner fractures," "bucket-handle fractures")

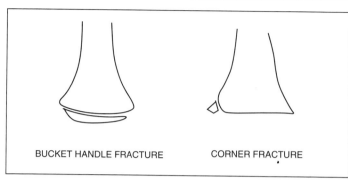

BUCKET HANDLE FRACTURE          CORNER FRACTURE

    **b.** Posterior rib fractures
    **c.** Diaphyseal fractures in pre-ambulatory infants
  **3.** Fractures at unusual sites (lateral clavicle, sternum, scapula, spine) or inconsistent with the reported mechanism of injury (e.g., spiral fracture from a fall) should also raise the question of abuse.
  **4.** Most skull fractures are linear and occur in the parietal bone. In general, sutures should be less than 3 mm wide at 2 years of age and less than 2 mm wide at 3 years of age.

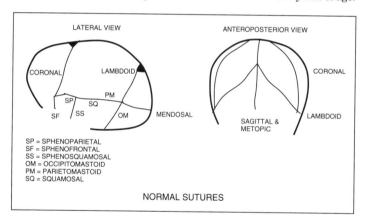

LATERAL VIEW               ANTEROPOSTERIOR VIEW

CORONAL   LAMBDOID

PM

SP   SQ

SF   SS   OM   MENDOSAL

CORONAL

SAGITTAL & METOPIC   LAMBDOID

SP = SPHENOPARIETAL
SF = SPHENOFRONTAL
SS = SPHENOSQUAMOSAL
OM = OCCIPITOMASTOID
PM = PARIETOMASTOID
SQ = SQUAMOSAL

NORMAL SUTURES

  **5.** Subperiosteal hemorrhage
  **6.** The **differential diagnosis** of abuse includes uncommon disorders such as osteogenesis imperfecta, Menkes' kinky hair syndrome, leukemia, periostitis of infancy, infantile cortical hyperostosis, and congenital insensitivity to pain. The first two entities are associated with wormian bones. The vast majority of battered children will not have evidence of underlying bone disease.
**B. Head CT**
  **1.** Findings are nonspecific and include:
    **a.** Subdural hematoma (acute or chronic)—often interhemispheric
    **b.** Parenchymal contusion or hematoma

    **c.** Cerebral edema
  **2.** A few rules of thumb to remember are that:
    **a.** A fall from a height of 3 feet or less (e.g., falling out of bed) will **not** result in an intracranial injury.
    **b.** An interhemispheric hematoma should raise concern for abuse.
**C. Abdominal and pelvic CT**
  **1.** The findings are sequelae of blunt trauma:
    **a.** Duodenal hematoma
    **b.** Intestinal perforation (usually small bowel)
    **c.** Liver contusions and lacerations
    **d.** Pancreatic transections and traumatic pancreatitis

# Airway

**I. Clinical history**
  **A. Age of the patient.** Epiglottitis is usually caused by *Haemophilus influenzae* and generally affects children age 3–6 years, whereas croup occurs in younger patients (6 months to 3 years).
  **B. Foreign-body ingestion** is a very common cause of breathing difficulty in the first few years of life.
  **C. Supervision.** Any child who has difficulty breathing **must** be closely monitored, preferably by experienced personnel who are capable of intubation if necessary. **Avoid** manipulation of the neck, which can precipitate complete airway obstruction.
**II. Imaging**
  **A. Plain films**
    **1.** Upright AP and lateral views of the neck
    **2.** Lateral decubitus views (if air trapping is suspected)
  **B. Fluoroscopy:** performed on inspiration and exhalation
**III. Interpretation**

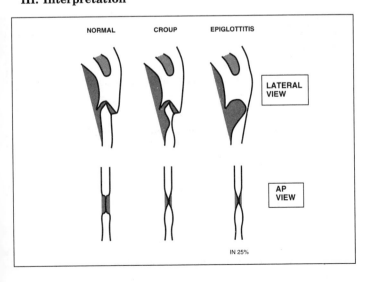

NORMAL    CROUP    EPIGLOTTITIS

LATERAL VIEW

AP VIEW

IN 25%

**A. Epiglottitis**
1. Symptoms: fever, sore throat, dysphagia, stridor, drooling; not usually preceded by upper respiratory infection
2. Findings
   **a.** "Thumb sign": thickened epiglottis and aryepiglottic folds
   **b.** Ballooning of hypopharynx
   **c.** Vallecula not well seen
   **d.** Subglottic edema that mimics croup (25%)
3. Treatment: intubation
4. **Pitfall: omega epiglottis.** The epiglottis appears enlarged but the aryepiglottic folds are normal.

**B. Croup**
1. Symptoms: "barking cough," often preceded by upper respiratory infection, inspiratory stridor
2. Findings: "steeple sign" (smooth conical narrowing of subglottic lumen)
3. Differential diagnosis: vocal cord paralysis, laryngeal webs

**C. Foreign-body aspiration: Findings**
1. Air trapping (affected side remains well inflated in decubitus views—90%)
2. Atelectasis (10%)
3. Fluoroscopy: air trapping (affected side remains overinflated during exhalation)

# Head Ultrasound

**I. Clinical history**
A. **Premature infant—rule out hemorrhage.** The germinal matrix is a fine network of vessels and neural tissue located along the walls of the lateral ventricles in the fetus that usually regresses by 34 weeks. At term, only a small portion is left along the caudothalamic groove. In premature infants, the germinal matrix is susceptible to rupture and hemorrhage since regression is incomplete. In babies born before 32 weeks' gestation or who weigh less than 1500 g, there is as much as a 70% chance of intracranial hemorrhage.
B. **Baby to be placed on extracorporeal membrane oxygenation (ECMO)—rule out hemorrhage.** When a child is placed on ECMO, anticoagulants are administered, which are contraindicated with a grade 2 or more severe intracranial hemorrhage.
C. **Child with high-output cardiac failure.** Vein of Galen aneurysms commonly present with high-output cardiac failure in neonates. Older children usually present with hydrocephalus and/or seizures.

**II. Imaging**
A. On any portable exam
1. Bring
   **a.** Gel
   **b.** Film (if needed)
   **c.** Previous exams to help guide your efforts

       **d.** Correct probe: sector 5 MHz

  **2.** Once at the intensive care nursery, have the nurse "make space" for the machine (we prefer to park the machine on the left side of the child since it allows us to scan with the right hand).

  **3.** Dim as many of the lights as possible. (Avoid the urge to increase the gray scale gain since this will overexpose the images.)

  **4.** Wash your hands and the probe before and after use.

**B. Scanning strategies**

  **1.** Use the 5-MHz sector probe and scan through the anterior fontanelle (hair usually won't interfere with the scan but abundant hair can create considerable air block and should be drenched with gel and smoothed down).

  **2.** The germinal matrix is located along the inferolateral walls of the lateral ventricles. Concentrate your efforts in this area.

  **3.** Adjust depth.

  **4.** Look for side-to-side symmetry on coronal images.

  **5.** Scan first with one focal spot and look for findings. When you want to take pictures, switch to multiple focal zones. Six images in the coronal plane and six in the sagittal plane will suffice. Remember to clean the transducer and wash your hands before and after scanning.

**III. Interpretation**

  **A. Hemorrhage**

    **1.** Grade 1

      **a.** Subependymal germinal matrix hemorrhage

      **b.** Increased echogenicity in the inferolateral wall of lateral ventricle anterior to the caudothalamic groove

    **2.** Grade 2

      **a.** Intraventricular hemorrhage

      **b.** Rupture through ependymal lining into the ventricle (may fill ventricle)

      **c.** Asymmetric choroid plexus with variable echogenicity. (Note that the choroid plexus **does not** extend into the frontal or occipital horns of the lateral ventricles; increased echogenicity in these areas implies hemorrhage.)

    **3.** Grade 3

      **a.** Intraventricular hemorrhage with ventricular dilatation

      **b.** May extend into third and fourth ventricles, basilar cisterns, and subarachnoid space

    **4.** Grade 4

      **a.** Intraparenchymal hemorrhage

      **b.** Usually unilateral in the frontoparietal region

  **B. Vein of Galen aneurysm.** The name is a misnomer. The vein is actually dilated due to draining a central arteriovenous malformation.

    **1.** Round, anechoic structure posterior to the third ventricle between the lateral ventricles.

    **2.** Swirling flow on color Doppler imaging

# Hip Ultrasound

**I. Clinical history. Painful hip—rule out septic joint.**
**Always** obtain plain films of the pelvis before embarking on
an adventure in hip ultrasound. A wide variety of disorders
can cause hip pain, such as Perthes' disease, fracture, slipped
capital femoral epiphysis, and arthritis.

**II. Imaging**
Place the patient supine with the hips in neutral position.
Using a 5-MHz **linear** probe, scan in a ventral oblique plane
along the axis of the femoral neck. Scan both the normal and
abnormal sides and compare.

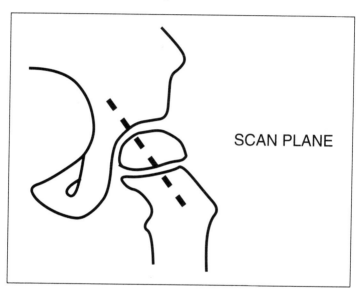

SCAN PLANE

**III. Interpretation**
  **A. Normal.** The joint capsule has a concave contour, and the
     thickness of the capsule from outer margins to cortex
     measures 2–5 mm. Both sides should be symmetric to
     within 2 mm.
  **B. Effusion.** The anterior recess of the joint capsule becomes
     distended with a convex outer margin. The most common
     cause of acute hip pain in the child with an effusion is
     **toxic synovitis,** not **septic arthritis.**

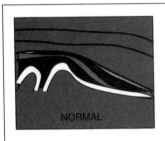
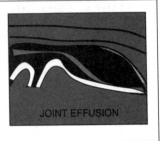

NORMAL          JOINT EFFUSION

# Intussusception

I. **Clinical history. Child 6 months to 4 years of age with abdominal pain, emesis, bloody ("currant jelly") stools, and right lower quadrant mass.** The constellation of these findings occurs in approximately 20% of cases. In children, the vast majority of intussusceptions are idiopathic and ileocolic; in fact, only 10% of **recurrent** intussusceptions are associated with a lead point. Air or contrast reduction is successful in approximately 75% of cases.

II. **Imaging**

   A. **Abdominal radiograph. Always** obtain an abdominal radiograph with a horizontal beam view to exclude **free air** before attempting a reduction. Look for:
   1. Absence of gas in the right lower quadrant
   2. Visualization of the head of the intussusception

   Note that gas filling the cecum and terminal ileum essentially excludes ileocolic intussusception. Always perform a **prone** view to preferentially fill the cecal tip with air.

   B. **Ultrasound:** Scan with either a 5- or 7-MHz linear transducer in the most suspicious area of the abdominal radiograph. Look for:
   1. "Pseudokidney": hypoechoic outer rim with central hyperechoic core with or without adjacent free fluid. Color flow may demonstrate central vessels.
   2. Target configuration on cross sectional imaging

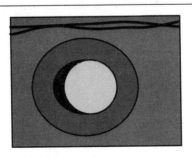

DOUGHNUT SIGN

### III. Contrast reduction

A. **Always** obtain an abdominal plain film before attempting a reduction. Free intraperitoneal air, peritonitis, and hypovolemic shock are absolute contraindications to contrast enema reduction.

B. Make sure that the child has IV access.

C. Call the pediatric attending on call.

D. Barium enema

1. Notify the **surgical service** that reduction of intussusception is being attempted. Perforation occurs in 1–3% of cases (most commonly in the normal distal bowel).

2. Prepare large volumes of gastrografin/dilute barium. Multiple attempts and/or soiling commonly occur.

3. Immobilize the child and place in a prone position.

4. Insert a Foley catheter and secure with **cloth adhesive tape,** attaching the buttocks together. Make sure that the anus is completely occluded.

5. Tubing should run unkinked straight from bag to table, not drape to floor.

6. The bag should be no higher than 3 feet above the table.

7. Manipulation or palpation of the intussusception is controversial. The classic teaching was that it should not be done due to an increased risk of perforation. Recent literature suggests otherwise.

8. Allow up to 15 minutes for the head of the intussusception to pass flexures or the ileocecal valve.

9. Up to 3–5 attempts can be performed.

10. Reduction is complete only when contrast is refluxed into the terminal ileum.

11. Take postevacuation abdominal x-ray and 24-hour abdominal x-ray to exclude recurrence (4–11% incidence). If intussusception recurs, you can redo air or contrast reduction but the presence of a lead point becomes more likely.

12. **Pitfalls**

a. Barium may fill a large appendix, mimicking the terminal ileum.

b. Occasionally there is a persistent filling defect representing an edematous ileocecal valve, which may mimic an unreduced intussusception even in complete reduction.

E. **Air reduction**

1. Notify the **surgical service** that reduction of an intussusception is being attempted. Perforation in air reduction is not as ominous a complication compared with contrast reduction if it is recognized and pneumoperitoneum is alleviated with a 14-gauge needle.

2. Immobilize the child.

3. Insert a Foley catheter and secure with **cloth adhesive tape,** taping the buttocks together. Make sure that the anus is completely occluded.

4. Tubing should run unkinked straight from machine to child.

5. Up to 120 mm Hg for up to 2 minutes can be used.

6. Manipulation or palpation of the intussusception is controversial. The classic teaching was that it should

not be done due to an increased risk of perforation. Recent literature suggests otherwise.

7. Reduction is complete when copious air reflux is seen in the terminal ileum. You may see sudden filling of the small bowel ("bunch of grapes").

8. If perforation occurs, relieve tension pneumoperitoneum with 14-gauge needle.

9. Take postevacuation abdominal x-ray and 24-hour abdominal x-ray to exclude recurrence (4–11% incidence). If intussusception recurs, you can redo air or contrast reduction but the presence of a lead point becomes more likely.

10. **Pitfalls**
   a. Always be cognizant of the possibility of perforation with pneumoperitoneum! If it is not recognized, large amounts of air in the peritoneal cavity could potentially limit diaphragmatic excursion and lead to respiratory depression.
   b. If the child has a small-bowel obstruction, reflux into the terminal ileum may be difficult to visualize.
   c. Reflux may occur before complete reduction.
   d. An edematous ileocecal valve may appear as a persistent filling defect.
   e. Lead points are usually **not** visualized.

# Pediatric and Neonatal Intensive Care Unit Radiography

I. **Clinical history. Check status.** Most pediatric ICU and neonatal intensive care unit (NICU) patients receive routine chest x-rays (at least daily), and often, little or no clinical information is provided. In general, the after-hours evaluation of these studies should be directed toward detection of findings that will acutely affect patient management. Although in many cases the physician will review all films on his or her patient, never assume that an abnormality, no matter how obvious, has been detected. Always **telephone** the physician taking care of the patient.

II. **Checklist**
   A. **Tubes and wires**
   B. **Lungs**
   C. **Heart**
   D. **Abdomen**

III. **Interpretation**
   A. **Tubes and catheters**
      1. **Endotracheal tube**
         a. The ideal location is approximately 1.0–1.5 cm above the carina. It moves in the same direction as the chin (i.e., moves caudad with neck flexion).
         b. Complications
            (1) Too high: cuff in hypopharynx or at vocal cords, which can result in air leak, aspiration, and gastric distention

**(2)** Too low: usually in right mainstem bronchus (may see left lung collapse)

**(3)** Overinflation of cuff (greater than 1.5 times tracheal diameter): predisposes to tracheal necrosis/stenosis

2. **Chest tube.** The ideal location is with both the side hole and end hole in the pleural space. Many are located in pleural fissures (usually of no consequence).

3. **Nasogastric tube**
   **a.** Ideal location is in the body of the stomach with the side hole distal to the gastroesophageal junction
   **b.** Complications
      **(1)** Too high: may cause aspiration pneumonia
      **(2)** Wrong location: may enter trachea and bronchi—should always be checked before feeding is initiated

4. **Percutaneous central venous catheter**
   **a.** Ideal location is in distal superior vena cava or right atrium
   **b.** Complications
      **(1)** Tip embolus to right heart or pulmonary artery: often best seen on lateral view
      **(2)** Improper location: can terminate in brachiocephalic veins or azygous vein (usually no consequence)

5. **Umbilical artery catheter**
   **a.** Ideal location is at the level of T6–10 or L3–5 (away from superior mesenteric artery, celiac axis, and inferior mesenteric artery)

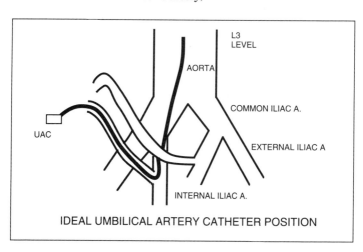

L3
LEVEL

AORTA

COMMON ILIAC A.

EXTERNAL ILIAC A

UAC

INTERNAL ILIAC A.

IDEAL UMBILICAL ARTERY CATHETER POSITION

   **b.** Complications
      **(1)** Wrong location: may terminate at the wrong level or in major aortic vessels such as the celiac axis, renal artery, or subclavian artery, where it can incite thrombosis
      **(2)** Perforation: rarely, the catheter can perforate the artery, resulting in major hemorrhage.

**6. Umbilical vein catheter**
  **a.** The ideal location is in the right atrium.

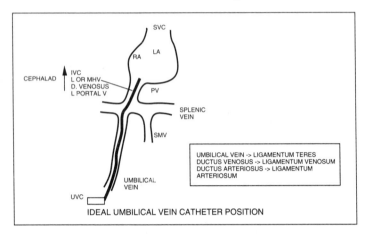

IDEAL UMBILICAL VEIN CATHETER POSITION

  **b.** Complications
    **(1)** Wrong location: can terminate in any structure depicted above (including the left atrium through a patent foramen ovale; the lateral view is helpful in locating the catheter tip).
    **(2)** Perforation: rarely, the catheter can perforate the vein, resulting in a major hemorrhage.
**B. Thorax**
  **1. Supine pneumothorax:** air in the pleural space that is often loculated anteriorly or medially in a supine neonate
    **a. Anteromedial (earliest location):** sharp delineation of mediastinal contours, outline of medial diaphragm under cardiac silhouette
    **b. Subpulmonic:** "deep sulcus sign"—costophrenic angle on the side of the pneumothorax unusually deep; may see sharp diaphragm despite left lower lobe infiltrate or lucent upper abdominal quadrant.
    **c. Apical/lateral (least common):** absence of lung markings peripheral to a sharp border.
    **d. "Tension":** shift of mediastinum and diaphragm away from affected side (ventilators)
    **e. Follow-up:** a decubitus film is helpful in clarifying equivocal cases.
  **2. Pneumomediastinum:** air in the mediastinum is usually due to positive pressure ventilation. Can occasionally lead to pneumothorax
    **a.** Subcutaneous emphysema in neck
    **b.** Air surrounding trachea and mainstem bronchi on lateral view
    **c.** Pneumopericardium: extends only to top of pericardium—very rare unless a pericardial tap performed
  **3. Opacification of hemithorax**
    **a.** Collapse/atelectasis: volume loss, rotation, and medi-

astinal shift (trachea) toward **affected** side (check endotracheal tube)

**b.** Effusion: mediastinal shift toward **unaffected** side
**c.** Consolidation
**d.** Agenesis/hypoplasia

**4. Pleural effusion**
**a.** Often seen at apex and laterally in lung fields
**b.** Myriad of etiologies—rarely seen in hyaline membrane disease

**C. Abdomen**
**1. Pneumoperitoneum.** Air in peritoneal space usually due to ruptured hollow viscus or recent abdominal surgery
  **a. Findings**
    **(1) Rigler's sign:** both sides of bowel wall visualized
    **(2) Air** under the right hemidiaphragm on **upright** chest radiograph (not portable)—both posterior-anterior and lateral views should be obtained
    **(3) Triangle sign:** gas between three bowel loops or two bowel loops and parietal peritoneum
    **(4) Hyperlucent liver**
    **(5) Hepatic edge sign:** air outlining inferior portion of liver
    **(6) Anterior superior oval:** oblong air collection anterior to the liver
    **(7) Ligamentum teres sign:** sharply defined vertical slit or oval at the porta hepatis
    **(8) Doge hat sign:** triangle-shaped air collection in Morison's (hepatorenal) pouch
  **b. Pitfalls**
    **(1) Postoperative air** usually resolves within **7–10 days**
    **(2) Rigler's sign** may be mimicked by abundant omental or mesenteric fat or meteorism (air swallowing resulting in multiple dilated gas-filled loops apposing each other).
  **c. Follow-up**
    **(1)** Perform left side down decubitus plain film centering on liver to achieve horizontal beam. Do **not** request "upright" portable film.
    **(2)** Air usually collects between the right lateral liver margin and lateral hemidiaphragm.

# References

### Acute Abdomen

Ablow RC, Hoffer FA, Seashore JH, Touloukian RJ. Z-shaped duodenojejunal loop: Sign of mesenteric fixation anomaly and congenital bands. *AJR Am J Roentgenol* 141:461, 1983.

Alford BA, McIlhenny J. The child with acute abdominal pain and vomiting. *Radiol Clin N Am* 30:441, 1992.

Blickman JG. *Pediatric Radiology: The Requisites.* St. Louis: Mosby, 1994.

Johnson JF. The acute abdominal series in infants and children, Parts 1–3. *Applied Radiol* 4–6:23–34, 19–29, 21–31, 44, 1994.

Merten DF. Practical approaches to pediatric gastrointestinal radiology. *Radiol Clin N Am* 31:1395, 1993.

Swisschuk LE, Hayden CK. The Pediatric Gastrointestinal Tract. In CM Rumack, SR Wilson, JW Charboneau (eds), *Diagnostic Ultrasound*. St. Louis: Mosby–Year Book, 1991.

### Child Abuse

Chu LL, Sartoris DJ. Clinical quiz. *Applied Radiol* 24:20, 1995.

Kleinman PK. Diagnostic imaging in infant abuse. *AJR Am J Roentgenol* 155:703, 1990.

Kleinman PK, Belanger PL, Karellas A, Spevak MR. Normal metaphysical radiologic variants not to be confused with findings of infant abuse. *AJR Am J Roentgenol* 156:781, 1991.

### Airway

John SD, Swischuk LE. Stridor and upper airway obstruction in infants and children. *Radiographics* 12:625, 1992.

### Head Ultrasound

Sherman NH, Rosenberg HK. Ultrasound essential for imaging neonatal brains. *Diagnostic Imaging* Nov 1994, Pp 108–115, 164.

### Hip Ultrasound

Harcke HT, Grissom LE. The Pediatric Hip. In CM Rumack, SR Wilson, JW Charboneau (eds), *Diagnostic Ultrasound*. St. Louis: Mosby–Year Book, 1991.

### Intussusception

Alford BA, McIlhenny J. The child with acute abdominal pain and vomiting. *Radiol Clin N Am* 30:441, 1992.

Merten DF. Practical approaches to pediatric gastrointestinal radiology. *Radiol Clin N Am* 31:1395, 1993.

### Pediatric and Neonatal Intensive Care Unit Radiography

Narla LD, Hom M, Lofland GK, Moskowitz WB. Evaluation of umbilical catheter and tube placement in premature infants. *Radiographics* 11:849, 1991.

Tocino IM. Pneumothorax in the supine patient: Radiographic anatomy. *Radiographics* 5:557, 1985.

# 11

# Radiation Exposure

I. **Clinical history: pregnant woman in the emergency room. Request radiographic study.** An issue that arises with surprising frequency at night is radiation exposure—typically, what kind of studies can be performed "safely" on pregnant women. **In general, any study that does not directly irradiate the pelvis (including head CTs and chest x-rays [CXRs]) results in minimal radiation exposure to the fetus.** Many believe that any exposure below 5000 mR is negligible. The combined risk of fetal effects (mortality, malformation, childhood cancer) is estimated to be approximately 0.003 per 1000 mR; thus, the risk from most imaging studies compared to the spontaneous incidence of congenital anomalies (4–6%) is very small. Any study that is medically necessary should be done without hesitation.

II. **Imaging.** The table below lists "ballpark" estimates of radiation doses for various exams.

| Examination | Approximate skin dose (mR) | Approximate fetal dose (mR) |
|---|---|---|
| Chest x-ray (posteroanterior) | 30 | <1 |
| Chest x-ray (lateral) | 100 | <1 |
| Abdominal x-ray | 400 | 200 |
| Pelvis | 500 | 100 |
| Head CT | 4000–6000 | <1 |
| Abdominal/pelvic CT | 1000–4000 | 3000–10,000 |
| IV urogram (10 films) | 5000 | 1750 |
| Upper GI exam (16 films) | 8800 | 290 |
| Barium enema (17 films) | 14,000 | 5000 |
| Fluoroscopy (14 films) | 5000/minute | Variable |
| Lumbar myelogram | 55,000 | 20,000 |
| Living on earth | 360/year | — |

For both CXRs and head CTs, we tell the technician to place a lead apron over the lower abdomen and pelvis. Although most of the fetal dose in CXRs is due to scattered radiation from tissue within the beam, this maneuver will minimally decrease fetal dose and is beneficial for the **mother's mental well-being.**

There is very low risk associated with imaging studies performed on women in the third trimester of pregnancy. However, no amount of radiation is beneficial and even low radiation doses have been associated with an increased risk of childhood cancer in some studies. The National Council on Radiation Protection recommends that for occupational situations (excluding medical and natural background radiation), a total dose equivalent limit should be 500 mR for the fetus with no greater than 50 mR per month of gestation.

A point that is not intuitively obvious to the early first-year resident is that the radiation from a fluoroscopic table emanates from below the table, not from the image intensifier above the patient. Therefore, when shielding the gonads, the lead apron should be placed **between the table and patient,** not on top of the patient.

# References

National Council on Radiation Protection. Report No. 116: Limitation of exposure to ionizing radiation. March 31, 1993.

Rothenberg LN, Pentlow KS. AAPM tutorial: Radiation dose in CT. *Radiographics* 12:1225, 1992.

Ward WF. Course notes from physics review course. Loyola University Medical Center and Stan A. Huber Consultants, 1995.

# Index

# Dear Reader

*We are thrilled to present the fifth edition of our MICHELIN guide to Chicago.*

*Our dynamic team has spent this year updating our selection to reflect the rich diversity of Chicago's restaurants. As part of our meticulous and highly confidential evaluation process, our inspectors have anonymously and methodically eaten through all of the city's neighborhoods to compile the finest in each category for your enjoyment. While the inspectors are expertly trained food industry professionals, we remain consumer-driven and provide comprehensive choices to accommodate your comfort, tastes, and budget. Our inspectors dine, drink, and lodge as "regular" customers in order to experience and evaluate the same level of service and cuisine that you would as a guest.*

*We have expanded our criteria to reflect the more current and unique elements of the city's dining scene. Don't miss the tasty "Small Plates" category, highlighting places with a distinct style of service, setting, and menu; as well as the comprehensive "Under $25" list, which includes an impressive choice at great value.*

*Additionally, you may also follow our Inspectors on Twitter @MichelinGuideCH as they chow their way around town. They usually tweet daily about their unique and entertaining food experiences.*

*Our company's founders, Édouard and André Michelin, published the first MICHELIN guide in 1900, to provide motorists with practical information about where they could service and repair their cars, find quality accommodations, and a good meal. Later in 1926, the star-rating system for outstanding restaurants was introduced, and over the decades we have developed many new improvements to our guides. The local team here in Chicago eagerly carries on these traditions.*

*We truly hope that the MICHELIN guide will remain your preferred reference to Chicago's restaurants.*

# Contents

Where to **Eat**

10

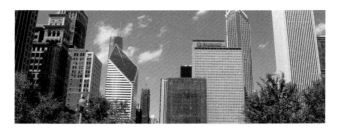

Contents

242

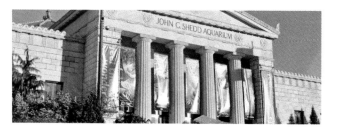

# The MICHELIN Guide

*"This volume was created at the turn of the century and will last at least as long".*

This foreword to the very first edition of the MICHELIN Guide, written in 1900, has become famous over the years and the Guide has lived up to the prediction. It is read across the world and the key to its popularity is the consistency in its commitment to its readers, which is based on the following promises.

### → Anonymous Inspections

Our inspectors make anonymous visits to hotels and restaurants to gauge the quality offered to the ordinary customer. They pay their own bill and make no indication of their presence. These visits are supplemented by comprehensive monitoring of information—our readers' comments are one valuable source, and are always taken into consideration.

### → Independence

Our choice of establishments is a completely independent one, made for the benefit of our readers alone. Decisions are discussed by the inspectors and the editor, with the most important decided at the global level. Inclusion in the guide is always free of charge.

### → The Selection

The Guide offers a selection of the best hotels and restaurants in each category of comfort and price. Inclusion in the guides is a commendable award in itself, and defines the establishment among the "best of the best."

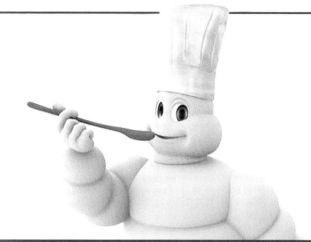

# How the MICHELIN Guide Works

### → Annual Updates

All practical information, the classifications, and awards, are revised and updated every year to ensure the most reliable information possible.

### → Consistency & Classifications

The criteria for the classifications are the same in all countries covered by the Michelin Guides. Our system is used worldwide and is easy to apply when choosing a restaurant or hotel.

### → The Classifications

We classify our establishments using XxXxX-X and 🏨🏨🏨-🏠 to indicate the level of comfort. The ✿✿✿-✿ specifically designates an award for cuisine, unique from the classification. For hotels and restaurants, a symbol in red suggests a particularly charming spot with unique décor or ambiance.

### → Our Aim

As part of Michelin's ongoing commitment to improving travel and mobility, we do everything possible to make vacations and eating out a pleasure.

7

# How to Use This Guide

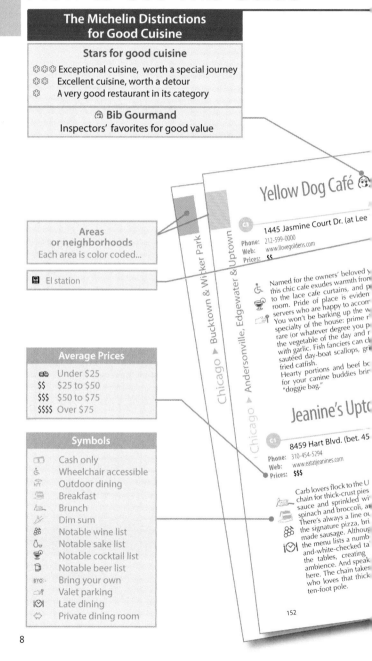

## The Michelin Distinctions for Good Cuisine

### Stars for good cuisine

❀❀❀ Exceptional cuisine, worth a special journey
❀❀ Excellent cuisine, worth a detour
❀ A very good restaurant in its category

### ⊛ Bib Gourmand
Inspectors' favorites for good value

**Areas or neighborhoods**
Each area is color coded...

🚇 El station

### Average Prices

| | |
|---|---|
| ⊜ | Under $25 |
| $$ | $25 to $50 |
| $$$ | $50 to $75 |
| $$$$ | Over $75 |

### Symbols

| | |
|---|---|
| ⌖ | Cash only |
| ♿ | Wheelchair accessible |
| 🌳 | Outdoor dining |
| 🍽 | Breakfast |
| 🍴 | Brunch |
| 🥟 | Dim sum |
| 🍷 | Notable wine list |
| 🍶 | Notable sake list |
| 🍸 | Notable cocktail list |
| 🍺 | Notable beer list |
| BYO | Bring your own |
| 🚗 | Valet parking |
| 🌙 | Late dining |
| ⟳ | Private dining room |

Chicago ▶ Andersonville, Edgewater & Uptown ▶ Bucktown & Wicker Park

## Yellow Dog Café ⊛

**G1** 1445 Jasmine Court Dr. (at Lee

Phone: 212-599-0000
Web: www.Ilovegoldens.com
Prices: $$

Named for the owners' beloved y
this chic cafe exudes warmth from
to the lace cafe curtains, and p
room. Pride of place is eviden
servers who are happy to accom
You won't be barking up the w
specialty of the house: prime r
rare (or whatever degree you p
the vegetable of the day and r
with garlic. Fish fanciers can ch
sautéed day-boat scallops, gr
fried catfish.
Hearty portions and beef bo
for your canine buddies brin
"doggie bag."

## Jeanine's Upto

**G1** 8459 Hart Blvd. (bet. 45

Phone: 310-454-5294
Web: www.eatatjeanines.com
Prices: $$$

Carb lovers flock to the U
chain for thick-crust pies
sauce and sprinkled wit
spinach and broccoli, an
There's always a line ou
the signature pizza, bri
made sausage. Althoug
the menu lists a numb
and-white-checked ta
the tables, creating
ambience. And speak
here. The chain takes
who loves that thick
ten-foot pole.

152

8

## Restaurant Classifications by Comfort

| More pleasant if in red | |
|---|---|
| X | Comfortable |
| XX | Quite comfortable |
| XXX | Very comfortable |
| XXXX | Top class comfortable |
| XXXXX | Luxury in the traditional style |
| 𝍢 | Small plates |

Map Coordinates

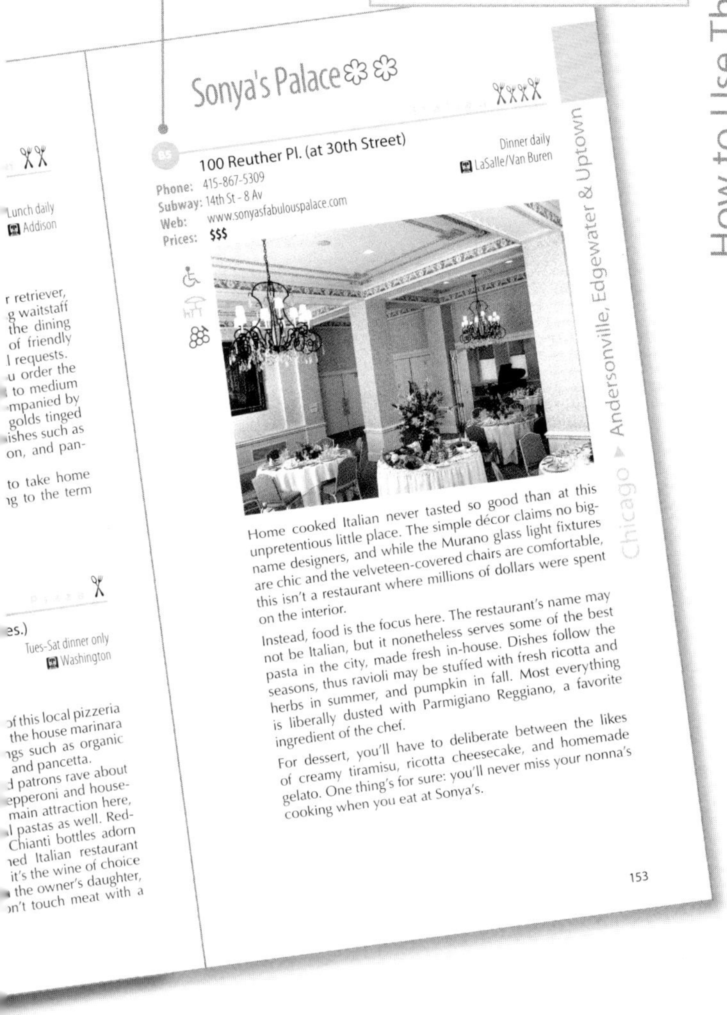
XX
Lunch daily
Addison

r retriever,
g waitstaff
the dining
of friendly
l requests.
u order the
to medium
mpanied by
golds tinged
ishes such as
on, and pan-
to take home
ng to the term

X
es.)
Tues-Sat dinner only
Washington

of this local pizzeria
the house marinara
ngs such as organic
and pancetta.
d patrons rave about
epperoni and house-
main attraction here,
l pastas as well. Red-
Chianti bottles adorn
ned Italian restaurant
it's the wine of choice
the owner's daughter,
n't touch meat with a

Sonya's Palace ✿✿

XXXX

B5

100 Reuther Pl. (at 30th Street)

Dinner daily
LaSalle/Van Buren

Phone: 415-867-5309
Subway: 14th St - 8 Av
Web: www.sonyasfabulouspalace.com
Prices: $$$

Home cooked Italian never tasted so good than at this unpretentious little place. The simple décor claims no big-name designers, and while the Murano glass light fixtures are chic and the velveteen-covered chairs are comfortable, this isn't a restaurant where millions of dollars were spent on the interior.

Instead, food is the focus here. The restaurant's name may not be Italian, but it nonetheless serves some of the best pasta in the city, made fresh in-house. Dishes follow the seasons, thus ravioli may be stuffed with fresh ricotta and herbs in summer, and pumpkin in fall. Most everything is liberally dusted with Parmigiano Reggiano, a favorite ingredient of the chef.

For dessert, you'll have to deliberate between the likes of creamy tiramisu, ricotta cheesecake, and homemade gelato. One thing's for sure: you'll never miss your nonna's cooking when you eat at Sonya's.

Chicago ▸ Andersonville, Edgewater & Uptown

153

# Where to Eat

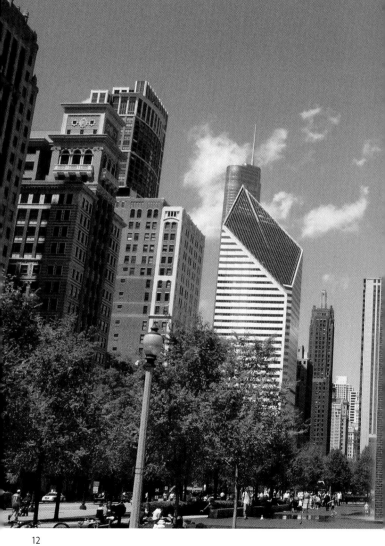

# Chicago

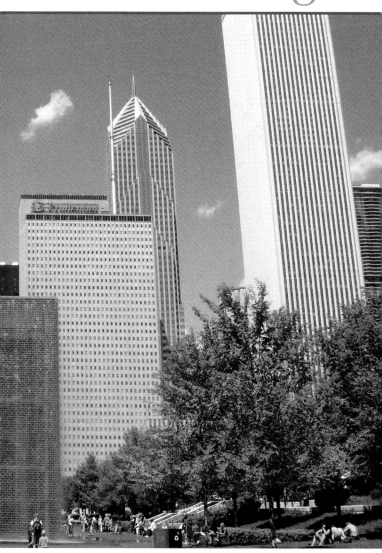

A walk through the neighborhoods of Chicago's North side, rich with culinary traditions from centuries of immigrant settlers, becomes a globetrotting voyage. Charming hotels and bed-and-breakfasts populate the quaint streets of Andersonville, while architecture buffs keep their eyes peeled for the art deco buildings along Bryn Mawr Avenue and Lake Michigan's beaches.

## HOW SWEDE IT IS

A water tower emblazoned with the blue-and-yellow Swedish flag rises above Clark Street, proudly representing Andersonville's Nordic roots. Stop into the Swedish-American Museum for a history lesson or go straight to its gift shop for a bag of old-school red Swedish fish. Take-home treats also abound here, with homey meatballs, herring, and lingonberry preserves starring as part of a smorgasbord of packaged goods available online at **Wikstrom's Gourmet Foods**—one of the last extant Swedish emporiums in the area. Locals line up for cinnamon-streusel coffeecake and other European pastries at the **Swedish Bakery**, and leave with boxes piled high or stay at the counter for an individually sized treat with a complimentary cup of coffee. For the heartiest appetites, a Viking breakfast at **Svea Restaurant** with Swedish-style pancakes, sausages, and toasted limpa bread fits the bill.

Beyond the well-represented Scandinavian community, Andersonville brings the world to its doorstep thanks to those amply stocked shelves at **Middle East Bakery & Grocery**. Their deli selection features a spectrum of spreads, breads, olives, and hummus making it entirely feasible to throw a meze feast in minutes. Adventurous home cooks also depend on the grocery section to keep their pantries full of fresh spices, dried fruits, rosewater, nuts, and teas.

## AN ASIAN AFFAIR

Across town, the pagoda-style roof of the Argyle El stop on the Red Line serves as another visual clue to the plethora of eats below: in this case, an East Asian lineup of Chinese, Thai, and Vietnamese restaurants, noodle shops, delis, bakeries, and even herbalists. Platters of lacquered, bronzed duck and pork make **Sun Wah BBQ** an inviting and popular spot for Cantonese cuisine. Served over rice, these glistening barbecued meats make for a royal feast. Andersonville's charming and family-run **Sunshine Café** specializes in Japanese noodles and potato croquettes, but sushi lovers will need to content themselves with just one, very delicious maki. For those less inclined to cook for themselves, a new generation of casual eateries is booming throughout these streets—**bopNgrill** is one such jewel, which specializes in Korean fusion items like *loco moco* or fantastically messy burgers including the "Umami" featuring truffled mushroom duxelle, sun-dried tomato confit, bacon, smoked Gouda, and spicy-creamy *togarashi* mayo.

## MEAT AND POTATOES —AND MORE

Chicagoans can't resist a good sausage, so find them giving thanks regularly to the German immigrants who helped develop Lincoln Square and whose appreciation for fine meats still resonates in this neighborhood. Old World-inspired butchers ply their trade, stuffing wursts and offering specialty meats and deli items at **Gene's Sausage Shop**. For a more refined carte of chops, steaks, free-range poultry, and more, head to **Lincoln Quality**

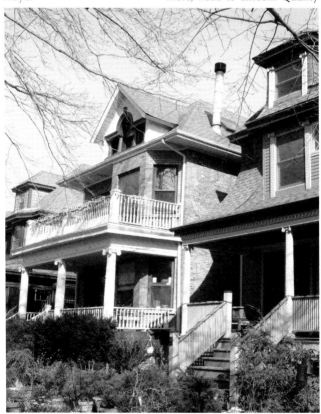

**Meat Market**. Speaking of meat treats, **Wolfy's** serves one of the best red-hots in Uptown, pilling its hot dogs with piccalilli, pickles, peppers, and other impossibly colored condiments. Its iconic neon sign (a crimson frankfurter jauntily pierced by a pitchfork) intensifies the urge to stop.

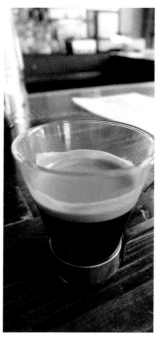

For fresh vegetables, fruits, flowers, and local baked goods, Chicago boasts a farmer's market in most neighborhoods, most days of the week. The **Andersonville Farmer's Market** (held on Wednesdays) houses a cluster of bakeries and an orchard's worth of Asian fruit. Meanwhile, the **Lincoln Square Farmer's Market** throws its booths open on Tuesdays and hosts live music during its Thursday evening market hours. Also in Lincoln Square, **HarvesTime Foods** wears its sustainability on its sleeve, with a solar-paneled roof and vast selection of local produce and goods.

A collaboration between beloved artisans Co-op Sauce and Crumb Chicago, Edgewater's **Sauce and Bread Kitchen** brings two of the city's favorite local products together at one café. Made-to-order breakfast and lunch sandwiches filled with delectable maple sausage or applewood-smoked turkey are lovingly lavished with house-made condiments like tomato sauce (a fan favorite for good reason). Crowds also come in droves for other party treats like tangy hot sauces and pickled vegetables.

## RAISE A GLASS

Critically acclaimed as one of the country's best boutique coffee shops, **The Coffee Studio** pours a mean cup of joe. Their locally roasted brews pair exceedingly well with a pre-ordered box of the "glazed & infused" doughnuts and are known to bring about ever-lasting enjoyment. In Edgewater, the creative community convenes at **The Metropolis Café**, an offshoot of Chicago's own **Metropolis Coffee Company**. Searching for something stronger than caffeine to bring to your next reservation? As the name suggests, family-owned producers and small-batch offerings are the focus at **Independent Spirits Inc.**, an Edgewater wine and liquor shop replete with global selections.

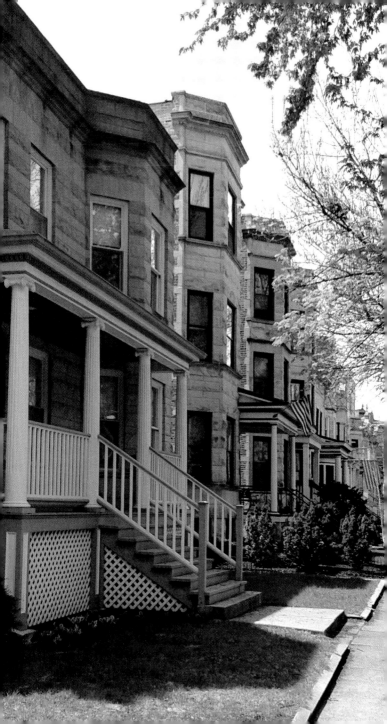

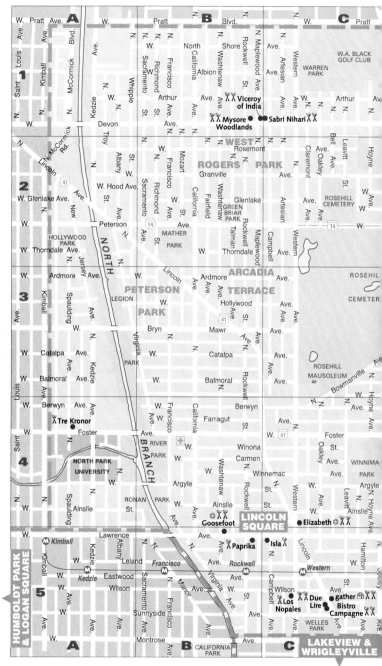

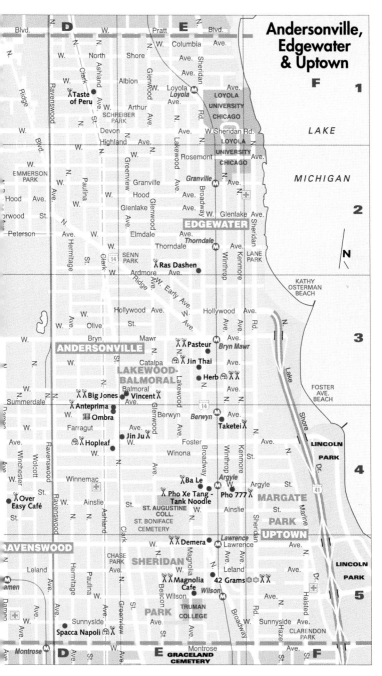

# Andersonville, Edgewater & Uptown

Blvd. **D** W. Pratt **E** W. Blvd. **F** 1

W. Columbia Ave.

N. North Shore Ave.

Albion W. Sheridan Rd.

Ⅹ**Taste of Peru** Loyola *Loyola* Ave. **LOYOLA UNIVERSITY CHICAGO**

Arthur W. *LAKE*

SCHREIBER PARK

Devon Ave. W. Sheridan Rd.

Highland **LOYOLA UNIVERSITY CHICAGO** Ave. *MICHIGAN*

EMMERSON PARK Rosemont

Granville *Granville* Ⓜ Ave.

Hood Ave. Hood Ave. 2

Peterson Glenlake Ave. W. Glenlake Ave.

**EDGEWATER**

Elmdale

Thorndale *Thorndale* Ave.

SENN PARK

Ⓧ**Ras Dashen**

Ardmore Ave.

Ridge *Early* Ave.

KATHY OSTERMAN BEACH

Hollywood Ave. Hollywood Ave. 3

Olive *Mawr*

Bryn ⅩⅩ**Pasteur** *Bryn Mawr* Ⓜ

**ANDERSONVILLE** Catalpa Ⓜ Ⅹ**Jin Thai** Ave.

**LAKEWOOD-BALMORAL** Ⓜ**Herb** ⅩⅩ

Balmoral FOSTER AVE. BEACH

Summerdale ⅩⅩ**Big Jones** **Vincent**Ⅹ

Ⅹ**Anteprima** Ave.

▤**Ombra** Berwyn *Berwyn* Ⓜ Ave.

Farragut Ⅹ**Jin Ju**Ⅹ

ⓂⅩ**Hopleaf** Foster **Taketei**Ⅹ 4

Ave. Winona LINCOLN PARK

Winnemac

Over Easy Café Ⅹ**Ba Le** *Argyle* Ⓜ

Ⅹ Pho Xe Tang - Argyle St.

Ainslie Tank Noodle **Pho 777**Ⅹ *MARGATE*

**RAVENSWOOD** Ⅹ Ⅹ**Demera** Ⓜ *Lawrence* **PARK**

CHASE PARK Lawrence **UPTOWN**

Leland **SHERIDAN** W. Leland Ave. LINCOLN PARK

ⅩⅩ**Magnolia Cafe** **42 Grams**❄ⅩⅩ 5

Wilson *Wilson*

**PARK** TRUMAN COLLEGE

Sunnyside Sunnyside Ave.

Ⅹ**Spacca Napoli**Ⓜ CLARENDON PARK

*Montrose* Ⓜ **D** Montrose **E** Ave. **F**

GRACELAND CEMETERY

19

# Anteprima

Italian

**D4**

### 5316 N. Clark St. (bet. Berwyn & Summerdale Aves.)

**Phone:** 773-506-9990
**Web:** www.anteprimachicago.net
**Prices:** $$

Lunch Sun
Dinner nightly
 Berwyn

Nestled into a vibrant strip of shops and eateries, this family-friendly gem is set apart by smart plate-glass windows and olive green-tinted woodwork. Inside, rusticity rules the roost with pressed-tin ceilings and intricate wood paneling. It's the kind of place where even solo patrons feel welcome, especially when perched on a window seat overlooking the bustling street.

Following its moniker, diners should "preview" the wide-ranging menu before opting for such delights as grilled sardines with sweet fennel, fragrant herbs, and fine olive oil. Delicious pastas include homemade ravioli—filled with a blend of crushed peas and mint—finished with a light, Parmesan-flecked sauce. For dessert, a rich, well-made panna cotta wobbles with lemon syrup and zest.

# Ba Le

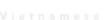 

**E4**

### 5014 N. Broadway (at Argyle St.)

**Phone:** 773-561-4424
**Web:** www.balesandwich.com
**Prices:** ⊜⊜

Lunch & dinner daily

 Argyle

Though the French influence on Vietnamese cuisine has been well-documented, Ba Le makes sure it's front and center, literally, with a mouthwatering display of baguettes, macarons, and chocolates at its clean, modern storefront in Little Saigon.

Take a seat at a table or the L-shaped bar overlooking Broadway before digging into a thrilling (and filling) *bánh mì* overflowing with lemongrass-seasoned sausage, homemade pickled daikon, and jalapeño on a crusty baguette. Get the most bang for your buck with crispy pork egg rolls which hit the spot perfectly, as do *pâté chaud* and *chao tom* from the grab-and-go coolers. Be warned, though: many a hungry patron stopping by to pick up a lunch sandwich has been swayed by the pastry case of impulse treats.

# Big Jones

**5347 N. Clark St. (bet. Balmoral & Summerdale Aves.)**

**Phone:** 773-275-5725
**Web:** www.bigjoneschicago.com
**Prices:** $$

Lunch & dinner daily

Berwyn

Big Jones has all the genteel charm you'd expect from a restaurant specializing in Southern cuisine. Green brocade wallpaper surrounds large framed prints of haunting low-country landscapes. Guests are greeted with a "Guide to Good Drinking" upon arrival, featuring barrel-aged punch selections and a lengthy roster of bourbon and whiskey.
Start with whole kernel-studded cornbread and honey butter, a fitting salvo for a meal steeped in Southern tradition. Sweet potato bisque is poured tableside over cornbread croutons, spicy apple chutney, and fried sage. Pickled pork shank and smoked jowl beef up red beans, braised voodoo greens, and aromatic Arkansas rice. An elderberry jelly roll sprinkled with benne seeds finishes the meal on a classic note.

# Bistro Campagne

**4518 N. Lincoln Ave. (bet. Sunnyside & Wilson Aves.)**

**Phone:** 773-271-6100
**Web:** www.bistrocampagne.com
**Prices:** $$

Lunch Sat – Sun
Dinner nightly
Western (Brown)

The romantic ideal of a French bistro is alive and well at Bistro Campagne. Light slants gently through wooden Venetian blinds, bouncing off cream-and-brick walls in the welcoming dining room. Choose a white cloth-covered table inside, under the red-golden soffit ceiling or outside under twinkling lights and green tree branches in the garden.
Inspired accompaniments make for memorable versions of rustic French standards. Meltingly tender *foie de veau* sparks happy sighs from calves' liver lovers, complemented by crisp bacon and Dijon mustard cream. House-made pappardelle and maitake mushrooms soak up the lavender-infused jus that finishes white wine-braised rabbit. Black figs are tucked into a moist brown butter *pain perdu* drizzled with caramel.

# Demera

Ethiopian

 E5

**4801 N. Broadway (at Lawrence Ave.)**

| | | |
|---|---|---|
| **Phone:** | 773-334-8787 | Lunch & dinner daily |
| **Web:** | www.demeraethiopianrestaurant.com | |
| **Prices:** | **$$** |  Lawrence |

Demera's well-lit corner location welcomes hungry Uptown residents looking to immerse themselves in Ethiopian cuisine. Colorful wicker seating at the dining room's communal table gives groups an authentic dining experience, while picture windows offer plenty of people-watching for everyone.

Vegetarian and omnivorous offerings abound on the menu, which features a small glossary of terms to help newcomers. Pleasantly spicy *ye-siga wot* combines tender chunks of beef with onions and ginger in a rich *berbere* sauce. Served with turmeric-infused split peas and jalapeño-laced collard greens, the stew is a hearty pleasure. Sop up extra sauce with piles of tangy and soft *injera*, presented in the traditional Ethiopian manner in lieu of silverware.

# Due Lire

Italian

 C5

**4520 N. Lincoln Ave. (bet. Sunnyside & Wilson Aves.)**

| | | |
|---|---|---|
| **Phone:** | 773-275-7878 | Dinner Tue – Sun |
| **Web:** | www.due-lire.com | |
| **Prices:** | **$$** |  Western (Brown) |

Naples native and gentleman's gentleman Massimo Di Vuolo welcomes guests from near and far to charming Due Lire. Smartly situated near the Old Town School of Folk Music, the dining room is often dotted with locals taking in dinner and a show. Understated khaki-colored walls, dark woods, and rustic ceiling beams keep the spotlight on the plate.

Comforting but refined modern Italian dishes warm up Lincoln Square residents on those cold Chicago nights. Sample braised chicken thighs and roasted fennel with a root vegetable ragù; saffron-hued *arancini* stuffed with asparagus and fontina; or fresh, made-to-order short rib ravioli nestled with porcini and *Parmigiano*. Pair the simple, seasonal fare with a selection from the Italian-dominated wine list.

# Elizabeth

XX

**4835 N. Western, Unit D (bet. Ainslie St. & Lawrence Ave.)**

| | |
|---|---|
| **Phone:** | 773-681-0651 |
| **Web:** | www.elizabeth-restaurant.com |
| **Prices:** | $$$$ |

Dinner Tue – Sat

Western (Brown)

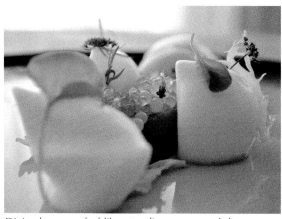

Dining here can feel like attending a very cool dinner party with strangers.

Maybe it's a nod to this former "underground" Chef Iliana Regan's humble beginnings in Chicago, but this unmarked building with neither address number nor sign is easily missed. Once inside, the hosts and servers are gracious and welcoming from start to finish. The décor conveys homey appeal, with thick wooden tables, comfy mismatched chairs, and an ornate white-tiled ceiling.

The chef herself may participate in the careful presentation of dishes, sharing anecdotes and purveyor stories. Every local-sustainable-foraged buzzword may be in play, but these ingredients are used with intelligence. "Elizabeth's Staples" begins with a deep, pink spoon filled with shrimpy noodles, intense kale, and a shard of Parmesan. This is paired with a demitasse of bitter cocoa nibs and chamomile flowers topped with an astonishingly good mushroom consommé. "Bread and celery root" may arrive as a bowl of green shavings, leaves, and gelée with roasted and chilled celery root balls in a silky celery root soup, served with a roll made with goat's milk and cattail pollen alongside pancetta-butter and whisky-spiked caramel.

# 42 Grams ✿ ✿

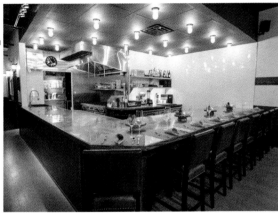

**Contemporary** 🍴🍴

**4662 N. Broadway (bet. Clifton & Leland Aves.)**

**Phone:** Not listed

Dinner Wed – Sun

**Web:** www.42gramschicago.com

**Prices:** $$$$

🚇 Wilson

To know the name refers to the supposed weight of two souls is to also know that this is not your usual restaurant. In fact, it's hardly a restaurant at all and more like a dinner party with strangers—you even need to arrive with a bottle or two of wine under your arms. There are two sittings: the first is at the counter where you watch Chef/owner Jake Bickelhaupt and his two colleagues in action; for 8.30 P.M. arrivals, it's the large communal table. For both, you'll be sharing your dinner with people you don't know, but the ice is usually broken by someone asking where their fellow diners have eaten recently.

The set menu offers no choice but any allergies are discussed during the bothersome flurry of emails that follow the initial impersonal booking process. Then it's over to Jake's charming wife, Alexa, to guide diners through the multiple dishes.

The cooking is clever and contemporary and the ingredients superlative, whether that's the Miyazaki Wagyu or Santa Barbara uni. Dishes are wonderfully well-balanced and the modern techniques are used to great effect to deliver superb flavors.

# gather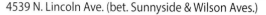

ℂ5     ✗✗

## 4539 N. Lincoln Ave. (bet. Sunnyside & Wilson Aves.)

| | | |
|---|---|---|
| Phone: | 773-506-9300 | Lunch Sun |
| Web: | www.gatherchicago.com | Dinner nightly |
| Prices: | $$ | 🚇 Western (Brown) |

A chic, cozy space allows guests to get up close and personal at gather. Barstools at the open kitchen's polished granite counter offer front row seating for diners seeking dinner and a show, while tall communal tables fill with patrons enjoying bites served on long boards from the menu's "gather and share" section. Rear dining rooms offer more solitude and romance.

American farm-to-table dishes are elevated with unexpected ingredients and preparations. Half chicken showcases two techniques—slices of juicy, pan-seared breast and a crunchy fried leg—over creamy polenta and delicate straws of fried onion. Tangy apple, celery leaf, and parsley slaw lightens the richness of a thick slab of crispy pork belly drizzled with sweet caramelized milk.

# Herb 😊

E3     ✗✗

## 5424 N. Broadway (bet. Balmoral & Catalpa Aves.)

| | | |
|---|---|---|
| Phone: | 773-944-9050 | Dinner Wed – Sat |
| Web: | www.herbrestaurant.com | |
| Prices: | $$ | 🚇 Bryn Mawr |

Thai street food reaches a fine dining pinnacle at Herb, where Chef/owner Patty Neumson delivers a transporting series of dishes in a smart and sophisticated setting. Natural materials and accents—stone, exotic plants, and wildflowers—offset taupe leather and a shimmering glass façade.

Unique ingredients scale sublime heights on the carefully curated menu, also available as three- or five-course prix-fixe offerings. A deep ceramic bowl holds a mound of king, enoki, and oyster mushrooms, dressed tableside with turmeric-infused curry broth. Raw shrimp salad showcases the vibrant flavors of Thai cuisine, with searingly hot chili, lime, fish sauce, and fragrant mint chiffonade. Smoked fish adds earthy funk to mild long beans and kabocha squash.

# Goosefoot ✿

✕✕

**2656 W. Lawrence Ave. (bet. Talman & Washtenaw Aves.)**

| | | |
|---|---|---|
| Phone: | 773-942-7547 | Dinner Wed – Sun |
| Web: | www.goosefoot.net | |
| Prices: | $$$$ | 🏛 Rockwell |

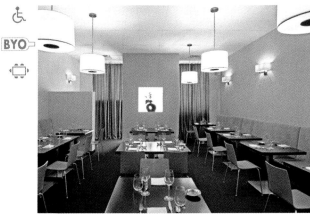

This understated plate-glass façade may seem lost in a sea of mediocrity, but the restaurant it houses is truly distinct. The décor combines mustard-colored banquettes, black lacquered tables, and modern artwork to fashion a space that is contemporary, energetic, and instantly likeable. Thoughtful details include a menu made of planting seed paper that guests are encouraged to take home, soak, and use to grow their own wildflowers. Dishes are intricate and take time for the charming staff to describe, which may explain the slow, steady pace of dining here.

The nine-course menu highlights the noteworthy skills of Chef Chris Nugent, combining a classical edge with contemporary artistry. Start with a pretty plum and butter scallop set over crab risotto, topped with a wafer of maitake. Angus beef is cooked here to perfection, with its superb crust and succulent pink meat set on a bed of rich lentils alongside glossy sauce Bordelaise and crisp balls of pickled apple.

End meals on an extraordinary note with the finely crafted chocolate egg filled with smooth banana mousse, set over blackcurrant sauce, coconut mousse, a cube of coconut jelly, and just a hit of sea salt to enhance each flavor.

# Hopleaf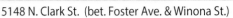

**D4**

## 5148 N. Clark St. (bet. Foster Ave. & Winona St.)

**Phone:** 773-334-9851
**Web:** www.hopleaf.com
**Prices:** $$

Lunch & dinner daily

Berwyn

Perfectly ordinary from the outside, Hopleaf thrives as a labor of love for owners, Michael and Louise. Named after a pale ale brewed in Malta, this serious tavern has beer and food fans in raptures over their stirring selection of sips, snacks, and serious eats. Dine comfortably amid exposed brick walls, steelwork, and shabby-chic furnishings whether seated at the traditional front bar, in the rear, or by the glassed-in kitchen. A great collection of enamel beer signs will put you in the mood for a brew with your Belgian or Thai-style mussels, followed by hearty shavings of porcetta folded into crusty ciabatta with tangy giardinera and creamy mayo. Dinner may flaunt extra variety—but for dessert, fix upon lavender-buttermilk panna cotta crowned with blackberry compote.

# Isla

**C5**

## 2501 W. Lawrence Ave. (bet. Campbell & Maplewood Aves.)

**Phone:** 773-271-2988
**Web:** www.islapilipina.com
**Prices:** @@

Lunch & dinner Tue – Sun

Western (Brown)

**BYO**

The two signs reading "Tuloy Po Kayo!" and "Salamat Po!" (*welcome* and *thank you* in Tagalog) say it all at this family-run favorite in Lincoln Square. The parking lot outside its small strip-mall exterior is always filled to capacity with locals ready for huge plates of authentic Filipino cuisine.
Regulars go with a side of garlic fried rice to pair with the kitchen's carnivorous specialties. Plan on indulging in hearty portions of pork and chicken *adobo* in traditional garlic-vinegar sauce; deep-fried slabs of pork belly, *lechon kawali*, with Filipino-style gravy; or onion- and tomato-stuffed whole squid. Come dessert, the vibrant purple *ube* ice cream, made from violet sweet potatoes and coconut, might be even more fun to look at than eat.

Chicago ▲ Andersonville, Edgewater & Uptown

# Jin Ju

Korean   ✕

**E4**

### 5203 N. Clark St. (at Foster Ave.)

**Phone:** 773-334-6377      Dinner Tue – Sun
**Web:** www.jinjurestaurant.com
**Prices:** $$

A sexy spot on a stretch of bustling Clark Street, Jin Ju spins out luscious Korean classics with aplomb. Inside, dim lighting, dark wood furnishings, and luxuriant red walls create a sophisticated coziness, while servers are gracious and attentive.

The menu showcases a range of specialties to start, like plump *mandoo*, batter-fried spicy chicken wings, or *pajun*, a savory Korean-style pancake filled with the likes of kimchi, served sliced in wedges with a tangy soy- and rice-vinegar dipping sauce. The *dak dori tang* could warm the coldest day in the Windy City—its fiery red pepper broth is brought to the table bubbling and brimming with braised chicken, potato, carrots, and leafy herbs accompanied by sticky rice, along with a tasty assortment of *banchan*.

# Jin Thai

Thai   ✕

**E3**

### 5458 N. Broadway (at Catalpa Ave.)

**Phone:** 773-681-0555      Lunch & dinner daily
**Web:** www.jinthaicuisine.com
**Prices:**     🚇 Bryn Mawr

   ♿   🏠  

As if Jin Thai's location in the shadow of Edgewater's Saint Ita bell tower isn't holy enough, Buddhist monks blessed this small restaurant before it opened in 2011. Owners Chai and Jin Roongseang keep the front and back of the house in harmony, while Buddha statues perched around the black-and-gray room maintain watch over the spicy, crispy, and tangy dishes cooked to order.

Guests looking to expand their repertoire beyond satay and pad Thai will find new favorites among such vibrant dishes as tempura chicken pieces with house-made lime sauce; and boneless catfish fillets floating in a spicy curry studded with Thai eggplant and green beans. Chicken noodle soup bobbing with rice vermicelli and chopped scallions does more than soothe—it transcends.

# Los Nopales

✂

**4544 N. Western Ave. (bet. Sunnyside & Wilson Aves.)**

Phone: 773-334-3149          Lunch & dinner Tue – Sun
Web: www.losnopalesrestaurant.com
Prices: ⊜⊜          Western (Brown)

**BYO**

Behind the lone hunter-green awning on Western Ave. hides a large and bright fiesta for the senses at Los Nopales. Namesake cacti decorate the space, along with framed paintings and wooden sculptures of the same subject. Avocado- and lemon-hued walls twinkle with holiday lights and flutter with Dia de los Muertos flags. The steady pulse of trumpets streams through the softly lit room.

Classic Mexican dishes are augmented with nopales, cooked and sliced in dishes like crunchy jicama salad. Three petite quesadillas stuffed with sautéed spinach and mushrooms are a filling starter, surrounded by a mound of creamy guacamole. Fresh green and orange salsas, packed with *chile de arbol*, cilantro, tomatillo, and garlic, are silky and worth every drop.

# Magnolia Cafe

✗✗

**1224 W. Wilson Ave. (at Magnolia Ave.)**

Phone: 773-728-8785          Lunch Sun
Web: www.magnoliacafeuptown.com      Dinner Tue – Sun
Prices: $$          Wilson

Uptown residents turn to Magnolia Cafe for chic comfort in a homey neighborhood standby. Close-knit tables covered in kraft paper and tasseled lampshades hanging from exposed wood beams create a warm atmosphere for dining, while a small bar near the entry stands at the ready for creative pre-dinner cocktails and brunch mimosas.

Chef/owner Kasra Medhat's menu incorporates a melting pot's worth of ingredients into American bistro standards. *Huevos rancheros* are filling enough to soak up the excesses of Saturday night, with two sunny side-up eggs layered with homemade salsa and guacamole over a mix of black beans, sweet corn kernels, and crumbled chorizo. Composed salads and dishes like applewood-smoked chicken pappardelle round out a roster of dinner options.

# Mysore Woodlands

XX

Indian

**B1**

**2548 W. Devon Ave. (bet. Maplewood Ave. & Rockwell St.)**

**Phone:** 773-338-8160                                                      Lunch & dinner daily
**Web:** www.mysorewoodlands.info
**Prices:** ☕☕

**BYO**

There is no lack of authentic Indian food in Chicago, but Mysore Woodlands stands out from the pack thanks to its focus on South Indian vegetarian cooking. Bold, intense flavors make up for the basic banquet hall-style décor at this orange-hued venue set on a restaurant-heavy stretch of Devon.

The Woodlands special *thali* lets diners sample a swath of delicacies without breaking the bank—platters are laden with metal bowls of crunchy *poriyal* like okra with mustard seeds and chilies; and soups like peppery *rasam* with basmati rice. Mysore masala *dosas* filled with spiced potatoes, or pancake-like *uthappams* with tamarind-infused *sambar* and coconut chutney, offer a whirlwind culinary tour; while cashew- and cardamom-flecked rice pudding delivers a rich finale.

# Ombra

Italian

**D4**

**5310 N. Clark St. (bet. Berwyn & Summerdale Aves.)**

**Phone:** 773-506-8600                                                          Dinner nightly
**Web:** www.barombra.com
**Prices:** ☕☕                                                                    🚇 Berwyn

Ombra may share a main entry with nearby cousin Acre, but its seasonal menu—focused on Italian small plates—is all its own. Raised booths upholstered with old leather jackets, orbital lights papier-mâchéd with weathered strips of newsprint, and wooden plank dividers telegraph a casual-cool mood.

Peruse the *salumi*, cheese, wine, and daily specials listed on the chalkboard, or pick from the dozens of *cicchetti* displayed behind glass at the dining counter. Panko-crusted pork trotter terrine set over an acidic arugula salad is at once rich and crunchy; while cold composed salads with grilled chicken, olives, and raisins are antipasti on steroids. Negronis, Bellinis, and pours of house-made grappa or limoncello keep the bar hopping.

# Over Easy Café

✗

**4943 N. Damen Ave. (bet. Ainslie & Argyle Sts.)**

**Phone:** 773-506-2605　　　　　　　　　　　Lunch Tue – Sun
**Web:** www.overeasycafechicago.com
**Prices:** ⊜⊜　　　　　　　　　　　 Damen (Brown)

Ravenswood residents get cracking early, lining up regularly for a warm breakfast and friendly brunch at Over Easy Café. An egg motif dominates the cheerful space while keeping things tasteful. Tightly nested tables foster a friendly communal vibe. Hot complimentary Julius Meinl coffee makes waiting in the foyer almost a pleasure.

As expected, the menu doesn't yolk around, with eggs playing a central role in nearly every dish. Overstuffed sandwiches feature scrambled eggs mixed with chopped truffled-pheasant sausage, parsley pesto, and wild mushrooms spilling out of toasted telera rolls. Green goddess egg salad bridges the gap between brunch and lunch. Blueberry crunch pancakes or French toast with an eggy crust keep sweet cravings at bay.

# Paprika

✗

**2547 W. Lawrence Ave. (bet. Maplewood Ave. & Rockwell St.)**

**Phone:** 773-338-4906　　　　　　　　　　　Dinner Tue – Sun
**Web:** www.paprikachicago.com
**Prices:** $$　　　　　　　　　　　 Rockwell

Chef Shah Kabir and his family know hospitality. Prepare to be swept up in their warmth and care (with maybe a splash of kitsch) the minute you enter this richly colored space, adorned with artifacts. Even the chef himself is at the door welcoming guests to sit and sip a cool, refreshing *lassi*.

From aromatic, homemade curries to tasty twists on *dahls* (*turka dahl ki shabzi* is a revelation), everything is fresh and fragrant. Bengali fish curry is a notable attraction—its flavors mild yet lively with mustard seeds, firm and fresh green beans, and silky-sweet onions. A very nice selection of vegetarian dishes might include the veggie samosa: its soft, light shell is stuffed with spiced potatoes, peas, cauliflower, and served with a trio of tangy chutneys.

# Pasteur

Vietnamese XX

**5525 N. Broadway (bet. Bryn Mawr & Catalpa Aves.)**

Phone: 773-728-4800                     Lunch & dinner Tue – Sun
Web: www.pasteurrestaurantchicago.com
Prices: ⊜⊜                              🚇 Bryn Mawr

The newest incarnation of the Vietnamese restaurant that originally opened in 1995 is named after Saigon's Avenue Pasteur. The inside features an attractive layout that is fresh looking yet heavily influenced by colonial design with its bright white façade topped by ornate black lacquered roof work. Tablecloths dress the tables in the airy room where beveled mirrors and painted scenes adorn the walls.

Items to be enjoyed include *nem*, skewers of ground chicken and pork seasoned with lemongrass, wrapped around sugarcane and grilled; or *ga kho gung*, claypot ginger chicken. *Tom xao sa-te*, wok-tossed shrimp with dried red peppers and a bright assortment of vegetables, is nestled in a flavorful and aromatic sauce with subtly sweet-funky undertones.

# Pho 777

Vietnamese X

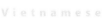

**1063-65 W. Argyle St. (bet. Kenmore & Winthrop Aves.)**

Phone: 773-561-9909                     Lunch & dinner Tue – Sun
Web: N/A
Prices: ⊜⊜                              🚇 Argyle

A market's worth of fresh ingredients make Pho 777 stand out in a neighborhood where Vietnamese restaurants—and their signature soup—seem to populate every storefront. Bottles of hot sauce, jars of fiery condiments, and canisters of spoons and chopsticks clustered on each table make it easy for regulars to sit down and start slurping.

Add choices like meatballs, tendon, flank steak, and even tofu to the cardamom, ginger, and clove-spiced beef broth, which fills a bowl the size of a bathroom sink, then throw in jalapeños, Thai basil, and mint to your liking. If you're not feeling like *pho* this time around, snack on spring rolls with house-made roasted peanut sauce; or a plate of lacy *banh xeo* stuffed with shrimp, sprouts, and herbs.

# Pho Xe Tang - Tank Noodle

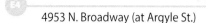

🍴

**E4**

4953 N. Broadway (at Argyle St.)

**Phone:** 773-878-2253     Lunch & dinner Thu — Tue
**Web:** www.tank-noodle.com
**Prices:** 😋     🚇 Argyle

**BYO**

A stone's throw from the Little Saigon El stop, this humming corner spot keeps *pho*-enthusiasts slurping and satisfied. Join the crowds during prime meal times at the large communal, cafeteria-style tables displaying caddies stocked with soup spoons, chopsticks, and deeply spiced, umami-rich sauces. Service is basic and the simple room lacks charm, but no one seems to notice.

The massive, hardcover menu offers all manner of goodies, like noodle plates, *báhn mì*, DIY wraps, and *congee*, along with an impressive array of bubble teas and fruity drinks. However, nearly every place is set with small plates brimming with heaps of fresh herbs, sprouts, and lime wedges to garnish the myriad *pho* options, all made with an alluring, sweetly spiced broth.

# Ras Dashen

🍴

**E2**

5846 N. Broadway (bet. Ardmore & Thorndale Aves.)

**Phone:** 773-506-9601     Lunch & dinner daily
**Web:** www.rasdashenchicago.com
**Prices:** $$     🚇 Thorndale

Take the hostess up on her offer to sit at a traditional table and enjoy Ras Dashen's Ethiopian fare in a truly authentic environment. Cushioned rattan chairs surrounding low *mossab* tables with conical domed lids await communal trays arriving from the kitchen. The bar serves Ethiopian honey wine, African beers, and cocktails like the rosy champagne *qay arafa* for those who want to fully immerse themselves in the culinary culture.

Delicately crisp lentil-stuffed *sambusas* whet the appetite for *doro wat*, the national dish of Ethopia, which does its country proud with aromatic and tender braised chicken in a sumptuous *berbere* sauce. Sides of warm *ib* cheese, freshly made from buttermilk, and spongy *injera* cool the palate from the creeping heat.

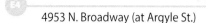

*Chicago ▶ Andersonville, Edgewater & Uptown*

33

# Sabri Nihari

Chicago ▶ Andersonville, Edgewater & Uptown

Indian

 C1

### 2502 W. Devon Ave. (bet. Campbell & Maplewood Aves.)

**Phone:** 773-465-3272    Lunch & dinner daily
**Web:** www.sabrinihari.com
**Prices:** 💶

Named for both a signature stew and a famous shop in Pakistan, Sabri Nihari does both inspirations justice within its colorful yet upscale space that's been serving Halal Pakistani, Afghan, and Indian specialties to the neighborhood since 1977. For newcomers to the world of Indo-Pak cuisine and culture, a stroll past the shops on Devon Avenue after lunch is a feast for the senses.

Oversized rounds of fluffy naan are key to sopping up the flavorful sauces of each dish such as the Nihari beef or lamb stew, loaded with crushed pepper and spices; frontier chicken in garlic- and ginger-infused tomato sauce; or fruity chutney served alongside crispy batter-dipped chicken *pakoras*. Traditional menu items also include hearty biryanis and *lahori boti haleem*.

# Spacca Napoli

Pizza

 D5

### 1769 W. Sunnyside Ave. (bet. Hermitage & Ravenswood Aves.)

**Phone:** 773-878-2420    Lunch Tue – Sun
**Web:** www.spaccanapolipizzeria.com    Dinner nightly
**Prices:** 💶    🚇 Montrose (Brown)

Long before Chicago deep-dish, Italy was famous for its Neapolitan pies. The "Vera Pizza Napoletana" sign at Spacca Napoli's door proclaims that this is the real deal, Naples-certified pizza, thanks to its authentic *pizzaiolo*, Jonathan Goldsmith. That glass-tiled custom Bisazza wood-burning oven in the center of the open kitchen is a tip-off, too.

The casual menu features a dozen varieties of red or white pizzas, along with antipasti and desserts for those who need more than a pie. Juice-glasses filled with wine served alongside crispy squash blossoms stuffed with ricotta and sweet peppers whet appetites. Pizzas arrive uncut, blistered, and charred, with just enough chewy bite to let the fresh mozzarella—cow's milk or *bufala*—and toppings shine.

# Taketei

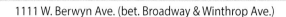

**E4**

## 1111 W. Berwyn Ave. (bet. Broadway & Winthrop Ave.)

**Phone:** 773-769-9292                                    Dinner Mon – Sat
**Web:** N/A
**Prices:** ⊜⊜                                                    Berwyn

**BYO**

Though it's a mere sliver of a space, Taketei's Japanese temple of fresh piscine makes a bold statement in this neighborhood, noted for its Vietnamese joints. The wee room, so small there's not even a true sushi counter, remains serenely bright but minimal, filled with a handful of white tables and chairs. A limited menu makes the most of shiny pieces of fish. With the majority of nigiri available for less than $3 each, regulars know to load up or go all out with a sashimi platter featuring a wide selection of generously sliced seafood like mackerel, octopus, and *maguro* with a bowl of rice. Manageably sized, non-gimmicky rolls along with appetizers like pert, crunchy *hiyashi wakame* salad or spinach with sweet sesame sauce supplement this appealing array.

# Taste of Peru

**D1**

## 6545 N. Clark St. (bet. Albion & Arthur Aves.)

**Phone:** 773-381-4540                                    Lunch & dinner daily
**Web:** www.tasteofperu.com
**Prices:** $$

**BYO**

Don't be put off by the plain-Jane exterior. Inside, wood masks mingle with posters of Peruvian destinations atop desert-toned walls; red tapestries cover the tables; and lively (sometimes live) music reveals the passion of Cesar Izquierdo. This chatty owner has been touting his peppery cuisine in East Rogers Park for eons.

The menu shows a range of Peruvian food, from the classic *papa rellena* stuffed with tender ribeye cubes, walnuts, and raisins, to a steamed rice- tomato- and onion-combo in *lomo saltado*. If the complimentary *aji verde* tingles the taste buds a little too much, take a swig of cold and refreshing Inca Kola. When choosing a sip to savor with your meal, take note that Chilean *pisco* won't be welcomed—this is a Peruvian place, after all.

35

# Tre Kronor

Scandinavian ✗

**A4**

### 3258 W. Foster Ave. (at Spaulding Ave.)

**Phone:** 773-267-9888
**Web:** www.trekronorrestaurant.com
**Prices:** 🍲

Lunch daily
Dinner Mon – Sat

BYO

This cheery corner cottage with its hand-painted fairy tale murals and chalet accents is an apt home for Swedish standby Tre Kronor. Named after a Stockholm castle and the three crowns on the Swedish national emblem, this restaurant's yellow-and-blue décor also shows off its Scandinavian heritage. The Sweden Shop across the street lets guests transport a bit of Nordic atmosphere back to their homes.

Breakfast is an all-day affair here, as the kitchen turns out batches of plump iced cinnamon rolls; thick waffles piled high with fruit and whipped cream; and airy Swedish pancakes with tart lingonberry sauce. Swedish meatballs with pickled cucumbers; Reuben sandwiches on toasted *limpa* rye bread; or salmon-and-dill quiche are among their savory standards.

# Viceroy of India

Indian ✗✗

**B1**

### 2520 W. Devon Ave. (bet. Campbell & Maplewood Aves.)

**Phone:** 773-743-4100
**Web:** www.viceroyofindia.com
**Prices:** 🍲

Lunch & dinner daily

The periwinkle and lavender walls, sky-blue ceiling painted with clouds, and steely booths lining the spacious dining room at Viceroy of India keep things cool, letting the spice-inflected cuisine churned out by the kitchen provide the heat. White linen-draped tables as well as a full bar and wine list make this West Rogers Park retreat a regal choice.

Though an à la carte menu is available for those who've got to get their fill of tandoori chicken, longtime patrons and lunch regulars make a beeline for the popular lunch buffet, stocked with North Indian standards like *pakoras*, samosas, *saag paneer*, chicken *makhani*, and goat curry. Complimentary naan is available by the basketful.

The grab-and-go café next door lets passersby get their sweet fix.

# Vincent

## 1475 W. Balmoral Ave. (bet. Clark St. & Glenwood Ave.)

Phone: 773-334-7168
Web: www.vincentchicago.com
Prices: $$

Lunch Sun
Dinner Tue – Sun
Berwyn

Go Dutch at Vincent, where traditional cuisine from the Netherlands meets a tried and true bistro menu. Tall votive candles, high-top marble tables, and gilded frames lining brocade-papered walls warm the dual rooms. While the interior is comfortably informal, a dog-friendly patio offers a warm-weather option for pooch-loving customers.

The juicy grilled lamb burger is a menu mainstay, though its toppings—perhaps Montchevre goat cheese, violet mustard, and arugula—change regularly. Five variations of *moules frites* range from the customary beer, garlic, and parsley to tangy tamarind, *sambal*, and lime leaf. Other standouts include a thick slice of crisped pork belly topped with tomato jam and drizzled with a warm bacon-garlic vinaigrette.

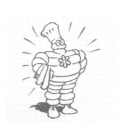

Remember, stars
(🏵🏵🏵 … 🏵) are awarded
for cuisine only! Elements
such as service and decor
are not a factor.

# Bucktown & Wicker Park

Like many of the Windy City's neighborhoods, Bucktown and Wicker Park have seen their residents shift from waves of Polish immigrants and the wealthy businessmen who've erected stately mansions on Hoyne and Pierce avenues, to the young, hip crowds introducing modern taquerias and craft breweries to these streets. Still, the neighborhood knows how to remain a beacon for trendsetters who love to be on the cutting edge of all things creative and culinary. Far from the internationally known boutiques along the Magnificent Mile, indie shops and artisan producers of Milwaukee and Damen avenues offer one-of-a-kind treasures for all the five senses.

Get a taste of Wicker Park's vast underground music scene by stopping at Reckless Records or at some of the city's largest music events: Wicker Park Fest is held each July and features no less than 28 bands; while the annual Green Music Fest draws every eco-minded local in town. Snap up funky

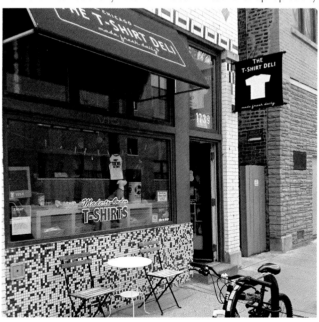

home accessories and original works at flea market-chic Penguin Foot Pottery, or wear art on your sleeve by designing your own Tee at the appropriately named T-shirt Deli.

## HOT DOGS AND HAUTE TREATS

It's a well-known saying that you don't want to know how the sausage is made, but the person who coined that famous phrase never visited the **Vienna Beef Factory**. Their popular workshop tour whets the appetite for a 1/3-pound Mike Ditka Polish sausage at the café, or a make-your-own-Chicago-dog kit with celery salt, sport peppers, and electric-green pickle relish from the gift shop. For more Eastern European flavor, **Rich's Deli** is the Ukrainian Village's go-to market for copious cuts of smoked pork, as well as *kabanosy, pasztet*, Polish vodka, Slavic mustard, and other fiery goods. Unlike many local markets, the staff here speaks English, so don't be afraid to ask. Any lingering questions on meat will be answered after talking with husband-and-wife team, Rob and Allie Levitt, the brains (and stomachs) behind Noble Square's **Butcher & Larder**. Combining the growing interest in whole animal butchery with the desire to support local farmers, the Levitts produce sausages, terrines, and house-cured bacon. They also conduct demos on how to break down whole animals. If "God is in the details," then **Goddess & Grocer** brings to life this turn of phrase. While it may be every serious cook's dream come true, even newbies flock here to stock up on soups, salads, chili,

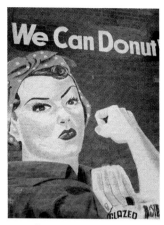

cupcakes, and haute, homemade treats better than what Mom used to make. They also cater, so go ahead and pretend like you crafted those delicate dinner party hors d'oeuvres all on your own!

## SUGAR RUSH

A world of hand-crafted goodies make this neighborhood a rewarding destination for anyone addicted to sweet. For nearly a century, family-run **Margie's Candies** has been hand-dipping its chocolate bonbons and serving towering scoops of homemade ice cream to those Logan Square denizens and dons (including Al Capone, that old softy). Equally retro in attitude, the lip-smacking seasonal slices and small-town vibe of **Hoosier Mama Pie Company** brings old-timey charm to this stretch of Ashland Avenue. From sumptuous tiered wedding cakes to spot-on replicas of Wrigley Field recreated in batter and frosting, the stunning selection of cakes displayed in the window at **Alliance Bakery** would make even Willy Wonka green with envy. For those who can't decide

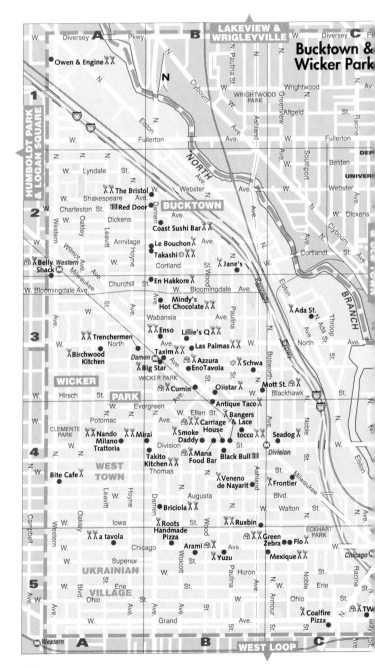

HUMBOLDT PARK & LOGAN SQUARE

Owen & Engine ✕✕

W. Diversey Pkwy. B W. Diversey C Pl.

N

WRIGHTWOOD
PARK

Wrightwood

Altgeld

N. Av

St.

Fullerton

Racine

N. Paulina St.

Greenview

N. Ashland Ave.

Clybourn Ave.

Elston Ave.

W. Fullerton Ave.

DEP

Belden

UNIVER

Southport

Webster

W. Lyndale St.

W. Webster Ave.

✕✕ The Bristol W.

Shakespeare Ave.

Red Door

W. Charleston St.

Dickens

Oakley Ave.

Western Ave.

Leavitt

Hoyne

Damen Ave.

BUCKTOWN

Ave.

W. Dickens

Clybourn Ave.

Coast Sushi Bar ✕✕

Le Bouchon ✕ Ave.

Takashi ❁✕✕

Cortland St.

Wood St.

✕ Jane's

Cortlandt St.

Ave.

W.

BRANCH

✕ Belly
Shack Ⓜ

Western Milwaukee Ave.

✕ En Hakkore ✕

W. Bloomingdale Ave.

Churchill St.

W. Bloomingdale Ave.

Mindy's
Hot Chocolate ✕✕

✕ Ada St.

Ada St.

Throop St.

Wabansia Ave.

Paulina

✕✕ Trenchermen

North

Enso ✕✕

Lillie's Q ✕✕

Bosworth

North Ave.

✕ Birchwood
Kitchen

Damen Ⓜ

Taxim ✕✕

Las Palmas ✕✕

✕ Big Star

Ⓐ Azzura
❁ EnoTavola

❁ Schwa

Expwy.

WICKER PARK

Ⓐ ✕ Cumin

Oiistar ✕

Mott St. Ⓐ ✕

W. Hirsch St.

PARK

Blackhawk

St.

WICKER

Antique Taco ✕

W. Evergreen

W. Ellen St. ✕ Bangers
& Lace

Ave.

Noble

W. Potomac

Ⓐ ✕✕ Carriage
House

CLEMENTE
PARK

✕✕ Nando ✕✕ Mirai
Milano ●
Trattoria

Smoke
Daddy ●

tocco ✕✕

Seadog ✕

Division St.

Division Ⓜ

Milwaukee

Elston

✕ Bite Cafe ✕

Takito
Kitchen ✕✕

Ⓐ ✕ Mana
Food Bar

Black Bull ▤

Thomas

WEST
TOWN

✕ Veneno
de Nayarit

✕ Frontier

Leavitt

Hoyne

Damen

Augusta

Blvd.

Campbell

Oakley

Western

Iowa

✕ Briciola ✕✕

W. Walton St.

Ave.

✕ Roots St.
Handmade
Pizza

✕✕ Ruxbin

ECKHART
PARK

✕✕ a tavola

Chicago

Arami Ⓐ ✕

Ⓐ ✕✕ Green
Zebra ●● Flo ✕

Chicago Ⓒ

W. Superior

Wolcott

Ave.

✕ Yuzu

Mexique ✕✕

St.

UKRAINIAN

St.

Paulina

Huron

Noble

Racine

W.

Erie

N. St.

Erie

St.

Blvd.

VILLAGE

Ohio

Armour

Ohio

St.

Ⓐ ✕ TW

✕ Coalfire
Pizza ●

Ⓜ Western

Grand Ave.

St.

A B WEST LOOP C

what pastry they'd like to sink their teeth into, Bucktown's **Red Hen Bread** doesn't make the choice any easier. Crusty baguettes and glistening braided challah compete for space with croissants, muffins, scones, cookies, tarts, and more. Looking for something less traditional? Unusual combinations are the norm at **Black Dog Gelato**, where goat cheese, cashew, and caramel come together for a uniquely satisfying scoop. But if in a rush, take your decadent dessert (maybe a bar of whiskey gelato dipped in chocolate and candied bacon) to-go.

## SUDS AND SPUDS

The craft beer movement has been brewing in Chicagoland for quite some time, where lovers of quality suds and superlative bar snacks find an array of both in Bucktown and Wicker Park. Regulars at Logan Square's **Revolution Brewing** snack on bacon-fat popcorn and sweet potato cakes while sipping on the in-house Double Fist Pale Ale or Anti-Hero IPA. Meanwhile, **Moonshine Brewing Company**, rife with a rare selection of draft beers, cans, cervezas, as well as domestic and imported macros, sees a habitual following of spirited locals and comfort food fans. Find these same devotees filling up the booths and sidewalk tables at **Silver Cloud**, for hearty servings of chicken pot pie, grilled cheese sandwiches, and cocktails that keep this diner hopping at all hours. This food-and-beer marriage reaches new heights at **Piece**, which not only serves up one of Chicagoland's most popular hand-tossed pizzas but also produces a roster of award-winning beers to accompany its crispy New Haven-style pies. For a master class on the wide and wonderful world of craft brews, the noted beer school at Wicker Park's **Map Room** gives students a greater appreciation for the art—though a self-taught tour of the bar's worldwide selection is indeed educational and perhaps more enjoyable?

## THE LUSH LIFE

Considering its dramatic role in the era of Prohibition, it's no surprise that speakeasy-inspired spots go over like gangbusters in Chicago. **The Violet Hour**, one of the pioneers of the bespoke cocktail trend, still shakes things up late into the night at its no-reservations temple. Pair your updated Old Fashioned with

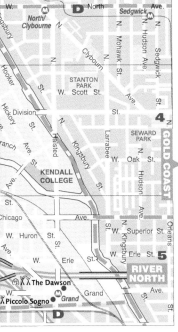

pickles and cheese or frites with aïoli for a truly pleasurable affair. The subterranean vaults of a former bank are now home to **The Bedford**, whose heavy steel doors, walls of shining safe deposit boxes, and marble and limestone accents lead the way to a warren of lounge-y areas and dining dens. If you are itching for some south-of-the-border flair on the later night, make a beeline for **Taco Burrito Express #3** on North Ashland. This fast, family-run, and cash-only favorite doles out *al pastor* and chorizo tacos until the party winds up at 11:00 P.M. For those who prefer their Mexican food handed to them by *luchadores* donning wrestling masks, the quirky **Tamale Spaceship** truck has touched down in these parts with an actual storefront. Sports of another sort take the spotlight at **Emporium Arcade Bar**. Here, rows of video games and pinball machines from the 1980s bring back memories for those who grew up hitting the arcade—which of course can be even more fun with a craft beer or whiskey pour.

## KITCHEN SKILLS

Meals at the **Kendall College Dining Room** let you brag about knowing future Michelin-starred chefs before they've hit it big. As one of Chicago's premier culinary institutions, the college gives its chef trainee's real-world guidance as they provide elegant lunch and dinner service. Floor-to-ceiling windows overlook the fully functioning professional kitchen, where instructors can be seen helping students tune their fine-dining skills. Reservations are required, but the experience is a must for home cooks looking to be inspired. For more hands-on experience, a class at **Cooking Fools** lets aspiring Food Network stars hone their knife skills or bake a batch of tamales from scratch.

When looking to strut your culinary stuff over a dinner party at home, it's easy to stock your pantry simply by swinging by the **Wicker Park & Bucktown Farmer's Market** (open on Sundays) for an impressive fleet of fresh produce, artisanal cheeses, and more. Then, peruse the shelves of **Olivia's Market** for painstakingly sourced specialty items and a vast wine and beer selection. **Local Folks Food** is a family-run enterprise whose chief mission is to develop natural gourmet condiments (mustard and hot sauce anyone?) tailor-made for slathering over burgers. Purchase these same tangy treats on the shelves at the lauded **Green Grocer** and make your next cookout the envy of everyone on the block. Finally feeling ready to grow your own vegetables? Sign up for a plot at **Frankie Machine Community Garden** and see if you've got a green thumb!

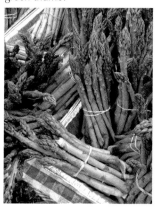

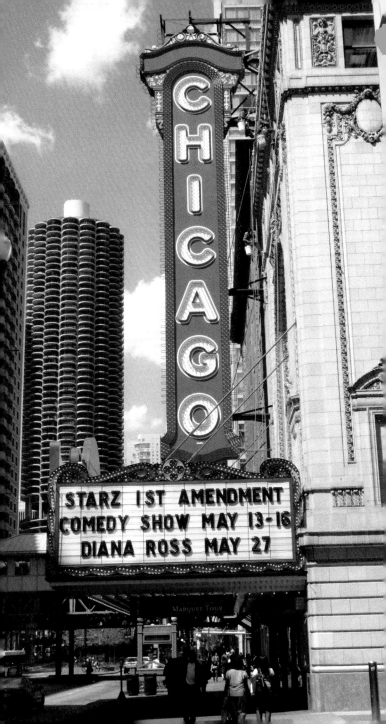

# Ada St.

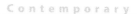

**C3**

Contemporary ✗

### 1664 N. Ada St. (bet. Concord Pl. & Wabansia Ave.)

**Phone:** 773-697-7069 — Lunch Sun
**Web:** www.adastreetchicago.com — Dinner Mon – Sat
**Prices:** $$

Despite its obscure location among the industrial warehouses of far-east Wicker Park, adventurous diners have no trouble seeking out Ada St. Reservations aren't accepted after 6:30 P.M., so the cozy, brick-walled lounge quickly becomes a party space where patrons peruse the wooden cubbies of vinyl to create their own soundtrack.

The menu of small plates is influenced by both hearty gastropub dishes and lighter Mediterranean fare. Tabasco mash ketchup heats up a plate of charred, tender octopus, while a poached egg gilds rich duck confit tossed with *cavatelli*. Even the snappy green beans need nothing more than Dijon butter to shine. Before you take off, show your appreciation by choosing the last item on the menu: a six-pack of beer for the kitchen staff.

# Antique Taco

**B4**

Mexican ✗

### 1360 N. Milwaukee Ave. (at Wood St.)

**Phone:** 773-687-8697 — Lunch & dinner Tue – Sun
**Web:** www.antiquetaco.com
**Prices:** ⊗⊗ — 🚇 Damen (Blue)

No reservations and walk-up counter service lead to an inevitable wait at Antique Taco (wear comfortable shoes). Ease the pain by browsing well-curated racks of knickknacks while awaiting market-fresh Mexican food, which arrives on *abuela*-worthy china plates. Place your order and score a wooden stool at a boxy plank table.

Antique Taco piles its corn tortillas with substantial and delicious fillings. Crispy battered fish is spiced up with *sriracha* tartar sauce and chilled smoked cabbage slaw. Shredded roast pork is rubbed with adobo, glazed in tamarind, and joined with creamy avocado and *queso fresco* for tasty carnitas. Pickled red onions add punch to chunky guacamole. Vodka-spiked *agua frescas* are nice, but the *horchata* milkshake is unmissable.

44

# Arami

**B5**

Japanese  ✗

## 1829 W. Chicago Ave. (bet. Wolcott Ave & Wood St.)

**Phone:** 312-243-1535
**Web:** www.aramichicago.com
**Prices:** $$

Dinner Tue – Sun

 Division

Window displays of dangling bamboo, moss, and soft river stones offer an inviting and very serene retreat at Arami. Inside, a long sushi bar and skylights cut into cathedral-like ceilings enhance the minimalist space framed with pale-green walls. Thrilling specialty cocktails with Japanese spirits complement an ample inventory of sake, Scotch, *sochu*, and beers.

Arami is not the destination for fat, gimmicky maki. Instead, fresh seafood spiked with garlic, truffle, and pickled items let flavors sparkle in a more subtle way. Toro tartare comes in a single bite of minced tuna with bonito-soy sauce, Asian pear, and black *tobiko*; while hamachi sashimi draped over black river rocks shine with pickled mushroom, truffle oil, and sprouts.

# a tavola

**A5**

italian  ✗✗

## 2148 W. Chicago Ave. (bet. Hoyne Ave. & Leavitt St.)

**Phone:** 773-276-7567
**Web:** www.atavolachicago.com
**Prices:** $$

Dinner Mon – Sat

Don't bother looking for a sign: a tavola takes up residence in a stately brick house on an otherwise storefront-lined block in the Ukrainian Village—an ivy-covered façade is a dead giveaway in the summer. Stepping inside is like arriving at Chef/owner Dan Bocik's home for a dinner party, where a convivial and gracious atmosphere reigns from the three-seat wine bar and gorgeous original wood floors, to a serene back patio.

The concise menu offers straightforward Italian food, though who needs frills when pillows of gnocchi with crispy sage and brown butter; or on-point beef tenderloin with roasted rosemary potato coins are so effective on their own? Dessert follows the same simple blueprint with a tangy lemon curd-filled shortbread tart.

# Azzurra EnoTavola

**B3**

### 1467 N. Milwaukee Ave. (at Honore St.)

**Phone:** 773-278-5959
**Web:** www.azzurrachicago.com
**Prices:** $$

Lunch Sat – Sun
Dinner nightly
 Damen (Blue)

If you squint your eyes upon entering this homage to Italy's edible and drinkable treasures, you can almost believe you're in Portofino. Clusters of Victrola phonograph horns-turned-light fixtures hang from pressed-tin ceilings, illuminating the warmly painted room, while a random smattering of azure-blue tables and chairs lend a seaside feel.

Indecisive guests will have a difficult time choosing from the lineup of shareable appetizers and mains. Friends may fight over a farro and mushroom arancini set upon rich porcini cream sauce; or two pounded, breaded, and crisply pan-fried pork cutlets served Milanese-style with arugula salad and shaved *Parmigiano*. For a sweet finish, a lemon panna cotta—spiked with *limoncello*—has just the right amount of wiggle.

# Bangers & Lace

**B4**

### 1670 W. Division St. (at Paulina St.)

**Phone:** 773-252-6499
**Web:** www.bangersandlacechicago.com
**Prices:** $$

Lunch & dinner daily

 Damen (Blue)

Despite the frilly connotations, this sausage-and-beer mecca's name refers not to doilies, but to the delicate layers of foam that remain in the glass after your craft brew has been quaffed. You'll also have lots of opportunity to study the lace curtains as you plow through their extensive draft beer menu, noted on blackboards in the comfortably worn-in front bar room.

Decadent foie gras corn dogs (actually French garlic sausage wrapped with soft-sweet brioche cornbread) and veal brats with melted Gouda elevate the humble sausage; while a slew of sandwiches suit simpler tastes. Grilled cheese gilds the lily with taleggio, raclette, and Irish cheddar; and dreamy house-made chips drizzled with truffle oil and malt vinegar are more than a bar snack.

# Belly Shack

Fusion

**A2**

### 1912 N. Western Ave. (at Milwaukee Ave.)

**Phone:** 773-252-1414     Lunch & dinner Tue – Sun
**Web:** www.bellyshack.com
**Prices:**      Western (Blue)

Belly Shack's concise menu is an eclectic Asian-Latin mash-up that reflects the Korean and Puerto Rican backgrounds of Chef Bill Kim and his wife, Yvonne Cadiz-Kim. Place your order and take a number—a metal stand that looks like it was made by a high school shop class—then wait for your dishes to arrive.

Korean barbecued beef is a favorite, but regulars enjoy new tastes from the roster of daily specials that can include the *lechon tostada*. This treat is comprised of thinly sliced, slow-roasted pork loin piled high onto a fried corn tortilla with grated sharp cheddar, mashed smoky black beans, and pineapple-cilantro salsa. For dessert, lick up peaks of creamy vanilla soft-serve with topping combos such as caramel and freshly grated Vietnamese cinnamon.

# Big Star

Mexican

**B3**

### 1531 N. Damen Ave. (bet. Milwaukee & Wicker Park Aves.)

**Phone:** 773-235-4039     Lunch & dinner daily
**Web:** www.bigstarchicago.com
**Prices:**     Damen (Blue)

Whiskey, rock and roll, and Mexican food—what else is there in life? Not much, apparently, at this jam-packed Wicker Park hipster haven where all are in affordable abundance. The crowd keeps the room pumping every night as they throw back shots, PBRs, and *micheladas*.

Despite the grungy décor, the food is as well-crafted as you'd expect from a Paul Kahan operation. Crispy braised pork belly drizzled with tomato-*guajillo* sauce and shredded spit-roasted pork shoulder in a pineapple marinade make for delicious tacos; while *salsa de frijole con queso* (a crock of pinto bean dip with lime salt-sprinkled chips) is a dish far better than a simple bar snack is ever expected to be. Need a taco fix stat? Hit up the cash-only taqueria window and walk away happy.

# Birchwood Kitchen

American

### 2211 W. North Ave. (bet. Bell Ave. & Leavitt St.)

**Phone:** 773-276-2100
**Web:** www.birchwoodkitchen.com
**Prices:**

Lunch Tue – Sun
Dinner Tue – Fri
Damen (Blue)

On a stretch of brick storefronts, Birchwood Kitchen's periwinkle façade stands out like a gem. Inside, the earthy café has a country feel, with old church pews lining exposed brick walls and daily specials cleverly written on aluminum baking pans. Peruse the offerings in the dessert case, since items like shortbread lemon bars and chocolate chip banana bread may affect how much you want to order from the walk-up counter.

Along with daily brunch offerings like Belgian waffles, lunch standards like sandwiches, soups, and salads are forever in demand. If the tuna melt on toasted multi-grain bread with roasted tomato slices and Gruyère isn't enough, try a side of satisfying chickpea salad tossed with creamy mayonnaise dressing spiked pink with chipotles.

# Bite Cafe

American

### 1039 N. Western Ave. (bet. Cortez & Thomas Sts.)

**Phone:** 773-395-2483
**Web:** www.bitecafechicago.com
**Prices:** $$

Lunch & dinner daily

This charming, slightly bohemian café looks unassuming, but its homey food and friendly service leave an indelible impression. Hipster locals grab the latest issue of *The Onion* and wait for their coffee at the small back counter, while others take the comfy banquettes or powder-blue metal chairs. An eclectic selection of artwork rotates gallery-style on the walls.

Simple diner fare gets a homestyle upgrade across the board, with a menu that puts new twists on familiar breakfast bites like blueberry bread with lemon butter; or poutine with smoked bacon gravy. Careful homemade details add oomph to savory lunch and dinner items like an open-faced fried chicken sandwich on a fresh and fluffy biscuit with green tomato jam and melted cheddar.

# Black Bull

Spanish

**B4**

## 1721 W. Division St. (bet. Hermitage Ave. & Paulina St.)

**Phone:** 773-227-8600      Lunch & dinner daily
**Web:** www.blackbullchicago.com
**Prices:**       🚇 Division

Like bulls, hungry foodies are drawn to the color red—at least that's what the thinking must be at this chic tapas spot dominated by a neon bull and candy-apple exterior. Inside, glasses of crimson and rosé sangria are in everyone's hands, helping the noise skyrocket as the night wears on.

Look at the colorful chalk-drawn mural above the kitchen, depicting Spanish scenes, products, and food terms, to get a sense of what's on offer. Shareable plates mix tradition with contemporary twists, like crispy hollowed-out *patatas bravas* filled with ketchup and aïoli. A half-dozen pickled mussels arrive in a tin beneath a layer of creamy potato foam; while an excellent consommé poured over a farm egg yolk and truffles is brightened by a dash of manzanilla sherry.

# Briciola

Italian XX

**B4**

## 937 N. Damen Ave. (bet. Augusta Blvd. & Iowa St.)

**Phone:** 773-772-0889      Dinner Tue – Sun
**Web:** www.briciolachicago.com
**Prices:** $$      🚇 Division

After decades of cooking and traveling, Chef/owner Mario Maggi was ready to open a small place—just a crumb, or "una briciola," of a restaurant. This tiny trattoria nestled between Ukrainian Village's brick buildings is indeed a speck of warmth and charm, festooned with party lights on the patio and mustard-toned walls inside.

Traditional Italian cuisine gets personalized tweaks from the chef. *Carpacci* may include paper-thin octopus, beets, or beef; *macaroncini alla Briciola* folds diced Tuscan sausage into a spicy garlic-sage sauce; and a hefty bone-in pork chop, pounded thin, breaded, and pan-fried until golden, is a house classic dressed with arugula and shaved Parmesan.

A bottle from the wine shop down the block makes the meal even more convivial.

49

# The Bristol

B2

American XX

### 2152 N. Damen Ave. (bet. Shakespeare & Webster Aves.)

**Phone:** 773-862-5555
**Web:** www.thebristolchicago.com
**Prices:** $$

Lunch Sat – Sun
Dinner nightly

Get to know your neighbors a little better at this dim, bustling haunt boasting a lineup of seasonal American fare with a Mediterranean twist. Regulars sit shoulder-to-shoulder at thick butcher block communal tables or at the concrete bar, squinting under filament bulbs to see the constantly changing menu's latest additions on chalkboards throughout the room. After sharing a Moscow Mule in a frosty copper mug, duck fat fries, or monkey bread with dill butter, it might be time for messy *elotes* tossed with sweet chili jam to be licked off each finger; or an heirloom tomato tart with a SarVecchio cheese crust and shaved onions. Do the right thing and save room for homemade Nutter Butter cookies with dark chocolate sabayon for dipping.

# Carriage House 🌶

B4

Southern XX

### 1700 W. Division St. (at Paulina St.)

**Phone:** 773-384-9700
**Web:** www.carriagehousechicago.com
**Prices:** $$

Lunch Sat – Sun
Dinner nightly
🚇 Division

Carriage House brings South Carolina hospitality to the heart of Wicker Park. Gauzy shades cover large windows in the understated dining room. Wire cage light fixtures lend farmhouse flair; bentwood bistro chairs and tufted leather ottomans add a contemporary touch.

The menu mixes traditional dishes with modern interpretations for a North-South blend of flavor and technique. Velvety Charleston she-crab soup is poured tableside over bright orange roe that bursts in the mouth. A scrumptious house-made garlic bologna and pimento cheese sandwich on brioche bridges the worlds of fine dining and country charm. Family-style suppers like a low-country boil with shrimp, clams, and rabbit *chaurice* sausage are meant to be shared around a table of friends.

# Coalfire Pizza

 **C5**

✕

### 1321 W. Grand Ave. (bet. Ada & Elizabeth Sts.)

**Phone:** 312-226-2625 Lunch Wed – Sun
**Web:** www.coalfirechicago.com Dinner Tue – Sun
**Prices:** 💿💿  Chicago (Blue)

Sure, you could come for a salad, but at Coalfire, the focus is rightly on pizza and yours should be too. Rust-red walls put diners in the mood, and in a playful bit of recycling, empty tomato sauce cans on each table become the perfect stand for sizzling pizzas churned straight from the 800-degree coal oven.

Coalfire has its ratio down to a fine art and knows not to burden its thin crust with too many toppings. Simple combinations like mortadella and garlic; Calabrese salami, Italian sausage and pepperoni; or a few top-quality anchovies pair sublimely with tangy tomato sauce and a chewy crust that's blackened and blistered in all the right spots. Not feeling the combos? Build your own pizza and pick your own trappings from Gorgonzola to goat cheese.

# Coast Sushi Bar

 **B2**

✕✕

### 2045 N. Damen Ave. (bet. Dickens & McLean Aves.)

**Phone:** 773-235-5775 Lunch Sat – Sun
**Web:** www.coastsushibar.com Dinner nightly
**Prices:** $$

Dimly lit but lively, this high-volume sushi bar cranks out a remarkable variety of rolls to keep up with demand especially on weekends from noon till night. Two spacious dining rooms and a narrow sushi counter armed with wood-framed chairs accommodate the chatty crowds. Bring your own sake, wine, and bottle opener to make the wait more tolerable.

The broad selection of Japanese dishes ranges from signature maki and nigiri to innovative appetizers like fried soft-shell crab with mango-shallot salsa. Miso soup spiked with jalapeño is served in a coffee cup for easy sipping. A deep bowl of boatman *chirashi* is laden with orange *tobiko*, pickled veggies, shiso leaves, and an array of sashimi. Dig right in or grab a sheet of toasted nori for a custom-wrapped hand roll.

# Cumin

**B3**

### 1414 N. Milwaukee Ave. (bet. Evergreen & Wolcott Aves.)

Phone: 773-342-1414
Web: www.cumin-chicago.com
Prices: 

Lunch Tue – Sun
Dinner nightly
Damen (Blue)

This proudly-run blend of Nepalese and Indian eats sits among a plethora of bars, coffee shops, and vintage stores in boho-centric Bucktown. While fans of the sub-continent love Cumin for its clean and modern surrounds, linen-lined tables struggle to contain the myriad plates that pile up during its ubiquitous lunch buffet.

Paintings of mountain scenes frame crimson-red walls and prep diners for an authentic range of flavorful food hailing from the Northeast. Nibble on crispy samosas or onion *bhajis* (finely shredded onion fritters) teamed with mint chutney, then soak pieces of buttery naan in rich and vibrant *saag* bobbing with soft chunks of chicken. For a sweet finale, dig into a creamy pistachio *kulfi* or opt for a light and fruity mango *lassi*.

# The Dawson

**D5**

### 730 W. Grand Ave. (at Halsted St.)

Phone: 312-243-8955
Web: www.the-dawson.com
Prices: $$

Lunch Sat – Sun
Dinner nightly
Chicago (Blue)

"See and be seen" should be the motto of this hip spot, where globe lights shine like beacons through the façade's towering windows. Inside, a wraparound bar attracts spirited guests like moths to a flame. A lengthy communal table and open kitchen with chef's counter offer myriad opportunities for meeting, greeting, and eating.

Cocktails like the Surfer Rosa, which balances tequila and mezcal with blood orange and chilies, loosen-up diners jonesing for big flavors. When hunger strikes, caramelized onion sabayon, potato confit, and garlicky pea shoots add depth to an Arctic char fillet. And lest you forget dessert, bourbon-pecan bread pudding set upon flash-frozen vanilla cream and drizzled with sea salt-butterscotch sauce, is meant for sharing—or not.

# En Hakkore

 Korean

### 1840 N. Damen Ave. (bet. Churchill & Moffat Sts.)

**Phone:** 773-772-9880                     Lunch & dinner Mon – Sat
**Web:** N/A
**Prices:**                            Damen (Blue)

Healthy doesn't have to be humdrum. This simple little Korean eatery, run by a husband-and-wife team and decorated with more than a hint of whimsy, specializes in big bowls of *bibimbap*. You choose your rice and protein, be it pork or barbecue beef, decide on the heat level and then dive straight in—up to 16 different vegetables are used and they're as tasty as they are colorful. Also worth trying are the steamed *mandoo* (pork dumplings) and the curiously addictive tacos made with *paratha*.

Simply place your order at the counter, grab a plastic fork and, if you're with friends, commandeer the large communal table. There's no alcohol (and it's not BYOB) so instead take advantage of an invigorating soft drink from the fridge. You'll feel so virtuous.

# Enso

Japanese

### 1613 N. Damen Ave. (bet. North & Wabansia Aves.)

**Phone:** 773-878-8998                          Lunch & dinner daily
**Web:** www.ensochicago.com
**Prices:** $$                               Damen (Blue)

All bases are covered at Enso, from tempura to ramen and *chirashi* to teriyaki, but it's mostly about maki. There are fairly classic combinations of ingredients on offer, but also more challenging blends of flavor. If you can't decide then you can always "make your own maki"—but you'll only have yourself to blame should the memory of your chosen flavors return to haunt you at a later date. The homemade steamed buns are also good; a filling of roasted pork belly with pickled vegetables inside one of these little pillows of delight is hard to beat.

The vaulted room looks like a Goth's cellar, all black and moody, with the open kitchen at the far end shining like a beacon of hope. Larger parties should try to snare one of the low-slung booths.

# Flo

**C5**

### 1434 W. Chicago Ave. (bet. Bishop St. & Greenview Ave.)

**Phone:** 312-243-0477     Lunch Tue – Sun
**Web:** www.flochicago.com     Dinner Tue – Sat
**Prices:** 💲     Chicago (Blue)

It's not Santa Fe, but the Southwest is well represented in West Town through the chili-packed flavors at Flo. This early meals joint cranks out a variety of spicy and tasty Tex-Mex dishes for diners crowded into the sunlight-dappled dining room. Pressed-tin ceilings, mirrors mounted on exposed brick, and narrow plank floors add quaint appeal.

Made-to-order breakfast and brunch is served until 2:30 P.M., allowing ample time for Fruity Pebbles French toast or breakfast burritos. *Pollo picante* quesadillas get a kick from pickled jalapeños and Jack cheese. *Sopapillas* come in sweet as well as savory varieties like house-made chorizo with scrambled eggs and cheddar. As in the Southwest, fresh red or green chili sauce is always offered as an option.

# Frontier

**C4**

### 1072 N. Milwaukee Ave. (bet. Noble & Thomas Sts.)

**Phone:** 773-772-4322     Lunch Sat – Sun
**Web:** www.thefrontierchicago.com     Dinner nightly
**Prices:** $$     Division

If Davy Crockett is king of the wild frontier, then chances are he'd be smitten by this stylish, modern-day saloon. To start, a taxidermied grizzly bear, wolf, and bison head hang among football-flaunting flat-screens behind the 40 foot-long bar. And even Frontier's menu drives home the hunt-and-gather theme, with dishes divided into three sections: "Fried," "Foraged," and "Whole Animal Service."

Carnivores revel in the chef's signature duck tacos juiced with salsa verde, while pescetarians beg for crab Benedict—a superb staple of toasted muffins with sweet crabmeat, soft poached eggs, and spicy Hollandaise. Calorie-counters love the well-dressed house salad, but for dessert, there is no passing up on crispy sugar doughnuts—gently caressed with a rum-apple sauce in true Crockett fashion.

# Green Zebra

 **C5**

Vegetarian

**1460 W. Chicago Ave. (at Greenview Ave.)**

| | | |
|---|---|---|
| **Phone:** | 312-243-7100 | Dinner nightly |
| **Web:** | www.greenzebrachicago.com | |
| **Prices:** | $$ |  Chicago (Blue) |

Named after a popular heirloom tomato variety, Chef/owner Shawn McClain's vegetarian standby is beloved among Chicagoans looking for an upscale meat-free experience. Japanese minimalism inspires the small space's décor, with palms and bamboo lining the entry and earthy tones throughout the room.

Diners graze on shared small plates paired with organic and biodynamic wines. Creamy hen of the woods mushroom pâté, served with caramelized Vidalia onion marmalade and toasted bread, ensures that no one misses the meat. Peppery arugula purée and a dollop of crème fraîche balance silky celery root soup. Thin shards of dark chocolate and dense peanut mousse with currant coulis are a match made in vegan heaven; a crushed pretzel garnish gilds the lily.

# Jane's

**B2**

American

**1655 W. Cortland St. (bet. Marshfield Ave. & Paulina St.)**

| | | |
|---|---|---|
| **Phone:** | 773-862-5263 | Lunch Fri – Sun |
| **Web:** | www.janesrestaurant.com | Dinner Tue – Sun |
| **Prices:** |  | |

Jane's is nearly as much of an historic fixture as the well-kept 19th century building in which it resides, having made its name as a neighborhood favorite since 1994. Vaulted ceilings with chunky wood beams hover over claw-foot tables, thereby complementing exposed brick walls hung with artwork while emphasizing a rustic and homey vibe.

Global accents and vegetarian specialties on the menu showcase the kitchen's wide-ranging definition of comfort food. If the freshly ground half-pound sirloin burger topped with pancetta, grilled pineapple, mozzarella, and chipotle aïoli isn't enough, mashed potatoes and salad on the side should leave you fulfilled. Lighter fare like an Asian chicken salad, or a bowl of Jane's corn chowder are ideal taste bud teasers.

# Las Palmas

**B3**

### 1835 W. North Ave. (at Honore St.)

**Phone:** 773-289-4991

**Web:** www.laspalmaschicago.com

**Prices:** $$

Lunch Sat – Sun

Dinner nightly

 Damen (Blue)

Vivid décor complements the spirited flavors on the menu at Las Palmas, from the colorful Mexican artwork on adobe-style walls to exposed ductwork welded to resemble a scaly dragon winding through the deceptively large space. If the weather suits, the outdoor garden or glassed-in atrium beckon; if not, a cozy fireplace in the front room keeps things intimate.

The cocktail menu draws inspiration from both South and Central America, featuring myriad capirinhas and mojitos alongside inventive cucumber-lime and pineapple margaritas. Vibrant and modern Mexican dishes like crispy *taquitos* with chicken *barbacoa*, pickled red onion, and tangy salsa *cruda*; and seafood-filled cornmeal empanadas with peanut-jalapeño relish showcase the kitchen's flair.

# Le Bouchon

**B2**

### 1958 N. Damen Ave. (at Armitage Ave.)

**Phone:** 773-862-6600

**Web:** www.lebouchonofchicago.com

**Prices:** $$

Lunch & dinner Mon – Sat

 Damen (Blue)

Pressed-tin ceiling? Check. Brick-and-Dijon color scheme? Check. Close-knit tables in a snug space? Check. A warm welcome from an actual Frenchman? Check. Owner Jean-Claude Poilevey has fashioned the quintessential bistro experience at Le Bouchon, where straightforward French fare never goes out of style. The informal atmosphere gets convivially raucous as the night goes on with regulars lining the bar and petite dining room.

Familiar, approachable favorites rule the menu: *soupe à l'oignon*, wearing its traditional topper of broiled Gruyère on a moist crouton, oozes and bubbles over the sides of a ramekin; and an ample fillet of *saumon poche* napped in beurre blanc is the essence of simplicity. A lunch prix-fixe keeps the wallet light but belly full.

# Lillie's Q

**B3** B a r b e c u e ✖️✖️

## 1856 W. North Ave. (at Wolcott Ave.)

**Phone:** 773-772-5500         Lunch & dinner daily
**Web:** www.lilliesq.com
**Prices:** $$        Damen (Blue)

This self-described "urban barbeque" is a honky-tonk celebration of smoked meats rubbed in "Carolina dirt" (their own recipe) and down-home sides in a rustic setting. Leather belts hold cushions on the banquettes in a room filled with iron light fixtures, exposed brick, and white subway tiles. Servers in modern mechanic's shirts hoist metal trays and carry Mason jars filled with "moonshine" whiskey cocktails. The bar is big on beer.

Tri-tip is tender and pink-tinged after its time in the smoker with the joint's signature dry rub, improved only by a squirt of one of Lillie's five sauces, like mustardy Carolina Gold or Hot Smoky. Smoked-fried chicken gets a drizzle of Tupelo honey over its peppery breading from a tableside ceramic honey pot.

# Mana Food Bar

**B4** V e g e t a r i a n ✖️

## 1742 W. Division St. (bet. Paulina & Wood Sts.)

**Phone:** 773-342-1742        Lunch Sat
**Web:** www.manafoodbar.com      Dinner nightly
**Prices:** 🪙        Division

Feeling like your body needs a jump-start? Mana, whose name translates to "the life force coursing through nature," is a good place to get your mojo back. Though welcoming to vegans, vegetarians, gluten-free diners, and anyone who's looking for a nutrient boost, it's not just a health bar: the small space also offers a full bar with sake cocktails, smoothies, and freshly squeezed juices.

Mana may be a tiny spot, but its diverse menu of vegetarian dishes is big on taste—and spice. Korean *bibimbap* mixes a roster of vegetables like pea pods, roasted carrots, and pickled daikon with a fresh sunny side-up egg; while horseradish and cracked black pepper sneak into macaroni and cheese. House-made hot sauce with serranos and jalapeños adds extra pep to any dish.

57

# Mexique

**C5**

Mexican XX

1529 W. Chicago Ave. (bet. Armour St. & Ashland Ave. )

**Phone:** 312-850-0288
**Web:** www.mexiquechicago.com
**Prices:** $$

Lunch & dinner Tue – Sun

Chicago (Blue)

Close quarters don't stop Mexique from packing 'em in. Large groups fill most of the banquettes in the slender space, but a bar stretching half the length of the room makes it easy for smaller parties to stop in for a glass of sangria. A large rear window offers a glimpse of Chef Carlos Gaytan at work in the kitchen, and congratulatory graffiti from visiting chefs provides distraction on the way to the restroom.

Many of the contemporary Mexican dishes are inspired by classic French techniques. Tried-and-true starters include seafood-stuffed *pescamal* with preserved lemon garnish and a bold chili-infused bouillabaisse, and traditional Mexican accompaniments like nopales and watermelon radish add crunch to smoky scallops and hibiscus-glazed pork belly.

# Mindy's Hot Chocolate

**B3**

Contemporary XX

1747 N. Damen Ave. (bet. St. Paul Ave. & Willow St.)

**Phone:** 773-489-1747
**Web:** www.hotchocolatechicago.com
**Prices:** $$

Lunch Wed – Sun
Dinner Tue – Sun
Damen (Blue)

Rich temptations—and savory bites to complement those sweets—are found behind the floor-to-ceiling glass doors of this lofty, industrial Bucktown dessert bar. Chocolate-toned leather banquettes, sleek dark wood chairs, and caramel-brown walls drive the point home.

Savory dishes are straightforward and good, like a BLET that tweaks the typical BLT formula by adding an over easy egg to herb mayo-slathered and grilled brioche. But the sweets are pure decadence. A trio of profiteroles are filled with coffee cocoa nib ice cream, frozen hot chocolate, and banana sherbet, then topped with shards of toffee brittle and drizzled with Moloko stout hot sauce. Too much? Simple but comforting snickerdoodle cookies or hot chocolate with fresh marshmallows satisfy.

# Mirai

Japanese ✗✗

**B4**

### 2020 W. Division St. (bet. Damen & Hoyne Aves.)

| | | |
|---|---|---|
| **Phone:** | 773-862-8500 | Dinner nightly |
| **Web:** | www.miraisushi.com | |
| **Prices:** | $$ | Damen (Blue) |

Mirai is a bit like Disney World. You know it's not real, but who cares? The Japanese food is westernized and by no means traditional, but unless you're dining out with Mr. Shinzo Abe, rest assured that nobody will cry foul.

Bold and appetizing flavors beg to take center stage. It's really all about the fish at this spot—just look around and you'll find most devotees feasting on sashimi, *unagi*, and maki. If raw fish doesn't float your boat, take a shot at one of the house specialties like *kani nigiri*, a baked king crab concoction. There is also a surfeit of hot dishes—think chicken *togarashi* with spicy, sweet, and tangy flavors. Affable and alert service combined with a relaxed atmosphere, especially on the front patio, make this a hit among area residents.

# Mott St.

Fusion ✗

**B3**

### 1401 N. Ashland Ave. (at Blackhawk St.)

| | | |
|---|---|---|
| **Phone:** | 773-687-9977 | Dinner Tue – Sat |
| **Web:** | www.mottstreetchicago.com | |
| **Prices:** | $$ | Division |

New Yorkers know Mott Street as the bustling artery in the heart of Chinatown, but to Chicagoans the name connotes something off the beaten path. Inspired by the night stalls of Asia, this funky joint set in a red building incorporates a chicken wire-caged pantry stocked with jars of red pepper, black vinegar, and other pungent edibles—all of which appear again in the food on your plate.

Offerings crisscross the globe from Korea, Latin America, and all the way back to India, melding diverse ingredients in spring rolls stuffed with minced kimchi and melted Oaxaca cheese; or layers of spicy fermented Napa cabbage, tender shredded pork, and seared sticky rice with kimchi broth. A frozen, chocolate-covered and peanut-coated baby banana cools things down.

Chicago ▲ Bucktown & Wicker Park

# Nando Milano Trattoria

Italian

 **A4**

**2114 W. Division St. (bet. Hoyne Ave. & Leavitt St.)**

**Phone:** 773-486-2636 | Dinner nightly
**Web:** www.nandomilano.com
**Prices:** $$ | Division

A corner bar television constantly tuned to (European) football, vintage *aperitivo* posters, and a welcoming patio tailor-made for afternoon glasses of prosecco: charismatic host Dario Vullo has installed his own little slice of Milan in Wicker Park. The chic trattoria offers an intensely Italian menu and wine list to match the authentic accents of Vullo and family.

A trio of *arancini* are playfully prepared, with each rice ball sporting a unique shape—sphere, triangle, and cube—to denote a special filling like Bolognese ragù and smoked mozzarella; or mascarpone and spinach. House-made pastas like beet gnocchi in saffron sauce steal the show from equally flavorful and fresh focaccia sandwiches layered with creamy burrata and *Prosciutto di Parma*.

# Oiistar

Asian

**B3**

**1385 N. Milwaukee Ave. (bet. Paulina & Wood Sts.)**

**Phone:** 773-360-8791 | Lunch & Dinner Tue – Sun
**Web:** www.oiistar.com
**Prices:** ⊜⊜ | Damen (Blue)

It's easy to mistake Oiistar for yet another trendy ramen joint—but don't. Sure, it's got all the design hallmarks—from a minimalist wood-planked dining room and industrial open kitchen, to a turned-up soundtrack; but the internationally influenced menu makes it much more than your average slurp shop.

In fact, "It's A Small World" could be the unofficial theme song for their lineup of steamed buns and comforting ramen bowls showcasing noodles hand-pulled in-house each day: *kochujang* sauce complements barbecue chicken on the *pollo* bun, while the saltimbocca bun goes Italian with sage, prosciutto, and mozzarella. Extra special is the *chadolmen*, which blends a tangle of delicate wheat noodles with brisket and ground pork in a spicy miso and kimchi broth.

# Owen & Engine

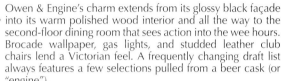

Gastropub XX

## 2700 N. Western Ave. (at Schubert Ave.)

**Phone:** 773-235-2930
**Web:** www.owenengine.com
**Prices:** $$

Lunch Sat – Sun
Dinner nightly

Owen & Engine's charm extends from its glossy black façade into its warm polished wood interior and all the way to the second-floor dining room that sees action into the wee hours. Brocade wallpaper, gas lights, and studded leather club chairs lend a Victorian feel. A frequently changing draft list always features a few selections pulled from a beer cask (or "engine").

British-inspired gastropub fare matches the impressive roster of brews and Pimm's cups. Bar nibbles like mustard-glazed soft pretzels with Welsh rarebit for dipping; or peanuts tossed in *sriracha*, Worcestershire sauce, and brown sugar cater to the snacking sort. Hearty entrées like bangers and mash feature house-made Slagel Family Farm's pork sausage and potatoes smothered in onion gravy.

# Piccolo Sogno

Italian XX

## 464 N. Halsted St. (at Milwaukee Ave.)

**Phone:** 312-421-0077
**Web:** www.piccolosognorestaurant.com
**Prices:** $$

Lunch Mon – Fri
Dinner nightly
 Grand (Blue)

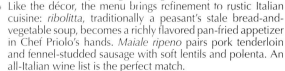

Power lunchers and socially minded dinner parties descend on this stately building, which stands out at its gritty intersection, for equal parts glad-handing and hearty eating. A labor of love for co-owners Tony Priolo and Ciro Longobardo, the swank space exudes conviviality and charm with brick archways and terrazzo floors. The obvious camaraderie between staff keeps things running efficiently.

Like the décor, the menu brings refinement to rustic Italian cuisine: *ribolitta*, traditionally a peasant's stale bread-and-vegetable soup, becomes a richly flavored pan-fried appetizer in Chef Priolo's hands. *Maiale ripeno* pairs pork tenderloin and fennel-studded sausage with soft lentils and polenta. An all-Italian wine list is the perfect match.

# Red Door

**B2**

### 2118 N. Damen Ave. (at Charleston St.)

**Phone:** 773-697-7221
**Web:** www.reddoorchicago.com
**Prices:** $$

Lunch Sat – Sun
Dinner Tue – Sun

 Even with no sign, it's easy to find this funky Bucktown bar: that red door is impossible to miss. Grab a metal barstool or a raised wooden banquette for an evening of seasonal cocktails, craft beers, and internationally inspired pub fare. On warm evenings, the backyard patio becomes romantic with candlelit communal tables and a canopy of twinkling lights overhead.

 Gastropub classics take a spin around the globe, while often featuring local ingredients (sometimes right from the patio). *Bulgogi*-glazed hanger steak and eggs is a weekend brunch favorite, layering tender chunks of hanger steak over scrambled eggs with a pile of spicy, hangover-busting kimchi on the side. Poutine boasts Wisconsin's Brunkow cheese curds and spicy curry gravy.

# Roots Handmade Pizza

 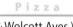
**B5**

### 1924 W. Chicago Ave. (bet. Winchester & Wolcott Aves.)

**Phone:** 773-645-4949
**Web:** www.rootspizza.com
**Prices:** $$

Lunch & dinner daily

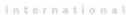 Division

  Quad Cities-style pizza may not be as famous as deep-dish, but its malted, slightly sweet crust is making a name for itself at Roots. Raised booths and a smattering of televisions serve up a sports bar vibe that's complemented by a multi-page selection of draft and bottled beer (to match the pies' provenance, the suds hail exclusively from the Midwest).

Starters like freshly fried hand-pulled mozzarella show more creativity than your typical Italian joint. Build your own pie or salad from a lengthy roster of ingredients, or veer off the beaten path with a bronzed crust piled with cheese, pickled jalapeños, avocado cream, and chorizo chili—an ode to neighboring Antique Taco. Tidy up with a most thoughtful amenity: a warm washcloth, presented tableside.

# Ruxbin

 American ✕✕

## 851 N. Ashland Ave. (at Pearson St.)

**Phone:** 312-624-8509  
**Web:** www.ruxbinchicago.com  
**Prices:** $$

Dinner Tue – Sun

🚇 Division

**BYO**

Refurbished and repurposed is the rationale behind Ruxbin's funky décor. In the tiny first-floor space, salvaged apple juice crates form wall panels and seat belts become chair backs. Up a few stairs, a stainless steel communal table offers a view into the semi-open kitchen.

Meals usually start with popcorn seasoned with changing flavors like sesame and seaweed—a preview of the menu's mix of American and international ingredients. A fresh oyster trio gets three distinct garnishes: *sambal*-pickled ginger, tangy apple mignonette, and pork belly with a smoked aroma revealed by lifting a glass cloche. Seared scallops and pork carnitas meld with black raisin emulsion. Rest easy that you won't miss the booze here after trying a house-made basil-hibiscus soda.

# Seadog

 Japanese ✕

## 1500 W. Division St. (at Greenview Ave.)

**Phone:** 773-235-8100  
**Web:** www.seadogsushibar.com  
**Prices:**

Dinner nightly

🚇 Division

**BYO**

Dim lighting, deep wood tones, and warm bronze hues set the stage for romance at this sexy little sushi bar just off the Division St. El stop. Not in the mood for love? Do not let that stop you from dropping in for a bite. Glazed brick walls and mosaic floors tiled with granite shards are as texturally interesting as the dishes turned out of the sushi counter.

Creative, contemporary appetizers and maki take center stage here, with a number of spicy options for the heat-seekers. Miso soup gets fresh jalapeños for a zesty kick; chopped scallop and wasabi *tobiko* tops crisp, light, and greaseless asparagus tempura; and dots of spicy *sriracha* and fried garlic adorn hamachi carpaccio.

Got cash in your wallet? Seadog will take 10 percent off your bill.

*Chicago ▲ Bucktown & Wicker Park*

# Schwa ✿

Contemporary ✕

**B3**

### 1466 N. Ashland Ave. (at Le Moyne St.)

| | | |
|---|---|---|
| **Phone:** | 773-252-1466 | Dinner Tue – Sat |
| **Web:** | www.schwarestaurant.com | |
| **Prices:** | **$$$$** | 🚇 Division |

BYO

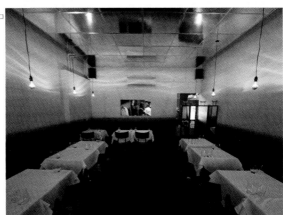

There comes a point when pared-down style jumps from being easy-to-miss and becomes hard-to-forget (think security grills on the façade). When a utilitarian and self-consciously bare interior seems modern and industrial. When temporarily disconnected phone lines and full mailboxes make every hipster in the room feel like he hit the jackpot to score this reservation. The booming hip-hop peppered with expletives reflects the deeply talented chefs' ethos, going well beyond laissez-faire to reach the point of "we don't give a damn." That said, you probably won't either. The food really is that good.

The 14-course nightly tasting has no menu, but there are plenty of tattooed servers ready to describe each dish with details that come at you like machine-gunfire.

Some courses show nuance and delicacy, like the smooth and fine rosewater sorbet topped with a thin round of cucumber. Others are wow-inducing and present extraordinary depth of flavor, as in the beautifully crafted quail egg raviolo with its unctuous sauce. Dessert can be pure genius that begins by placing a menthol crystal on the tongue for a tingly fresh prelude to lemongrass and coconut snow covered with intense passion fruit sauce.

# Smoke Daddy

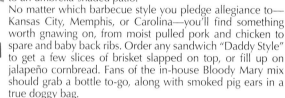

American ✗

**1804 W. Division St. (at Wood St.)**

**Phone:** 773-772-6656        Lunch & dinner daily
**Web:** www.thesmokedaddy.com
**Prices:**       Division

After a renovation doubled the size of this barbecue joint and live music venue, it's easier to grab a bite of burnt ends and a touch of the blues. The original room still oozes soul and smoke from its brick walls and vinyl floor, while the new space is bright and airy with a retractable glass door leading to an umbrella-shaded patio.

No matter which barbecue style you pledge allegiance to—Kansas City, Memphis, or Carolina—you'll find something worth gnawing on, from moist pulled pork and chicken to spare and baby back ribs. Order any sandwich "Daddy Style" to get a few slices of brisket slapped on top, or fill up on jalapeño cornbread. Fans of the in-house Bloody Mary mix should grab a bottle to-go, along with smoked pig ears in a true doggy bag.

# Takito Kitchen

Mexican ✗✗

**2013 W. Division St. (bet. Damen & Hoyne Aves.)**

**Phone:** 773-687-9620        Lunch & dinner Tue – Sun
**Web:** www.takitokitchen.com
**Prices:** $$      Division

Chicago's upscale taco circuit gets a new contender with Takito, where fresh ingredients make Latin-inspired food sing. Tequilas take pride of place in the front dining room, waiting for their moment in a chile-salted margarita, while skylights and mirrors make the narrow, modern-industrial space seem even brighter and larger.

Sure, you can get a corn tortilla here, but sesame and hibiscus options let the kitchen get creative as evident in tacos filled with cornmeal-crusted redfish, beef *barbacoa,* or tamarind-chayote *pequin.* Shared plates like *sope de carne asada* blur culinary boundaries with the addition of Brunkow cheddar and green onion kimchi. It's an across-the-board mishmash of colorful flavors, but it's a good way to go over the top.

Chicago ▶ Bucktown & Wicker Park

65

# Takashi ✿

Fusion XX

B2

1952 N. Damen Ave. (at Armitage Ave.)

**Phone:** 773-772-6170
**Web:** www.takashichicago.com
**Prices:** $$$

Lunch Sun
Dinner Tue – Sun
Damen (Blue)

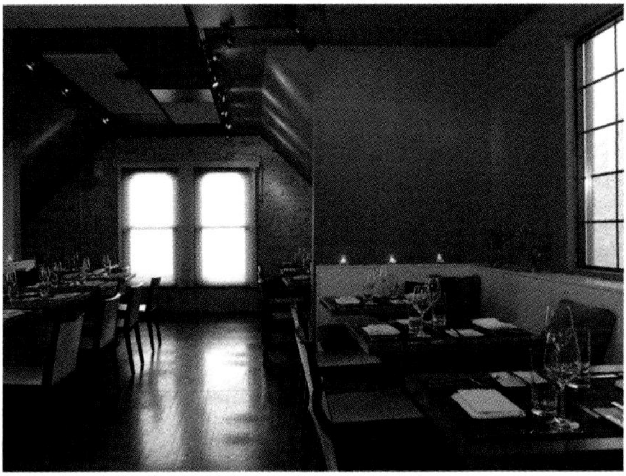

Bucking the trend of whisper-quiet, formal temples to Japanese cuisine, Takashi sports the liveliness of an intimate French bistro. Housed within a red brick townhouse on Damen Avenue's shop-lined thoroughfare, this bi-level space is minimally embellished in warm neutral tones.

Despite the elegant surrounds, an informal friendliness prevails at each meal. When the tables are full—of locals, couples, and business diners—the rooms take on a soulful vibe. And on less crowded evenings, servers go to great lengths to ensure the mood stays breezy and welcoming.

Chef Takashi Yagihashi melds Japanese flavors with seasonal ingredients and European techniques. *Mugifugi* pork loin two ways is emblematic of his style: roasted with ginger and soy, and prepared Cordon Bleu-style with pancetta and Brie. Tart *tobanjan* vinaigrette spices up a crudo trio of tender hamachi, meaty whelk, and thinly shaved Hokkaido scallops. A marriage of whimsy and refinement comes through in desserts like eggshells filled with milk chocolate crème brûlée or graham cracker ice cream with Valrhona sticky cake. Tables can order the six-course omakase with wine pairings, or call in advance for the chef's seven-course kaiseki menu.

# Taxim

**B3**

Greek

### 1558 N. Milwaukee Ave. (bet. Damen & North Aves.)

**Phone:** 773-252-1558      Dinner nightly
**Web:** www.taximchicago.com
**Prices:** $$      Damen (Blue)

Though Taxim channels the spirit of Greece in its food, its Moroccan-esque décor takes inspiration from Turkey and other Mediterranean coastal neighbors. The large room glints with light from hanging Moorish lanterns and copper-topped tables. Share small plates on the sidewalk patio to take full advantage of Wicker Park people-watching.

Many of Taxim's dishes get a modern twist while remaining respectful to the islands' traditional cuisine. Wild Greek oregano and ouzo-preserved lemon offer a perfect balance to roasted Amish Miller Farms chicken; while *loukoumades* prove that no one can resist fried dough, especially when tossed in wildflower honey and topped with rosewater-infused pastry cream. The all-Greek wine list is an adventure for oenophiles.

# tocco

**B4**

Italian

### 1266 N. Milwaukee Ave. (bet. Ashland Ave. & Paulina St.)

**Phone:** 773-687-8895      Dinner Tue – Sun
**Web:** www.toccochicago.com
**Prices:** $$      Division

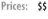

Are we in Milan or Wicker Park? Tocco brings haute design and fashion to the table with such upscale textural touches as polished resin, faux ostrich skin, and bubblegum-pink accents in this sleek black-and-white space. Don your catwalk best before visiting: a fashion-centric display near a long communal table hints at the chichi theme present throughout.

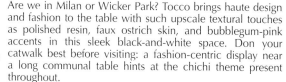

The décor is cutting-edge, but the menu respects and returns to Italian standbys. *Gnocco fritto*, a dough pillow served with charcuterie, is irresistible to even the most willowy fashionistas; while cracker-crisp artisan pizzas from wood-burning ovens are equally pleasing. Traditional *involtini di pollo*, pounded thin and rolled around prosciutto, gets a hit of brightness from lemon and white wine sauce.

# Trenchermen

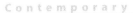 Contemporary

 **A3**

### 2039 W. North Ave. (bet. Hoyne & Milwaukee Aves.)

**Phone:** 773-661-1540
**Web:** www.trenchermen.com
**Prices:** $$

Lunch Sat – Sun
Dinner nightly
Damen (Blue)

In old-timey slang, a trencherman is a hearty eater and drinker, a definition that lets you know what you're in for at this glossy but comforting Wicker Park gastropub. Housed in a former Russian bathhouse, the black-and-white tiles and notched brick walls dividing the eclectic warren of rooms give a nod to the former tenant of this 1920s building.

Bar snacks and weekend brunch are taken just as seriously as full-on lunch and dinner here. Corned beef adds a manly touch to eggs Benedict, especially when drizzled with piquant *choron* sauce. Dense pretzel cinnamon rolls straddle the salty-sweet line. A menu favorite at any time of day, fried pickle tots are served with kicky beet-tinged red onion yogurt and thinly sliced chicken breast *bresaola*.

# TWO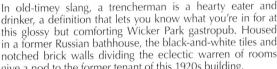

American

**C5**

### 1132 W. Grand Ave. (at May St.)

**Phone:** 312-624-8363
**Web:** www.tworestaurantchicago.com
**Prices:** $$

Dinner Tue – Sun
Chicago (Blue)

This urban interpretation of a Midwest tavern was set up by two owners, features two chefs, second-hand furnishings, and an address whose last digit is—you guessed it—the number two. Step past the vintage Toledo scales to arrive at this reclaimed wood-paneled space dressed with antique meat cleavers, quaint ceiling fans, and large barn doors.

If that doesn't scream farm-to-fork cuisine, consider what's being whipped up in the open kitchen (the banquette across from it affords the best view): a ramp *raviolo* filled with ricotta, a perfectly cooked hen's egg, and enhanced by brown butter and shiitakes; or a halibut fillet with cherry tomatoes and asparagus. On the sweet front, homemade puppy chow is chilled, crisp, and delicious with a uniform sugar dusting.

# Veneno de Nayarit

Seafood

## 1024 N. Ashland Ave. (at Cortez St.)

**Phone:** 773-252-7200

**Web:** N/A

**Prices:** $$

Lunch & dinner daily

 Division

 Roll up your sleeves, or even better, BYOB (bring your own bib) to this small but shining spot that sizzles with activity and intoxicating aromas. A sink in the corner of the vividly painted dining room lets diners wash up after cracking into crab legs and forking down ceviches, while buckets in the corner hint at the shells-on affair.

After the complimentary crab-and-shrimp tostada that's a vehicle for testing your taste buds against the house-made habanero salsa, it's time to dig into a seafood stuffed pineapple or oysters on the half shell. Langoustines split down their middle are broiled with garlic- and butter-soaked breadcrumbs, piled on a platter with salad, rice, seasoned fries, and garlic bread. It's meant for one, but cowards can share.

# Yuzu

Japanese

## 1715 W. Chicago Ave. (bet. Hermitage & Paulina Sts.)

**Phone:** 312-666-4100

**Web:** www.yuzuchicago.com

**Prices:** ⊖⊖

Lunch Mon – Sat

Dinner nightly

 Chicago (Blue)

 Ancient and modern accents work in harmony at Yuzu, where hand-painted anime murals catch the eye above weathered plank wainscoting. A century-old wooden slab finds new life as a sushi counter, where diners sip sodas from Ball jars and groove to hip tunes.

Whole ginger- and garlic-glazed grilled squid is sliced into rings, then sprinkled with scallions and creamy jalapeño sauce. Succulent *robata*-grilled skewers, purchased by the piece, arrive with specialized accompaniments like marinated pork shoulder with sweet chili sauce or *kalbi*-glazed short rib. The *tobiko*-topped Black Sea roll is one of a roster of quirky but manageably sized maki, all of which arrive with an artistic flourish—think: intricate, paisley-patterned sauces painted onto plates.

# Chinatown & South

For years, the Red Line was the only true link between Chinatown and the South Loop. They may be neighbors geographically, but continue to remain distinct opposites in the culinary, architectural, and demographic spheres. Recent development on both sides of the line has brought the two worlds closer together, combining old and new flavors that make them irresistible to Chicago food lovers.

## STROLL THE SOUTH SIDE

The Great Chicago Fire spared many of the South Loop's buildings, making this architecture some of the oldest in the city. Residential palaces like the Glessner House and Clark House are now open for tours, but a quick walk along Prairie Avenue gives a self-guided view of marvelous mansions. Further north, those massive former lofts along Printers Row have been converted into condos, hotels, bookstores, and restaurants, as has the landmark Dearborn Station—the oldest train depot in Chicago.

## SUN-UP TO SUNDOWN

The South Loop has the breakfast scene covered—literally—with dishes piled-high at casual neighborhood spots. Sop up an Irish Bennie adorned with corned beef hash or any

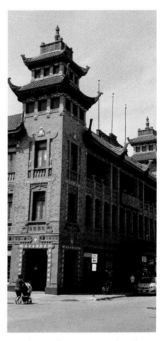

number of eggy entrées from frittatas to French toast at **Yolk**, located on the southern end of Grant Park. The aptly named **Waffles** smothers its signature squares with both savory and sweet flavors. Varieties like cheddar cheese are topped with coffee-braised short ribs, while red velvet waffles come with strawberry compote and whipped cream cheese. As long as you're adding to your cholesterol count, stop at one of the many locations of **Ricobene's** for a breaded steak sandwich or big slab of juicy barbecue ribs.

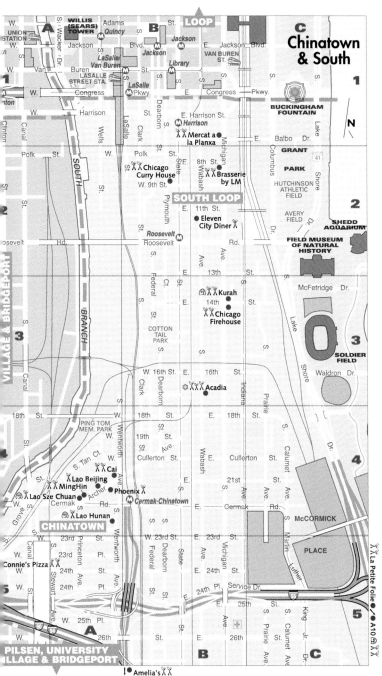

W. Wacker Dr.

WILLIS (SEARS) TOWER

UNION STATION

Adams

Quincy

St.

Jackson

Blvd.

Jackson

E. Jackson Blvd.

VAN BUREN ST.

LaSalle

Van Buren

LaSalle

Jackson

Library

Van Buren

St.

LaSalle STREET STA.

W. Congress Pkwy.

E. Congress Pkwy.

BUCKINGHAM FOUNTAIN

Clinton

Canal

W. Harrison

Harrison

St.

E. Harrison St.

Harrison

Balbo Dr.

Mercat a la Planxa

GRANT

41

PARK

Polk St.

W. Polk St.

St.

Polk St.

8th St.

Michigan

HUTCHINSON ATHLETIC FIELD

Chicago Curry House

W. 9th St.

Wabash

Brasserie by LM

AVERY FIELD

SHEDD AQUARIUM

Plymouth

E. 11th St.

SOUTH LOOP

Eleven City Diner

Columbus

Roosevelt

Roosevelt

Rd.

FIELD MUSEUM OF NATURAL HISTORY

osevelt

Rd.

Ave.

E. 13th St.

McFetridge Dr.

Federal

Ct.

Kurah

14th

St.

Chicago Firehouse

COTTON TAIL PARK

SOLDIER FIELD

Waldron Dr.

W. 16th St.

E. 16th St.

Clark

Dearborn

Acadia

Indiana

Prairie

Lake Shore

18th St.

18th

St.

E. 18th St.

PING TOM MEM. PARK

Wentworth

19th St.

Cullerton St.

Wabash

Cullerton St.

Calumet

Ave.

Cai

S. Tan Ct.

Lao Beijing

21st

St.

MingHin

Archer

Phoenix

Ave.

McCORMICK

Lao Sze Chuan

Cermak Rd.

Cermak-Chinatown

E. Cermak Rd.

PLACE

Lao Hunan

CHINATOWN

W. 23rd St.

E. 23rd St.

Canal

Princeton

Wentworth

Federal

Dearborn

Michigan

Martin Luther King

W. 23rd Pl.

Connie's Pizza

W. 24th St.

E. 24th St.

La Petite Folie

Stewart

24th Pl.

E. 24th Pl.

Service Dr.

25th St.

A10

W. 25th Pl.

King Jr. Dr.

Prairie

Calumet Ave.

90 94

W. 26th St.

26th St.

Amelia's

If you're strolling through the Museum Campus for lunch, grab cash for a bite at **Kim & Carlo's Hot Dog Stand** between the Field Museum and Shedd Aquarium. Vegetarians applaud their veggie dog with all the Chicago toppings, while everyone gets a taste of great skyline views from Grant Park. For a glimpse of real Windy City politics in action, grab a seat at **Manny's**, the venerable coffee shop and deli. Then sink your teeth into a giant pastrami on rye or a plate of crispy potato pancakes, while watching the city's wheelers and dealers do business.

When night falls, the South Loop really gets rocking. Buddy Guy himself often hits the stage at **Buddy Guy's Legends**, where live blues ring out nightly. Catch a set while digging into classic Southern soul food like fried okra, gumbo, or jambalaya. Similarly **The Velvet Lounge**, founded by late jazz legend Fred Anderson, moved from its original location in 2006, but still puts on a heckuva show. Other cutting edge and contemporary

musicians also perform here several times a week. For a blast from the past of a different sort, comedy and history combine at **Tommy Gun's Garage**. This dolled-up speakeasy hosts a riotous nightly dinner theater, allowing audiences to participate.

## CHINATOWN

That ornate and arched gate at Wentwoth Avenue and Cermak Road welcomes locals and visitors alike to one of the largest Chinatowns in America. This iconic structure is an apt symbol for the neighborhood, where the local population is still predominantly Chinese-American and history happily co-exists with contemporary life.

The two-story outdoor **Chinatown Square** mall encompasses everything from restaurants and small boutiques to big banks, thereby giving a buzzy culinary and cultural introduction to the community. Many of its restaurants offer classic Chinese-American fare that is an amalgam of Sichuan

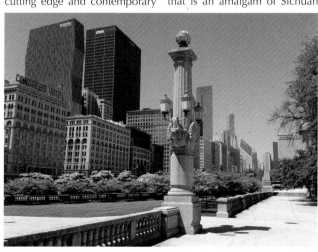

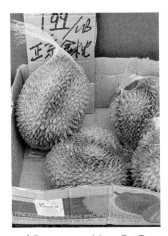

and Cantonese cuisines. But Tony Hu, the most prolific Chinese restaurateur in Chicago and the unofficial mayor of Chinatown, showcases the infinitely varied flavors and spices of regional Chinese cuisine from Beijing to Hunan at his fleet of local spots. Hint: If it starts with the word "Lao," he probably runs it. At the local standby **Go 4 Food**, a Sichuan beef lunch combo or wok-fried and hundred-spiced chicken continue to satiate pungent palates. Let the kids pick out a few intriguing Japanese sweets at **Aji Ichiban**, housed in the Chinatown Square mall, where bins filled with rainbows of foil-wrapped Japanese candy offer opportunities for tricks or treats. Unless you can read the characters on the wrappers, you're in for a surprise—though the store offers samples before charging by the pound.

Home cooks of every stripe know Chinatown isn't just a destination for dining out, but is also great for stocking up on good eats to bring to their own kitchens. In fact, the entire neighborhood is a specialty marketplace of sorts: find an impressive selection of fresh noodles at **Mayflower Food** before picking up wonton wrappers at **Hong Kong Noodle Company**. Aromatic teas of rare varieties fill the shelves at **Ten Ren Tea**; while freshly baked fortune cookies and almond cookies are a revelation at **Golden Dragon Fortune Cookies**. Those craving a wider range of sweets may pour over **Chiu Quon Bakery's** cases of cakes and other cream- or custard-filled pastries. But, for equipment and additional inspiration, grab a cookbook from the Chinese Cultural Bookstore and gear from **Woks 'n' Things**. Then pay homage to the perennial city pastime by watching the White Sox do their thing on U.S. Cellular Field, or the "Monsters of the Midway" take the gridiron inside Soldier Field's formidable walls.

Museums and learning centers showcase the Windy City's history from all angles. Apart from the stately collection of historic buildings in Grant Park's Museum Campus, this neighborhood is also home to Willie Dixon's Blues Heaven Foundation, whose mission is to preserve musical legacy. With its swooping green roof ornaments, the Harold Washington Library Center is impossible to miss, but an equally worthy site is the glass-ceiling winter garden hidden inside. **Iron Street Farm**, a seven-acre urban field in Bridgeport, is part of Chicago's focus on eradicating food deserts within city limits. There, local residents grow vegetables, raise chickens, and cultivate bees as part of the farm's educational programs.

# Acadia

Contemporary  XXX

**BS**

### 1639 S. Wabash Ave. (bet. 16th & 18th Sts.)

**Phone:** 312-360-9500
**Web:** www.acadiachicago.com
**Prices:** $$$

Dinner Wed – Sun

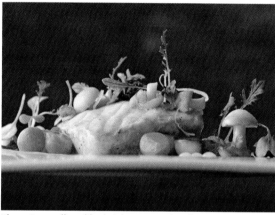

There is a gallery-like brightness to this dining room's white walls, silvery velvet chairs, and khaki carpeting. Bare tables are simply embellished with square slabs of slate for chargers and small stone vases holding fuzzy green moss. Busy evenings can be loud with voices bouncing off all those hard surfaces. Service is always smart, courteous, and very proficient.

Decorative accents of cedar, walnut, maple, and saw grass reflect the kitchen's elemental style of cooking, which is on display through a knotty pine portal.

When presenting minimal ingredients, the impact of each needs to be big—and this is wonderfully clear in the mushroom consommé with sage oil. Flaky biscuits with squiggles of luxurious whipped butter and flecks of black Hawaiian lava salt mean that even bread service is far from typical. Whether dining à la carte or prix-fixe, highlights of any menu may include halibut, which arrives as a deconstructed plate of clam chowder starring the butter-poached fish and adorned with a single shelled clam. Pleasant and deeply warming ravioli might be stuffed with pheasant farce and swimming in an intoxicating jus, alongside shaved Burgundy truffle, chervil, and sautéed chanterelles.

# Amelia's

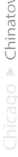

**4559 S. Halsted St. (at 46th St.)**

**Phone:** 773-538-8200
**Web:** www.ameliaschicago.com
**Prices:**

Lunch & dinner daily

Nods to traditional Mexican décor, such as white calla lilies and a terra-cotta roof-tiled awning, perk up the dining room of this South Side south-of-the-border standby just off the Dan Ryan. Ample seating at white linen-draped tables inside the unassuming corner restaurant welcomes neighborhood regulars and newcomers alike.

The menu names its inspiration as the cuisine of Central-Southern Mexico, but nonetheless, Amelia's feels free to incorporate global influences and techniques into its roll of dishes. Ash-layered tamales *judio* are steamed in banana leaves and topped with fruity sesame seed-infused *mole*; and Maine lobster empanadas join pleasantly with grapefruit salad. Homemade corn chips and fresh jalapeño-laced guacamole make a perfect couple.

# A10

**1462 E. 53rd St. (at Harper Ave.)**

**Phone:** 773-288-1010
**Web:** www.a10hydepark.com
**Prices:** $$

Lunch & dinner Tue – Sun

A10 is a highway that winds through the Italian Riviera, but its detour through Hyde Park comes courtesy of prolific restaurateur, Matthias Merges. University of Chicago students and staff populate this split space, building a buzz over marble-topped rounds in the low-key bar area or dark wood tables in the convivial dining room.

Like the décor, the menu deftly balances comfort and sophistication. A single fresh pasta ribbon folded back and forth becomes lasagna filled with succulent veal osso bucco, fresh baby oregano leaves, and both quark and *Parmigiano* cheeses tucked within each layer. Tender chunks of octopus, Niçoise olives, and saffron-tinged slaw dress a chickpea fritter; and rustic chocolate beignets with toasted meringue triangles sweeten the finish.

# Brasserie by LM

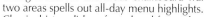

**800 S. Michigan Ave. (bet. 8th & 9th Sts.)**

| | | |
|---|---|---|
| **Phone:** | 312-431-1788 | Lunch & dinner daily |
| **Web:** | www.brasseriebylm.com | |
| **Prices:** | $$ |  Harrison |

From its prime Michigan Avenue location in the Essex Hotel, Brasserie by LM serves up French crowd-pleasers from morn to night. Cherner bentwood stools line the bi-level bar overlooking Grant Park, and frame tables in the more sedate dining room. An enormous chalkboard wall delineating the two areas spells out all-day menu highlights.

Classic bistro dishes from breakfast crêpes to steak frites deliver satisfying flavor. Slurpable French onion soup, served in a requisite ceramic lion's head bowl, is crowned with a moist baguette crouton and melted Gruyère. Herbed potato purée rests under a boneless salmon fillet crusted with Dijon-infused breadcrumbs. A bottomless mimosa brunch draws a crowd on weekends, as do prix-fixe menus for both lunch and dinner.

# Cai

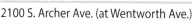

**2100 S. Archer Ave. (at Wentworth Ave.)**

| | | |
|---|---|---|
| **Phone:** | 312-326-6888 | Lunch & dinner daily |
| **Web:** | www.caichicago.com | |
| **Prices:** |  | Cermak-Chinatown |

Cai rolls out the red carpet for a lavish dim sum banquet on the second floor of Chinatown Square. Under crystal chandeliers, tuxedoed servers navigate carts through a sea of silk-covered chairs and round banquet tables. With almost 100 choices of rolled, steamed, fried, crimped, and folded dim sum illustrated neatly on a single menu page, simply pointing to an order makes perfect sense.

Bamboo steamers may contain a bevy of buns and dumplings including *xiao long bao*; crisply baked green chive puffs; tender shrimp-filled *har gow*; or fluffy dessert tarts with creamy, sweet egg yolks inside. When the dim sum parade ends at 4:00 P.M., the menu shifts to Cantonese specialties and entrée choices nearly as numerous as the earlier menu.

Chicago ▶ Chinatown & South

# Chicago Curry House

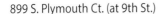

XX

 **899 S. Plymouth Ct. (at 9th St.)**

**Phone:** 312-362-9999
**Web:** www.curryhouseonline.com
**Prices:**

Lunch & dinner daily

 Harrison

Maybe you sniff the wafting aromas of ginger, garlic, and cumin first; maybe you hear the sitar tinkling its welcoming notes as you enter. Either way, you know immediately that Chicago Curry House is a worthy showcase of Indian and Nepalese cuisine.

The lunch buffet lets you eat your fill for under $12, with crispy *pappadum*, baskets of fresh naan, and must-have curries like the Nepalese *khasi ko maasu* with chunks of bone-in stewed goat in a velvety cardamom- and black pepper-sauce. Indian butter chicken, creamy and rich in a tomato- and *garam masala*-spiced stew, is equally sumptuous. À la carte offerings are even more extensive.

The staff has helpful suggestions for dealing with the area's draconian parking restrictions, so call ahead for tips.

# Chicago Firehouse

XX

 **1401 S. Michigan Ave. (at 14th St.)**

**Phone:** 312-786-1401
**Web:** www.chicagofirehouse.com
**Prices:** $$

Lunch & dinner daily

Roosevelt

Built in 1905 with yellow brick and limestone, this firehouse served the community for years. It then lay dormant for a couple of decades before being reborn as a restaurant at the turn of this century and is once again doing its bit for the locals. It's full of character, from the original, ornate tin ceiling and poles in the bar, to the captain's old office upstairs and the cellar downstairs—both now private dining rooms.

The place has quite a masculine feel but is comfortable and charmingly run. And you just know their smoke alarms work. The menu offers a roll-call of reliable American classics, all prepared in an unshowy way. Oysters and crab cakes are popular starters. Then meat takes center stage, from the rack of lamb to chateaubriand for two.

# Connie's Pizza

*Pizza* ✗✗

**2373 S. Archer Ave. (at Normal Ave.)**

**Phone:** 312-326-3443 · Lunch & dinner daily
**Web:** www.conniespizza.com
**Prices:** $$ ·  Halsted

No one knows who Connie was, but the name happened to be on the building bought by Jim Stolfe in 1963, and it stuck. Even Chicagoans who've never set foot in this spacious location know about its near-monopoly at White Sox games (including a complimentary shuttle to U.S. Cellular Field) and constant presence at citywide festivals. Those who do step inside the flagship come for the convivial vibe and, of course, pizza.

Of the many options, the deep-dish is Miss Popularity, but it's fun to go one further with a stuffed pizza topped with a buttery crust. The garlic- and oregano-laced sauce is pleasantly tangy, and carnivores sing the praises of Connie's plump fennel sausage. Call ahead to forego the 45-minute cooking time and pick your pie up at the drive-thru.

# Eleven City Diner

*Deli* ✗

**1112 S. Wabash Ave. (bet. 11th St. & Roosevelt Rd.)**

**Phone:** 312-212-1112 · Lunch & dinner daily
**Web:** www.elevencitydiner.com
**Prices:**  · Roosevelt

Nosh on a mile-high sandwich or chocolate malt at Eleven City Diner, a modern revival of the classic Jewish deli. Gleaming subway tiles play off retro leather booths and swiveling barstools, while jazz in the background keeps things moving with chutzpah and finesse.

Diner standards include patty melts, sandwiches piled with corned beef or pastrami, knishes, and latkes. Bubbie's chicken soup comes bobbing with a fluffy matzo ball the size of a baseball; while Junior's cheesecake from Brooklyn or a triple-decker wedge of red velvet cake sates all the sweet-loving guests. A full-service deli counter offers salamis and smoked fish to-go. For a true blast from the past, stop by the candy stand near the entry stocked with Bazooka Joe and other favorites.

# Kurah

XX

## 1355 S. Michigan Ave. (at 14th St.)

**Phone:** 312-624-8611
**Web:** www.kurahchicago.com
**Prices:** $$

Lunch & dinner daily

 Roosevelt

A glossy corner space on Michigan Avenue's South Loop stretch is now an inviting destination for Kurah's eclectic spread, also billed here as "Mediterranean tapas." Diners nibble flavorful bites near the stunning Moorish-mirrored bar, accompanied by other delightful touches like floor-to-ceiling windows and Edison bulbs dangling from soaring ceilings which add a romantic glow at dusk.

The menu, proudly stocked with organic meats and produce, skews Middle Eastern with small plates like rosemary-infused baba ghanoush served over roasted eggplant; or pine nut-stuffed beef *kubbeh* in a tart yogurt-dill dressing. Lamb abounds in racks and shanks as well as in shawarma and kebab platters; rose-infused flan with candied figs and pistachios is a refined finish.

# Lao Beijing

X

## 2138 S. Archer Ave. (in Chinatown Sq.)

**Phone:** 312-881-0168
**Web:** www.tonygourmetgroup.com
**Prices:** ⊚⊚

Lunch & dinner daily

 Cermak-Chinatown

Part of the Chinatown Square collection of shops and restaurants, Lao Beijing is a no-frills favorite among local business folk. The spare room matches its red and yellow color scheme to the spicy chili oil that is drizzled tableside over most plates. Journey through hundreds of regional dishes like Beijing duck or Northern-style pancakes in the encyclopedic menu, packed with color photographs for those who like to point and order.

Sichuan dumplings arrive with a dark red slick of chili oil, complementing the well-seasoned pork inside each of the half-dozen soft pillows. Lamb sautéed with cumin powder lives up to its name, featuring tender slices tossed with whole red chilies and cumin seeds, drenched in more chili oil over fluffy white rice.

79

# Lao Hunan

 **A4**

🍴

**2230 S. Wentworth Ave. (bet. Alexander St. & 22nd Pl.)**

**Phone:** 312-842-7888                    Lunch & dinner daily
**Web:** www.tonygourmetgroup.com
**Prices:** 💰💰                    🚇 Cermak-Chinatown

A quote from infamous Mao Zedong, "Serving the People," acts as Lao Hunan's unofficial motto. Servers in Red Army uniforms patrol the dining room displaying images of The Chairman. This unapologetic homage is off-putting to some, but doesn't keep crowds from rushing to sample their authentic Hunanese specialties.

Politics aside, aromatic dishes from the extensive hardcover menu showcase fiery flavors. Juicy stir-fried lamb in a memorable spicy sauce mixes with a mélange of tastes and textures: dry-roasted red chilies for heat; bell peppers, scallions, and Chinese celery for crunch; and cilantro for a cooling counterpoint. Twice-cooked duck tossed with chilies and vegetables is first roasted, then breaded and fried for a succulent, meaty finish.

# Lao Sze Chuan

 **A4**

🍴

**2172 S. Archer Ave. (at Princeton Ave.)**

**Phone:** 312-326-5040                    Lunch & dinner daily
**Web:** www.tonygourmetgroup.com
**Prices:** 💰💰                    🚇 Cermak-Chinatown

 One of the most adored spots in Chicago for tongue-tingling, lip-numbing, and belly-warming Sichuan dishes, Lao Sze Chuan is perpetually jammed with chili fiends craving that fiery, tingling sensation of "*ma la*." Even the décor screams "hot, hot, hot" with crimson tablecloths, waiters donning red aprons, and plastic chairs emblazoned with a bright curvy chili.

Mongolian beef tenderloin in a brown sauce with mushrooms is sweetened by onions and beloved by those who can't handle the heat. But, spice devotees should try the chef's special dry chili chicken, flash-fried with garlic, scallions, and heaps of dried red chilies. Even simple vegetables like crunchy cabbage get a piping dose of Sichuan heat when massaged with chili paste and chili oil.

# La Petite Folie

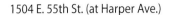

**1504 E. 55th St. (at Harper Ave.)**

Phone: 773-493-1394
Web: www.lapetitefolie.com
Prices: **$$**

Lunch Tue – Fri
Dinner Tue – Sun

Though its tree-lined courtyard off 55th Street may not be as picturesque as the Tuileries, La Petite Folie remains a transporting Gallic hideaway in Hyde Park. The graceful lace-curtained dining room and curvaceous wood bar draws scholarly types from nearby University of Chicago, with prices that satiate student budgets.

A retinue of French classics like whole trout Grenobloise are refreshed by seasonal market ingredients at the hands of Chef/co-owner Mary Mastricola. Slices of smoked duck drizzled with black currant vinaigrette get an earthy touch from apple-walnut compote in an elegant lunch salad. Even the wine list chosen by Mastricola's husband Michael is an all-French affair, with numerous by-the-glass choices from Bordeaux to Chablis.

# Mercat a la Planxa

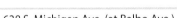

**638 S. Michigan Ave. (at Balbo Ave.)**

Phone: 312-765-0524
Web: www.mercatchicago.com
Prices: **$$**

Lunch & dinner daily

Harrison

Sit back and let executive Chef Jose Garces take you on a culinary tour of Barcelona by way of this operation in the Renaissance Blackstone Hotel. While he may not be a daily fixture here, his take on Catalan food will satisfy the most ardent fan. Climb a staircase to arrive in Mercat's earthy space, where bulbs hang from a cavernous ceiling and cast a radiant glow upon the gourmet fare.

For all-out satisfaction, share tapas like *pimentos de padron* (fried peppers with *salbitxada*) or spinach tossed with speck and fig. Savory palates enjoy charcuterie or cheese, while *croquetas de xocolata* set atop torched banana marshmallows are a fun finish.

"The Catalan Express"—a two-course lunch with iced tea for under $18—offers good value.

Chicago ▲ Chinatown & South

# MingHin

 Chinese XX

**A4**

### 2168 S. Archer Ave. (at Princeton Ave.)

**Phone:** 312-808-1999     Lunch & dinner daily
**Web:** www.minghincuisine.com
**Prices:** 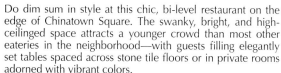    Cermak-Chinatown

Do dim sum in style at this chic, bi-level restaurant on the edge of Chinatown Square. The swanky, bright, and high-ceilinged space attracts a younger crowd than most other eateries in the neighborhood—with guests filling elegantly set tables spaced across stone tile floors or in private rooms adorned with vibrant colors.

Drool over the kitchen's glistening slabs of ribs, pork belly, and roast duck hanging on hooks. Then, sip a cup of jasmine tea while checking off a multitude of dim sum choices on the menu board. Crispy-skinned braised pork belly Macau-style, served with a bowl of sugar for sprinkling and dipping, is a must. That said, no trip here is complete without seafood selections like glossy shrimp dumplings filled with sweet green pea pod tips.

# Phoenix

Chinese X

**A4**

### 2131 S. Archer Ave. (bet. Princeton & Wentworth Aves.)

**Phone:** 312-328-0848     Lunch & dinner daily
**Web:** N/A
**Prices:** 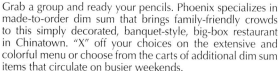    Cermak-Chinatown

Grab a group and ready your pencils. Phoenix specializes in made-to-order dim sum that brings family-friendly crowds to this simply decorated, banquet-style, big-box restaurant in Chinatown. "X" off your choices on the extensive and colorful menu or choose from the carts of additional dim sum items that circulate on busier weekends.

A boneless, red-stained slab of moist and tender barbecue pork gets even better when dipped into hot Chinese mustard. *Har gao* and *siu mai* are delicately steamed and filled with whole rock shrimp, fragrant ginger, and garlic. Potstickers are expertly fried and juicy.

À la carte menu items also offered for dinner include the chef's special crispy beef tenderloin, Peking duck, and traditional Sichuan dishes.

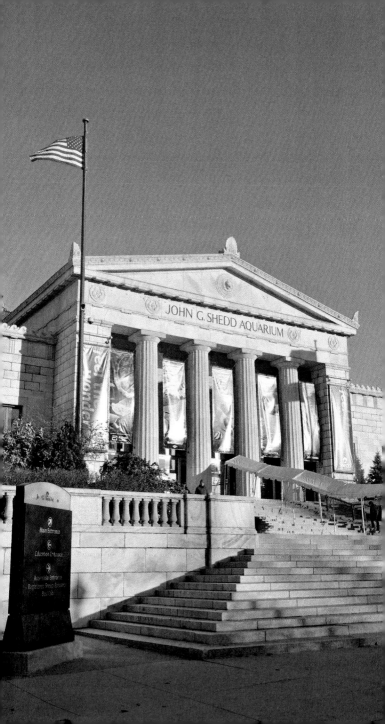

# Gold Coast

## GLITZ & GLAMOUR

The moniker says it all: the Gold Coast is one of the Windy City's most posh neighborhoods, flaunting everything from swanky high-rises along Lake Shore Drive to dazzling boutiques dotting Michigan Avenue. Stroll down the Magnificent Mile to discover that money can indeed buy it all, after which a spree at Oak Street will reveal millionaires mingling over Manolos and heiresses rummaging for handbags.

## APPLAUDING THE ARTS

Through the glamor, Gold Coast architecture is not just notable but stunning; and mansions crafted in regal Queen Anne, Georgian Revival, as well as Richardsonian Romanesque styles are unequivocally breathtaking. However, this neighborhood is not all about the glitz; it is also deeply committed to the arts, housing both the Museum of Contemporary Art as well as the world-leading Newberry Library. Culture vultures are sure to uncover something edgy and unique at A Red Orchid Theater, after which the exotic lunchtime buffet at **Gaylord** seems not only opportune, but also obligatory. This prized subterranean Indian location, with its spelled-out menu items and fully-stocked bar, is sought by both aficionados as well as anyone hungering for free appetizers during happy hour. Nearby, Le Cordon Bleu College of Culinary Arts houses **Technique**, a student-run restaurant where diners get to glimpse the next food fad in Chicago kitchens.

## RAUCOUS NIGHTS

Art and history notwithstanding, the Gold Coast also knows how to party. Visit any pub, club, or restaurant along Rush and Division streets to get a sense of how the cool kids hold it down. Opened in 2007, **The Drawing Room** is an upscale cocktail lounge complete with small plates of bar-style food. Given their vast lineup of grand libations, this sleek spot keeps the crowds entertained well into the wee hours of the morning. By then, breakfast should be on the burner at the **Original Pancake House**. This may seem like a lowbrow treat for a high-brow neighborhood, but few things are more satisfying than their fluffy pancakes, towering waffles, and sizzling skillet eggs. Another perfect place to start your day is at Italian deli **L'Appetito** with its heartwarming breakfasts, baked goods, and Italian- or American-style sandwiches. But, there is also some darn good junk food in this white-gloved capital of prosperity. American comfort classics like sliders, burgers, and mac and cheese find their way into the menu at **LuxBar**, a dynamic lounge and bar scene, favored for people-watching. For sweets after your savories, head over to **Teuscher's** for decadent dark chocolate or **Corner Bakery Cafe** for a fleet of bakery fresh sweets—the golden-brown cinnamon crème cake topped with crumbles of cinnamon streusel and powdered sugar has been drawing neighborhood residents for over two decades now and is a signature for good reason.

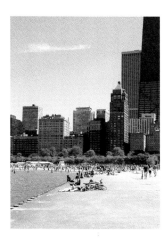

outside **Downtown Dogs**. Need a cup that revives after all these robust treats? **TeaGschwendner** is a lovely boutique where locals lose themselves in a world of exotic selections. But, if you don't feel like steeping your own "Sencha Claus" blend, then snag a seat at **Argo Tea** where clouds of whipped cream and flavorful iced drinks are part of the scene. It's just like Starbucks without the coffee! Serious cooks and gourmands make a beeline for **The Spice House**, where a vast spectrum of high quality and often esoteric spices, seasonings, and rubs (ground and blended in-house) make for an integral part of any delightful dinner party at home.

## HEAVEN ON EARTH

In keeping with its quintessentially elegant and old-world repute, the Gold Coast allows you to don Grandma's pearls for afternoon tea at **The Drake's Palm Court**. Daintily sip your tea while listening to the gentle strumming of a harp and sampling a tasty selection of sandwiches, pastries, and scones. If it's good enough for the Queen, it will certainly do. Also housed in The Drake Hotel, warm and luxurious **Cape Cod Room** is sublime for seafood specials and old-world cocktails, presented in oversized brandy snifters. Over on Delaware Pl, first-class wines and cocktails aren't the only thing heating up the scene at **Drumbar**—a rooftop hot spot at the Raffaello Hotel that lets the fashionable crowd frolic alfresco at night (and during the day on Sunday).

## A QUICK FIX

With many awards under its belt and boasting the best ingredients in town, **Gold Coast Dogs** is packed to the gills (er, buns). Inside, everyone is either a regular or about to become one; irrespective, they are all here for the same deliciously charred creation, perhaps topped with gooey cheddar cheese. Alternatively, humor your hot dog hankering by joining the endless queue

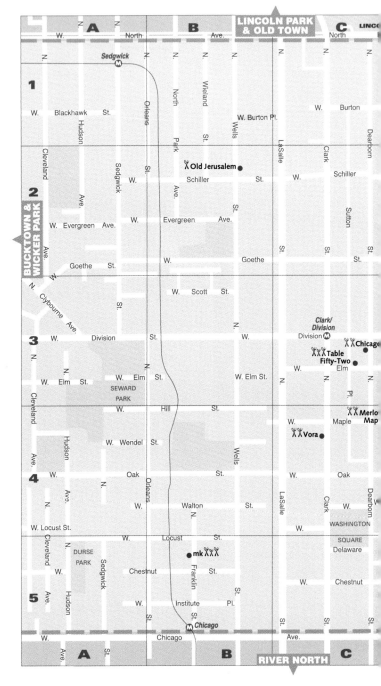

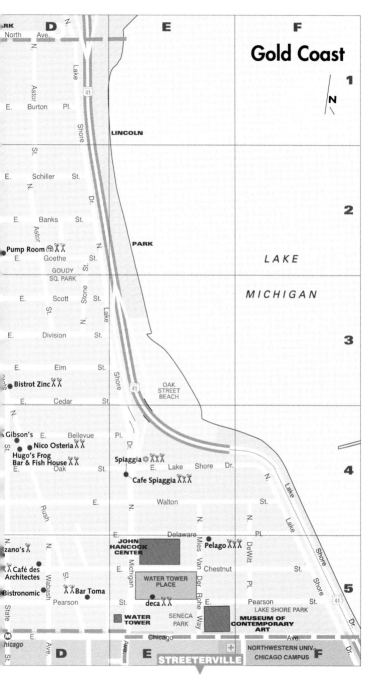

# Gold Coast

**LAKE**

**MICHIGAN**

Pump Room 🍸 ✕✕

Bistrot Zinc ✕✕

Gibson's
Nico Osteria ✕✕
Hugo's Frog
Bar & Fish House ✕✕
Spiaggia ✿ ✕✕✕

Cafe Spiaggia ✕✕✕

zano's ✕

✕✕ Café des
Architectes

Bistronomic

✕✕ Bar Toma

Pelago ✕✕✕

deca ✕✕

OAK
STREET
BEACH

JOHN
HANCOCK
CENTER

WATER TOWER
PLACE

WATER
TOWER

SENECA
PARK

LAKE SHORE PARK

MUSEUM OF
CONTEMPORARY
ART

NORTHWESTERN UNIV.
CHICAGO CAMPUS

STREETERVILLE

87

# Bar Toma

 **D5**

Italian

## 110 E. Pearson St. (bet. Michigan Ave. & Rush St.)

**Phone:** 312-266-3110
**Web:** www.bartomachicago.com
**Prices:** $$

Lunch & dinner daily

Chicago (Red)

Before Eataly came to town, Tony Mantuano was giving Chicagoans a whirlwind tour of Italian cuisine at Bar Toma. Stomachs growl at the sight of the pizza, gelato, pastry, and espresso stations ringing the room, and the family-style menu encourages sharing, with plates arriving from the kitchen as they're ready.

Hand-tossed thin-crust pizzas come in interesting varieties such as *merguez* sausage with olives and pistachios, as well as the classic Margherita. Burgers like the Bomba are a knife-and-fork deal: a juicy veal and beef patty with tomato jam, *fior di latte* mozzarella, and a handful of arugula in a pita-style bun. Gorgonzola gelato, served with warm roasted apple halves and crumbled amaretti cookies, is a delightfully rewarding dessert.

# Bistronomic

**D5**

French

## 840 N. Wabash Ave. (bet. Chestnut & Pearson Sts.)

**Phone:** 312-944-8400
**Web:** www.bistronomic.net
**Prices:** $$

Lunch Wed – Sun
Dinner nightly

 Chicago (Red)

Tucked away from the buzz of Magnificent Mile, Bistronomic is a great place to cool your (tired) heels. At first, its exterior may look a little unloved, but enter through its revolving door to arrive at a warm room that's focused on the bonhomie of dining with friends. Oxblood walls, grey banquettes, and a central bar give it a bistro feel, while the kitchen exudes creativity via fresh and tasty classics.

A modern interpretation of Niçoise salad with seared tuna, chopped olives, and baby potatoes is full of flavor—and perfectly coupled with crusty ciabatta slathered with cornichons and homemade pâté. Dinner may up the ante, but dessert rules at all times: imagine a homey poached Bosc pear glazed with vanilla ice cream and almond flakes.

# Bistrot Zinc

 French

**D3**

### 1131 N. State St. (bet. Elm & Cedar Sts.)

**Phone:** 312-337-1131                           Lunch & dinner daily
**Web:** www.bistrotzinc.com
**Prices:** $$                                     Clark/Division

 If you couldn't tell from the bright red exterior and hand-painted windows, Bistrot Zinc is indeed a classic dressed in mosaic-tiled floors, lemon-tinted walls hung with mirrors, woven rattan chairs, and yes, that curvaceous zinc bar. Suits, locals, and Gold Coast power shoppers populate the tables from lunch through dinner, as white-aproned waiters happily uncork bottles of *rouge et blanc*.

Don't look for modern surprises on the menu; contentment here is attained through uncomplicated but expertly prepared French dishes from frites to frisée. Whole trout, pan-fried until golden and napped with butter sauce, hits all the right notes; while daily standards like croque monsieur or French onion soup are enhanced by more ambitious monthly specials.

# Café des Architectes

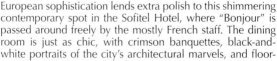 Contemporary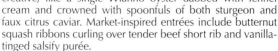

**D5**

### 20 E. Chestnut St. (at Wabash Ave.)

**Phone:** 312-324-4063                           Lunch & dinner daily
**Web:** www.cafedesarchitectes.com
**Prices:** $$$                                    Chicago (Red)

 European sophistication lends extra polish to this shimmering contemporary spot in the Sofitel Hotel, where "Bonjour" is passed around freely by the mostly French staff. The dining room is just as chic, with crimson banquettes, black-and-white portraits of the city's architectural marvels, and floor-to-ceiling windows with striking steel accents.

 The seasonally shifting lineup of small plates is simple but creative, like a single Wianno oyster dabbed with fennel cream and crowned with spoonfuls of both sturgeon and faux citrus caviar. Market-inspired entrées include butternut squash ribbons curling over tender beef short rib and vanilla-tinged salsify purée.

 For a more casual, small bites affair, move to Le Bar, the hotel's chic watering hole.

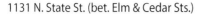

# Cafe Spiaggia

**E4**

### 980 N. Michigan Ave. (at Oak St.)

**Phone:** 312-280-2750  
**Web:** www.spiaggiarestaurant.com/cafe  
**Prices:** $$

Lunch & dinner daily

 Chicago (Red)

Time for a Roman holiday? Loosen your tie at Cafe Spiaggia, which offers all the Italian romance of its sophisticated next-door sibling in a more relaxed setting. Romanesque *trompe l'oeil* murals and gladiatorial torch lights enliven the long space. Take a table by the window for Oak Street Beach and Lake Michigan views—not quite the Amalfi coast, but close enough.

As with the flagship restaurant, each dish showcases top-notch ingredients. Ethereally crisp batter envelops sweet prawns and squid in *fritto misto*. Silky handmade ravioli are tenderly tucked with fresh ricotta, the season's pungent ramps, and crunchy hazelnuts for contrast. Tiramisu is a delight; light and creamy layers are dusted with luxe cocoa and topped with a delicate tuile.

# Chicago Q

**C3**

### 1160 N. Dearborn St. (bet. Division & Elm Sts.)

**Phone:** 312-642-1160  
**Web:** www.chicagoqrestaurant.com  
**Prices:** $$

Lunch & dinner daily

 Clark/Division

Banish all pre-conceived notions of rustic, honky-tonk shacks and smoky barbecue joints before you lay eyes on Chicago Q. Dolled-up in gleaming white subway tiles, glass enclosures, and shiny dark wood accents, this elegant bi-level row house nestled between buildings fits the prosperous atmosphere of nearby Rush Street to a T.

Chef/pitmaster Lee Ann Whippen, also the reigning queen of Chicago's barbecue scene, turns out lusciously tender Kobe brisket, pulled pork, and chicken that begs for a bourbon flight or maybe a Q martini with smoked olives. Pony up for the competition-style ribs, rubbed with a secret concoction that puts other 'cue to shame. Watermelon salad with grapes and balsamic glaze is a fittingly refined side for such superb slabs.

# deca

 Contemporary

**160 E. Pearson St. (at Water Tower Place)**

Phone: 312-573-5160  
Web: www.decarestaurant.com  
Prices: **$$**

Lunch & dinner daily

 Chicago (Red)

Part of the Ritz-Carlton's expansive 12th floor lobby, deca is a casual haunt that still keeps a few high-end accents around. Paintings hung in gilded frames add to the attractiveness in the seated dining area; and a gently trickling sculptural fountain (illuminated by a skylight) offers an auditory escape from the lobby's background buzz.

The well-edited menu features light, seasonal dishes that are skillfully prepared. Two large pillows of freshly made squash ravioli are garnished with hearty kale pistou, pickled wild mushrooms, and toasted pepitas. Wild salmon with a crunchy mustard crust is bathed in luxurious garlic-red wine jus. Finish in style with a wedge of tangy lemon tart decorated with fresh raspberries and set atop a neat pool of coulis.

# Gibson's

Steakhouse

**1028 N. Rush St. (at Bellevue Pl.)**

Phone: 312-266-8999  
Web: www.gibsonssteakhouse.com  
Prices: **$$$**

Lunch & dinner daily

 Clark/Division

Gibson's is the George Clooney of Chicago steakhouses: a little grey at the temples (it's been around since 1988), but still undeniably appealing to ladies and gents alike. Its sidewalk and atrium seating provide prime people-watching for the attractive locals gathered here, while a sultry, wood-paneled interior exudes timeless masculinity where white-jacketed waiters recite nightly specials.

The menu doesn't need to deviate from the classics—thick and juicy bone-in steaks charred expertly to medium-rare get a punch from creamy horseradish sauce; while raw bar grub like Alaskan king crab cocktail or lobster bisque are the real deal, served simply but flavorfully letting the seafood shine. The bar is a lively destination of its own.

# Hugo's Frog Bar & Fish House

**D4**

### 1024 N. Rush St. (bet. Bellevue Pl. & Oak St.)

**Phone:** 312-640-0999
**Web:** www.hugosfrogbar.com
**Prices:** $$

Lunch Sat – Sun
Dinner nightly
 Clark/Division

Housed in a sprawling setting adjacent to big brother Gibson's, Hugo's always seems packed. The vast dining room sets white linen-topped tables amidst dark polished wood and pale walls decorated with a mounted swordfish, fish prints, and model ships. Hugo's bar draws its own crowds with abundant counter seating.

The menu focuses on a selection of fish preparations as well as steaks and chops. These are supplemented by stone crab claws, oysters, crab cakes, chowders, and sautéed frog's legs. Speaking of frog's legs, the restaurant takes its name from the nickname of owner Hugo Ralli's grandfather, General Bruce Hay of Her Majesty's Imperial Forces.

Bring a football team to share a slice of the Muddy Bottom Pie, a decadent (and enormous) ice cream cake.

# Merlo on Maple

**C4**

### 16 W. Maple St. (bet. Dearborn & State Sts.)

**Phone:** 312-335-8200
**Web:** www.merlochicago.com
**Prices:** $$$

Dinner nightly

 Clark/Division

The multi-level Victorian brownstone that houses Merlo on Maple retains its turn-of-the-century charm, but the food speaks with an Italian accent. Hand-carved banisters lead to a second-floor dining room next to the animated kitchen. More subdued revelry can be found on the lower level, where servers light candles at each linen-covered table.

Chef/owner Luisa Silvia Marani brings a bit of her heritage to every dish, and many recipes come from her grandmother's archives in Emilia-Romagna. As such, no meal here would be complete without a bowl of delicate handmade tagliatelle tossed with meaty ragù Bolognese. Slices of warm *tarta di carciofi* stuffed with artichokes, mortadella, creamy eggs, and *Parmigiano Reggiano* showcase a host of quality ingredients.

# mk

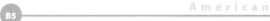

American ✗✗✗

**B5**

## 868 N. Franklin St. (bet. Chestnut & Locust Sts.)

**Phone:** 312-482-9179     Dinner nightly
**Web:** www.mkchicago.com
**Prices:** $$$     Chicago (Brown)

The larger than life "mk" emblazoned on the side of the former paint factory remains, but after 16 years on the western edge of River North, Chef Michael Kornick's eponymous flagship celebrated with a face-lift. Rich, warm browns replace mustard tones within this lofty, skylit space, still a favorite for big nights and romantic evenings.

Fear not: mk's signature pommes frites with truffle cream have stuck around, but the new 40-seat bar features a revived lineup of bites as well as a hearty menu of mains like pan-roasted duck breast with anise-scented cherries and grilled Mission figs. Seasonal desserts such as the strawberry shorty are playfully named but gracefully constructed, pairing a lemon biscuit with pine nuts and white balsamic ice cream.

# Nico Osteria

Italian ✗✗

**D4**

## 1015 N. Rush St. (bet. Bellevue Pl. & Oak St.)

**Phone:** 312-994-7100     Lunch & dinner daily
**Web:** www.nicoosteria.com
**Prices:** $$$     Chicago (Red)

Buzz around Nico Osteria has already reached deafening levels, especially since this Paul Kahan spot isn't tucked into a gentrifying corner of the city, but situated smack dab in the center of the chic Gold Coast. Communal bar seating keeps the space humming with energy, but moody lighting conspires to keep the vibe relaxed.

Though billed as Italian-inspired cooking, the kitchen takes liberties with traditional dishes on the seafood-heavy menu. Well-grilled and generously-oiled sourdough fett'unta topped with combinations like baccalà and Dungeness crab are rustic introductions to the meal. Ask for more bread to soak up the Neapolitan-style ragù—a skillet bubbling with goodies like a swordfish meatball and slabs of grilled pork belly in a tomato gravy.

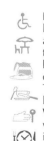

# Old Jerusalem

**Middle Eastern** ✗

### 1411 N. Wells St. (bet. North Ave. & Schiller St.)

**Phone:** 312-944-0459                                          Lunch & dinner daily
**Web:** www.oldjerusalemchicago.com
**Prices:** 😋                                                          🚇 Sedgwick

Set on a charming and centrally located stretch of Old Town, this family-run Middle Eastern favorite has been eagerly accommodating its happy customers for years.

The menu focuses on Lebanese classics, such as tabbouleh with cracked wheat, scallions, and tomatoes, seasoned with lemon, olive oil, and plenty of crisp, green parsley. Hummus arrives rich with tahini, perhaps accompanying the likes of grilled chicken kebabs and traditional flatbreads. Finish with flaky-sweet baklava.

While the décor may not impress, Old Jerusalem manages to make its well-worn looks feel cozy and comfortable for everyone. Very reasonable prices, family-friendly service, and generous portions make this *the* neighborhood go-to spot, whether dining in or taking out.

# Pelago

**Italian** ✗✗✗

### 201 E. Delaware Pl. (at Mies van der Rohe Way)

**Phone:** 312-280-0700                                          Lunch & dinner daily
**Web:** www.pelagorestaurant.com
**Prices:** $$$                                                          🚇 Chicago (Red)

Adjacent to Hotel Raffaello, the elegance of this brick structure is accentuated by large arched windows. Inside, the bi-level room wears a crisp style à la high ceilings, eminently comfortable leather seats, and a soft azure-blue color scheme.

If the décor doesn't transport you to the Mediterranean in a flash, look to the regional Italian menu with ingredients imported directly. A salad of plum tomatoes topped with creamy burrata and fragrant basil in a light dressing is as inherently satisfying. So, too, are pasta signatures including rich *risotto alle verdure* or creamy ricotta-filled ravioli swimming in a vibrant sauce of spinach and showered with slivers of nutty Parmesan. Swap dessert for a fine selection of imported cheeses, and never look back.

# Pizano's

P i z z a

 **D5**

## 864 N. State St. (bet. Chestnut St. & Delaware Pl.)

**Phone:** 312-751-1766        Lunch & dinner daily
**Web:** www.pizanoschicago.com
**Prices:**        Chicago (Red)

While Chicago may be hailed as home of the deep-dish pizza, the thin-crust pies at Pizano's have justly earned their own devoted following. This refreshing and cozy local spot recalls Italian-American style without feeling like a chain-restaurant cliché; even the waitstaff's genuine warmth is palpable.

Of course, the crowds come for the crust—here it is flaky, buttery, thin (by local standards), and perfectly crisp. As unexpected as it sounds, their pizzas are some of the best in town. And yet, it should be no surprise as pizza has long been the family calling: owner Rudy Malnati's father founded Pizzeria Uno.

The "thinner" offspring at Pizano's sates its growing fan-base from three locations, and even ships to those far from the Second City.

# Pump Room

 **D2**

C o n t e m p o r a r y

## 1301 N. State Pkwy. (at Goethe St.)

**Phone:** 312-229-6740        Lunch & dinner daily
**Web:** www.pumproom.com
**Prices:** $$       Clark/Division

Back when the Public Hotel was known as the Ambassador East, scores of celebrities clinked glasses and forks in the Pump Room. Though these memories are preserved in black-and-white photos hung throughout the hotel, today the sunken dining room is a classy, updated space where cushy circular booths, mod orbital lights, and brown kraft paper placemats meld flawlessly.

Under the direction of Jean-Georges Vongerichten, the seasonal American menu is as casually riveting as the décor. An amply sized boneless fried chicken breast is moist and flavorful beneath its shatteringly crisp coating, ready to sop up habanero-infused butter sauce. In an elegant sundae, handfuls of candied peanuts and caramel popcorn top three neat quenelles of salted caramel ice cream.

# Spiaggia

E4

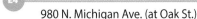

**980 N. Michigan Ave. (at Oak St.)**

| | | |
|---|---|---|
| **Phone:** | 312-280-2750 | Dinner nightly |
| **Web:** | www.spiaggiarestaurant.com | |
| **Prices:** | $$$$ | 🚇 Chicago (Red) |

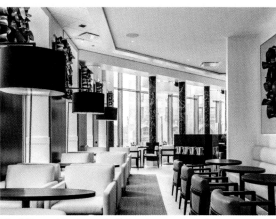

Chef Tony Mantuano's Spiaggia once again welcomes a rush of canoodlers and celebrants following a thorough renovation aptly timed to commemorate his 30th year in operation. This sterling Gold Coast Italian is now an ethereal expanse where newly installed frosted glass panels, white leather furnishings, and a porcelain-tiled bar area are illuminated by sunlight streaming through a wall of windows looking out onto Lake Michigan. Dark oak tables and bronzed botanical sculptures, as well as those original marble columns are earthy aesthetic diversions.

A series of raw preparations comprise the antipasti selection and lead to an impressive pasta lineup, featuring a perfectly cooked tangle of dried *spaghetti alla chitarra* judiciously dressed with a knockout combination of grey mullet *bottarga*, fresh chickpeas, and finely ground breadcrumbs. Breast of guinea hen is wrapped in *guanciale*, cooked in the wood-fired oven, and paired with a plump confit leg in Wagyu beef fat. A pickled garlic scape nicely offsets the decadent flavors of this lovely entrée.

There is less cause for celebration come dessert time since the choice is limited to a selection of miniature pastries and sweets.

# Table Fifty-Two

 Southern

 C3

**52 W. Elm St. (bet. Clark & Dearborn Sts.)**

| | |
|---|---|
| **Phone:** | 312-573-4000 |
| **Web:** | www.tablefifty-two.com |
| **Prices:** | $$$ |

Lunch Sun
Dinner Tue – Sun
 Clark/Division

Chef Art Smith's drawl floats overhead like a warm breeze as he chats up guests inside Table Fifty-Two's cozy white row house, a stately survivor of the Great Chicago Fire. Southern charm permeates every inch of the room, from the pressed copper ceiling to the white sideboards to a wood-burning oven churning out the restaurant's signature biscuits.

The meal might get started with an amuse-bouche of deviled eggs topped with pickled mustard seeds, and if it's a Sunday or Monday, the famous fried chicken will be making an appearance on many plates. Plump fried green tomatoes and thick pork chops are on order, but for a true down-home taste, get a tall wedge of hummingbird cake, fragrant with banana and pineapple and slathered in cream cheese frosting.

# Vora

 Asian

C4

**1028 N. Clark St. (bet. Maple & Oak Sts.)**

| | |
|---|---|
| **Phone:** | 312-929-2035 |
| **Web:** | www.vorachicago.com |
| **Prices:** | $$ |

Lunch & dinner daily

 Clark/Division

Whether you're a carnivore, herbivore, or somewhere in between, Vora's plethora of Asian offerings aims to please. The modern space puts nature at the forefront with vine-like clusters of light bulbs snaking above bars, room dividers punctuated with floral cutouts, and sprightly lime-green banquettes.

Can't choose from the health-oriented lineup of Taiwanese dim sum, Indian curries, or Chinese classics? The dim sum box is actually a bento offering a dizzying array of multi-cultural tastes: soft shrimp *siu mai*, juicy *xiao long bao*, steamed pork buns, and miso soup, as well as other bites. Slices of Sichuan beef and vegetables stir-fried in chili sauce can be amped up to match Chinatown's level of heat, or toned down to suit milder tastes.

A fascinating pair of lively North Side neighborhoods, both Humboldt Park and Logan Square have for long been revered as Chicagoland's heart and soul. Yes, they may reside a few steps off the beaten path, but locals here still live to eat and can be found searching the wares at global grocers, secret bodegas, and quick falafel shops. **Smalls** is one such tasty little smoke hut packed with foodies yearning for familiar barbecue specialties presented alongside unique Asian comfort food. Here, hickory-smoked brisket on Texas toast with Thai-style "tiger cry" sauce has earned a cult following for good reason. **Koreatown** is another prized thoroughfare spanning miles along Lawrence Avenue and preparing faithful fare that commences with

*banchan*, followed by charred *galbi*, juicy and tender *bulgogi*, or heartwarming *bibimbap*. Then, stroll along tree-lined streets complete with quaint buildings and trendy shops, until you land upon **Bang Bang Pie Shop**. Here, handmade, buttery biscuits or sweet and savory pies are likely to keep you inside—indefinitely. Community gardens like **Campbell Co-op** and **Drake Garden** with their special harvest of vegetables and plants not only unite the neighborhood's diverse groups, but also ensure gorgeous greenery in the midst of this city.

Humboldt Park is also home to Chicago's vibrant Puerto Rican community—just look for Paseo Boricua, the flag-shaped steel gateway demarcating the

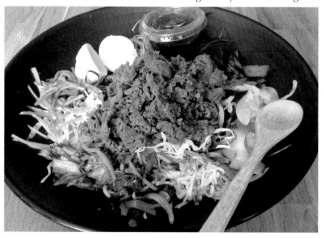

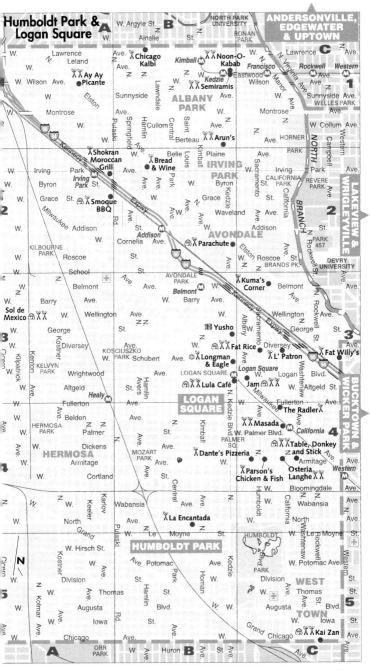

Humboldt Park & Logan Square

**A** | **B** | **C**

W. Argyle St. — NORTH PARK UNIVERSITY — RONAN PARK — ANDERSONVILLE, EDGEWATER & UPTOWN

W. Ainslie St.

W. Lawrence Leland Ave. — ✗ Chicago Kalbi — Kimball Ⓜ — ✗ Noon-O-Kabab — Francisco — Rockwell — Western Ave. — N. Virginia Ave. — W. Lawrence Ave. — **C**

W. Wilson Ave. — ✗✗ Ay Ay Picante — Eastwood — Wilson — Manor — Sunnyside Ave. — WELLES PARK — **1**

✗✗ Semiramis — Kedzie

Elston — Sunnyside — Lawndale — Springfield — ALBANY PARK

W. Montrose Ave. — Pulaski — Hamlin — Central — Saint — Montrose — W. Collum Ave. — HORNER PARK — Campbell — Western Ave.

Kennedy Expwy — I-90 — Cullom — Berteau — ✗✗ Arun's Ave.

W. Belle Louis Plaine Ave. — IRVING PARK — Sacramento — Irving Park — CALIFORNIA PARK — REVERE PARK

✗ Shokran Moroccan Grill — W. Irving Park St. — **Irving Park** — Ave. — Kimball — California St. — NORTH BRANCH

W. Irving Park

W. Byron — Byron — Ave. — Byron St. — **2**

W. Grace St. — Ⓜ✗ Smoque BBQ — Grace — Kedzie — Grace St. — PARK 2

W. Milwaukee — Waveland — California Ave.

W. Addison — Addison — St. — Addison — St. — PARK 457 — DEVRY UNIVERSITY

KILBOURNE PARK — St. — Addison Ⓜ — Elston — Roscoe St. — Rockwell St.

W. Roscoe — Cornelia Ave. — Ⓜ✗ Parachute — I-90 — Roscoe — BRANDS PK.

W. School — School — AVONDALE PARK — I-90 I-94 — Sacramento — ✗ Kuma's Corner — Belmont

W. Belmont Ave. — **Belmont** Ⓜ — W. Belmont Ave. — N. Rockwell Ave. — **3**

W. Barry — N. — W. Barry St.

Sol de Mexico ✗✗ — W. Wellington Ave. — Albany — Wellington Ave. — George St. — **3**

W. George St. — ZZ — N. Sacramento Expwy

W. Diversey — Kostner — KOSCIUSZKO PARK — ✗✗ Fat Rice — Diversey — ✗ L' Patron — ✗ Fat Willy's

Kilpatrick — Kenton — KELVYN PARK — W. Schubert Ave. — ⊛✗ Longman & Eagle — LOGAN SQUARE — Logan — Washtenaw

W. Wrightwood — LOGAN SQUARE Ⓜ — Logan Blvd. — St.

W. Altgeld — Hamlin — Ⓜ✗ Lula Café — ✗✗ Jam — Altgeld — St.

Healy Ⓜ — Ave. — Milwaukee — Fullerton — The Radler ✗ — BUCKTOWN & WICKER PARK

W. Fullerton Ave. — LOGAN SQUARE — Fullerton Ave.

W. Belden — Ave. — ✗✗ Masada — California — **4**

HERMOSA PARK — Palmer — St. — W. Palmer Blvd. — ⊛✗ Table, Donkey and Stick ✗ — Western

W. Dickens — MOZART PARK — PALMER SQ — Armitage Ave.

W. Armitage — ✗ Dante's Pizzeria — Osteria Langhe ✗✗

W. Cortland — St. — ✗ Parson's Chicken & Fish — Ave.

Keeler — Karlov — Wabansia — Ave. — Humboldt — Bloomingdale Ave. — California — Wabansia — Ave.

**N** — W. North Ave. — Grand — W. Le Moyne St. — ✗ La Encantada — North — W. Le Moyne St. — HUMBOLDT

W. Hirsch St. — Pulaski — **HUMBOLDT PARK** — Potomac Ave. — Homan — HUMBOLDT PARK — W. Potomac Ave. — Washtenaw — Rockwell — Western

Kostner — Kedzie

W. Division — Ave. — Thomas — Hamlin — St. — Division — WEST — Thomas — St.

Kolmar — W. Augusta — Blvd. — Augusta — TOWN — Blvd.

W. Iowa — Rd. — W. Iowa — St. — **5**

Kolmar Ave. — Chicago — W. Chicago — Grand — Chicago — ✗✗ Kai Zan — Ave.

ORR PARK — W. Huron — **B** — Ave. — Ave. — **C**

**A** | **B** | **C**

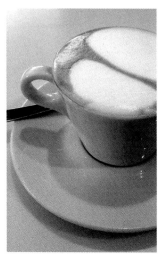

Bohemian-style coffee house and lounge flaunting the likes of excellent coffee, scones, and comfy couches. If that doesn't have you hooked for good, look to **Grandma J's Local Kitchen** bestowing folks with an abundant breakfast spread served alongside distinctive sides like French toast sticks and kale chips. Pastries take the cake at **Shokolad** and the staff at this Ukrainian gem makes sure you never lose sight of that fact: a stacked-to-the-top glass bakery case showcases its wares to great effect. Their signature cheesecake lollipops may not be from the old country, but rest assured that they are extraordinarily tasty.

## LOGAN SQUARE

An eclectic mix of cuisines combined with historic buildings and charming boulevards attracts everybody from hipsters and working-class locals, as well as artists and students to this lovely quarter. Within the culinary community, a blend of home chefs, star cooks, and staunch foodies can be found plunging into the shelves at **Kurowski's Sausage Shop**, a respected butcher specializing in handmade cuts of Polish meats. Novices take note: pair one of their flavorful sausages with toasted rye before picking up some pickles to-go from the very delicious and always reliable **Dill Pickle Food Co-op**. In line with this cultural explosion, Logan Square is also home to **4 Suyos**, a well-regarded Peruvian favorite cooking the classics with a creative twist. Find a plethora of regulars who practically live here for the soft, creamy tofu marinated in *anticuchos* sauce, coupled with quinoa, and crested with *queso*

district along Division Street. These storefronts are as much a celebration of the diaspora as the homeland, with an impressive selection of traditional foods, rare ingredients, and authentic *pernil*. In fact, the annual **Puerto Rican Festival** features four days of festivity, fun, and fantastic food. Get your fill of authentic Caribbean cuisine here, but for some marvelous Mexican feasting, make a dash for **Cemitas Puebla**—a mom-and-pop shop serving large, very satisfying *cemitas* slathered with meat, avocado, chipotles, and cheese.

Bill Dugan's **The Fishguy Market** has been serving Chicago's Michelin-starred restaurants for decades. However, if steaming hot dogs are a custom in Chicago, then **Jimmy's Red Hots** is the standard bearer of this neighborhood, and much to local pride they reaffirm the importance of purity here with "No freaking ketchup" and top-notch beef products. Also popular among residents is **KnockBox Café**, a *fresco*. Also of epicurean note is **Logan Square Farmer's Market** selling everything ingestible from raw honey to organic zucchini; while the uniquely sourced and beautifully packaged brews at **Gaslight Coffee Roasters** is a caffeine junkie's dream come true.

Just as kids delight in a day spent at **Margie's Candies** for their homemade chocolates, adults eagerly await a night out at **Scofflaw** for strong, gin-infused libations and secret menu combinations. Meanwhile, students prepare for an impromptu visit from *nonna* by stocking up on authentic eats from the **Half Italian Grocer**, but food wonks know to shop till they drop at **Independence Park Farmer's Market** for a divine dinner back home. Over in German-centric Lincoln Square, **Mirabell's** stays true to her Bavarian roots with plenty of big bites and bold brews. Less locally traditional but just as tantalizing is **Jimmy's Pizza Café**, justly mobbed for its mean rendition of a New York-style slice. Albany Park is another melting pot of global foods and gastronomic retreats minus the sky-high price. Plan your own Middle Eastern feast with a spectrum of cheeses, spreads, and flatbreads from **Al-Khyam Bakery & Grocery**, sealed by perfect baklava from **Nazareth Sweets**. But, if meat is what you're craving, then join the crowds of carnivores at **Charcoal Delights**, a time-tested burger joint. Otherwise, keep company with fish fans who are always in good hands at **Wellfleet**, a popular luncheonette named after the Cape Cod fishing town, and praised for instantly gratifying those crustacean cravings.

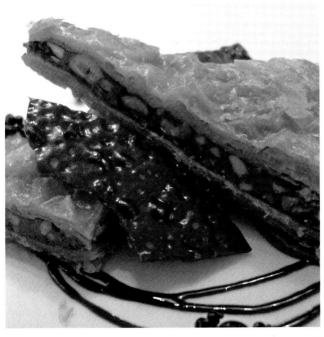

# Arun's

Thai XX

**4156 N. Kedzie Ave. (at Berteau Ave.)**

**Phone:** 773-539-1909

**Web:** www.arunsthai.com

**Prices:** $$$$

Dinner Tue – Sun

Kedzie (Brown)

Chef/owner Arun Sampanthavivat oversees every detail at this culinary mainstay, which has been serving a well-dressed, moneyed crowd since 1985.

No need to bring your reading glasses, since you won't need to fuss with a menu at Arun's. Instead, this upscale Thai restaurant treats its visitors to a 12-course prix-fixe of six appetizers, three entrées (served family-style), and three desserts. The dishes change regularly, but expect the likes of diced spicy pork served inside a grilled sweet pepper; or Panang beef curry with coconut milk. Carved vegetables shaped like butterflies and fish are memorable flourishes.

From the elegant setting and white-jacketed servers to the bountiful feast, it's no wonder people return so often for the princely experience.

# Ay Ay Picante

Peruvian XX

**4569 N. Elston Ave. (bet. Kennicott & Kiona Aves.)**

**Phone:** 773-427-4239

**Web:** www.ayaypicante.com

**Prices:**

Lunch & dinner daily

Irving Park (Blue)

Incans, Andeans, and conquistadors have shaped Peru's cultural and culinary history, and Ay Ay Picante celebrates them all, bringing flavor to an otherwise bland neighborhood. Murals of mysterious images of the Peruvian desert decorate the dining room, and pan flute melodies play in the background.

Leave the anti-carb at home; Peruvian staples of corn, potatoes, and rice are all over this six-page menu so vegetarians won't go hungry. Authenticity strikes a chord in classic dishes like crispy fried empanadas stuffed with hard-boiled egg and ground beef; or *tamal Peruano*, steamed banana leaves filled with chicken, nuts, and black olives, and paired with *salsa criolla*. Their signature *aji verde* is so much in demand it's now sold by the bottle.

# Bread & Wine

### 3732 W. Irving Park Rd. (at Ridgeway Ave.)

**Phone:** 773-866-5266
**Web:** www.breadandwinechicago.com
**Prices:** $$

Lunch Sat – Sun
Dinner Tue – Sat
 Irving Park (Blue)

Bread & Wine's mix of American bistro fare and international flair mirrors the cultural melting pot of surrounding nabe Humboldt Park, and the former laundromat's parking lot fills quickly. Solo diners perch at the 10-seat counter to watch the chefs at work, while groups crowd around tables made from cross-sections of fallen trees, snacking on barbecue *chicharrónes* or house-made charcuterie.

Plates like the mortadella sandwich smeared with olive pesto and stacked with tasso and pancetta further showcase the kitchen's prowess with cured meat. A substantial beet and barley salad is loaded with feta cheese and fresh arugula. Before you leave, browse the small market for bread, wine, and artisanal treats; diners receive a discount on same-day purchases.

# Chicago Kalbi

### 3752 W. Lawrence Ave. (bet. Hamlin & Lawndale Aves.)

**Phone:** 773-604-8183
**Web:** www.chicago-kalbi.com
**Prices:** $$

Dinner Wed – Mon

Take me out to the ballgame—or the Korean barbecue joint where a ballplayer would feel right at home. At this quirky spot, autographed baseballs line the shelves, while photographs and posters of ballplayers paper the walls. But the cluttered décor doesn't deter locals from frequenting this modest yet welcoming space.

Gas grills at each table give off an intoxicatingly savory perfume as patrons take their time searing their choice of well-marbled marinated beef, including the always-popular *bulgogi* or *kalbi*, and cool their mouths with a traditional array of *banchan*. For those who prefer their meat raw, beef tartare assumes an interesting twist of flavor and texture when folded with Asian pears, sesame seeds, and sesame oil.

# Dante's Pizzeria

Pizza ✕

C4

### 3028 W. Armitage St. (at Whipple St.)

**Phone:** 773-342-0002  
**Web:** N/A  
**Prices:** $$

Lunch & dinner daily

California (Blue)

Brush up on your knowledge of classic literature before heading to Dante's, where the Divine Comedy serves as inspiration. The no-frills décor, basic counter service, and metal soundtrack may seem like purgatory, but stay awhile as the pricey pies are pure paradise.

Each of the 20-inch pizzas—floppy and foldable in the classic New York-style—reference characters from this famous Italian epic. Try the Beatrice with garlic sauce and mushrooms; or the signature Inferno pie with nine rings of toppings like giardiniera, jalapeños, and pepperoni. It would be sinful not to share a starter of deep-fried poblano poppers oozing with cream cheese, bacon, and red onion; or deliciously rich mozzarella sticks. Not ready for such gluttony? Simply order by the slice.

# Fat Rice

Macanese ✕✕

C3

### 2957 W. Diversey Ave. (at Sacramento Ave.)

**Phone:** 773-661-9170  
**Web:** www.eatfatrice.com  
**Prices:** $$

Lunch Fri – Sun  
Dinner Tue – Sat

Logan Square

Not familiar with the food of Macau? Not to worry—Fat Rice turns the uninitiated into believers nightly. A wooden pergola shelters hardy souls braving the infamous wait for a table. Bar seating around the open kitchen gives a bird's eye view of the mélange of ingredients used in each dish, though servers are happy to walk any guest through the intoxicating mashup of Portuguese and Asian cuisine.

Sharing is recommended for platters like the namesake *arroz gordo*, a paella-esque blend of meat, shellfish, and pickles. Pillowy bread sops up chunky olive-and-*bacalhau* spread in a pool of verdant olive oil. Shredded dried pork and fried shallots are intriguing but successful dessert components when paired with salted caramel, sesame, and crispy rice.

# Fat Willy's

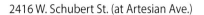

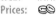  ✕

 **2416 W. Schubert St. (at Artesian Ave.)**

**Phone:** 773-782-1800        Lunch & dinner daily
**Web:** www.fatwillys.com
**Prices:** $$

Fat Willy's telegraphs an authentic and messy barbecue experience by luring all with its wafting scent of smoke, hickory, and applewood piles stacked at the entrance. This is only further teased by homemade sauces and paper towel rolls poised atop kraft paper-protected tables. With customers' doodles from the tables plastering the walls, it's a sign everyone comes and leaves happy here.

Crack through the charred surface on baby back and St. Louis-style rib slabs to devour the pink-tinged center, an indication of superior smoking. Brisket might verge on the dry side, but pulled pork sandwiches are juicy, while corn dogs are hand-dipped and fried. Root beer from Milwaukee's Sprecher Brewery adds a little Midwest taste to the bona fide Southern flavor.

# Jam

 ✕✕

 **3057 W. Logan Blvd. (at Albany Ave.)**

**Phone:** 773-292-6011        Lunch Thu – Tue
**Web:** www.jamrestaurant.com
**Prices:**  Logan Square

Hiding in plain sight on a residential Logan Square block, Jam remains the sweetheart of brunch-o-philes who won't settle for some greasy spoon. Clean white walls and gray stone tables punctuated by lime green placemats give a gallery-like feel to the space; a friendly welcome and wide-open kitchen keep it homey.

Their brunch standards like French toast are nothing short of luxurious: think brioche soaked in vanilla-and-malt-spiked custard cooked sous vide to absorb every drop, then caramelized in a sizzling pan and garnished with lime leaf-whipped cream and pineapple compote. Braised beef, tangy tomato *crema*, and smoked Gouda are rolled into lacy buckwheat crêpes and topped with a sunnyside egg for an elegant take on the breakfast burrito.

105

# Kai Zan

Japanese    🍴🍴

**2557 ½ W. Chicago Ave. (at Rockwell St.)**

Phone: 773-278-5776      Dinner Thu – Tue
Web: www.eatatkaizan.com
Prices: **$$**

A recent expansion has doubled the space of Kai Zan's tiny empire on far western Chicago Avenue, adding multi-rooms of wooden tables and benches next to the original sliver of marble sushi counter. Make a reservation to guarantee a spot at the counter, where it's a pleasure to watch chefs and twin brothers Melvin and Carlo Vizconde work in synchronicity. Though known for its sushi, grilled items like juicy beef tongue complement the roster of exceptionally fresh bites. Smoky seared saba and octopus sashimi are served with typically restrained seasoning, needing nothing more than dabs of soy and a dip in pickled wasabi sauce. Monthly specials may include Eskimo clouds, a poetic name for escolar-wrapped kushi oysters with Tabasco-ponzu foam.

# Kuma's Corner

American    🍴

**2900 W. Belmont Ave. (at Francisco Ave.)**

Phone: 773-604-8769      Lunch & dinner daily
Web: www.kumascorner.com
Prices:

Even vegans know the cult following of Kuma's Corner, though there's absolutely nothing for them on the menu at this heavy metal burger joint on an unassuming Avondale corner. It's not for the faint of heart: between the crowds, the crunching blasts of sound, and the NC-17 artwork, steady yourself with a beer or bourbon while waiting for a table and a juicy patty.

The lines wouldn't be stretching out the door if the kitchen weren't cranking out kick-ass burgers. The menu features more than a dozen options of 10-oz. monsters served on pretzel rolls with myriad toppings like roasted garlic mayonnaise, house-made hot sauce, and pepper jack cheese. Almost as famous, mac and cheese with add-ins offers a comparably artery-clogging change of pace.

# La Encantada

✂

**3437 W. North Ave. (bet. Homan & St. Louis Aves.)**

**Phone:** 773-489-5026                        Dinner Tue – Sun
**Web:** www.laencantadarestaurant.com
**Prices:** 💰💰

Run by the gracious Enriquez family, this *encantada* (enchanted) spot lives up to its name. Inside, royal blue, golden yellow, and exposed brick walls are hung with bright, gallery-style artwork (much of it is for sale), while contemporary Latin tunes waft through the air, creating a quixotic vibe. Culinary inspiration begins in the family's hometown, Zacatecas, but pulls from all around the country, with seriously delectable results.

Dig into the rich and cheesy *quesadilla de huitlacoche*; or the divine *chile en Nogada*, poblano peppers stuffed with tender ground beef, squash, fruit, and crunchy walnuts, topped with a creamy walnut sauce and pomegranate seeds. Match these delicacies with such decadent sides as chipotle-whipped potatoes.

# L' Patron

✂

**2815 W. Diversey Ave. (bet. California Ave. & Mozart St.)**

**Phone:** 773-252-6335                        Lunch & dinner daily
**Web:** www.lpatronchicago.com
**Prices:** 💰💰

Don't worry—the long line stretching past L'Patron's neon-bright façade isn't cause for concern. Counter service moves quickly at this affordable and popular Diversey Avenue taqueria, as staffers smoothly satiate customers with a concise but tasty array of tortas, tacos, and burritos wrapped in handmade tortillas. The interior décor is just as colorful as the outside, with pulsing Latin music to keep you moving as you munch.

Ultra-fresh dishes are cooked to order, like a grilled burrito stuffed with roasted poblanos, caramelized onion, and tomatillo-jalapeño salsa. Crisp tortilla chips, still warm from the fryer, are addictive companions for scooping chunky, garlicky guacamole, and many plates are accompanied by a generous scoop of homemade refried beans.

Chicago ▲ Humboldt Park & Logan Square

# Longman & Eagle ✿

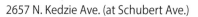
Gastropub ✕

B3

**2657 N. Kedzie Ave. (at Schubert Ave.)**

Phone: 773-276-7110
Web: www.longmanandeagle.com
Prices: $$

Lunch & dinner daily

🚇 Logan Square

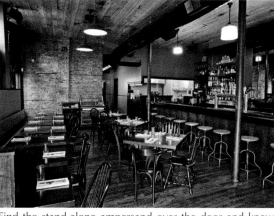

Find the stand-alone ampersand over the door and know that you have arrived at Longman & Eagle. The back room is more sedate than the bare-bones front bar, but by the time the night ends people will be packed in everywhere. This is the kind of place where the kitchen staff visibly prefers tattoos, beards, and bandanas to traditional chef toques. It's also where Millennials might bring their parents to enjoy haute cuisine without feeling as though they've sold out. The entire experience would seem a bit rough and tumble, but all that is kept in check by the outstanding food.

Aside from being delicious, the menu here is never boring so prepare yourself to want one of everything. Start with a decadent bowl of braised pork cheek and *cavatelli* in fontina-Mornay sauce, finished with grated black truffles and Parmesan. Hawaiian flavors are clear in every bite of the opah with griddled house-made sausage, pineapple relish, macadamia nut purée, and soy pudding.

Do not skip their beguiling desserts like apple pudding "pop tart" encased in tender pastry, dusted with vanilla sugar, and served alongside foie gras ice cream, poached pear, and jiggling cubes of vanilla "Jell-O."

# Lula Café

XX

**B3**

### 2537 N. Kedzie Ave. (off Logan Blvd.)

Phone: 773-489-9554

Web: www.lulacafe.com

Prices: $$

Lunch & dinner Wed – Mon

Logan Square

Simple furnishings and dim lighting provide all the ambience fans of this Logan Square hangout require, proving that Lula Café doesn't sweat the small stuff. In fact, the reclaimed bar still bears the signage of its previous life as a dry cleaner.

Thanks to the decadent likes of butterscotch bread pudding French toast, breakfast and brunch garner a cult following. The kitchen swings with the season to create dinnertime options like thinly sliced raw cobia arranged with diced Satsuma mandarin, charred kohlrabi, and slivers of Illinois gingerroot set off with Sichuan peppercorn and a drizzle of Sicilian almond oil. Chestnut *trofie* sauced with black olive-pocked wild boar ragù and sprinkled with smoked Gouda was a luscious wintertime offering.

# Masada

XX

**C4**

### 2206 N. California Ave. (bet. Lyndale & Palmer Sts.)

Phone: 773-697-8397

Web: www.masadachicago.com

Prices:

Lunch & dinner daily

California (Blue)

Masada Ramli, the mother of owner Shadi Ramli, is the inspiration of this richly adorned spot bedecked with metal lanterns and colorful glazed tiles. A collection of hamsas at the entrance wards off evil, and the lower level lounge pours a bevy of sprits including cocktails, crafts beers, and *arak*.

Although kebabs and wraps can be ordered, there's nothing commonplace about Masada's home-style cooking. Instead, imagine the likes of lamb's kidney and heart sautéed with onions and oyster mushrooms; or *fetit betinjan*, crunchy pita cubes and roasted eggplant dressed with tahini, pomegranate molasses, and lemon. A number of vegan options abound and attract, including *koshari*, a hearty mélange of rice, lentils, and gluten-free pasta, accompanied by spicy tomato sauce and tart pickles.

# Noon-O-Kabab

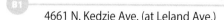

Persian ✗✗

**B1**

### 4661 N. Kedzie Ave. (at Leland Ave.)

**Phone:** 773-279-9309

**Web:** www.noonokabab.com

**Prices:** ⊖⊖

Lunch & dinner daily

🚇 Kedzie (Brown)

The uninitiated may read the name and envisage a fast-food kebab shop, but Noon-O-Kabab is a friendly neighborhood spot that takes their food seriously. The simple décor is nicely accented by walls painted with colorful murals, alcoves adorned with hand-painted tiles, and linen-topped tables conveying an authentic culinary experience.

Shakers of sumac set on each table in lieu of salt and pepper and plates of fresh pita with onion, radish, and herbs set the scene for a traditional Persian feast. Smoky, tender *koubideh* and *joujeh* skewers showcase marinated chicken and sirloin with heaping mounds of saffron-infused rice; while spicy pomegranate chicken wings do Chicago bar food one better. Close with creamy *bastani* crowned with crushed pistachios.

# Osteria Langhe

Italian ✗✗

**C4**

### 2824 W. Armitage Ave. (bet. Mozart St. & California Ave.)

**Phone:** 773-661-1582

**Web:** www.osterialanghe.com

**Prices:** $$

Dinner nightly

🚇 California (Blue)

A tapestry-length photograph of the Piemontese countryside is the only nod to tradition in Osteria Langhe's buzzy contemporary space. Lines of glowing bulbs hanging from a sculptural grid bring warmth to bare wood tables and metal chairs. A communal table at the restaurant's entrance, visible through the garage-like glass façade, shines like a beacon of conviviality.

Don't spoil your appetite by eating too many of the complimentary house-made black olive *grissini* before the entrées arrive. Regional specialties abound on the menu: rich, eggy strands of Piemontese *tajarin* pasta swirl around braised beef ragù or simple butter and sage. Use delicate crêpe-like *crespella*, filled with a variety of seasonal vegetables, to sop up spicy leek *fonduta*.

# Parachute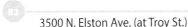

Chicago ▲ Humboldt Park & Logan Square

✕

**3500 N. Elston Ave. (at Troy St.)**

| | | |
|---|---|---|
| **Phone:** | 773-654-1460 | Dinnter Tue – Sat |
| **Web:** | www.parachuterestaurant.com | |
| **Prices:** | **$$** | |

A rollicking spin is given to Korean cuisine at Avondale's newfangled mom-and-pop operation. Chefs Beverly Kim and John Clark, aided by a talented support staff, apply their mutually impressive backgrounds to conjure up a creative carte.

Crisp slices of *chameh* melon are the foundation for a salad of mustard greens, crushed Manzanilla olives, and toasted buckwheat; while *dolsot bibimbap* gets a delish makeover. Here it is topped with line-caught albacore tuna, barbecued onions, preserved lemon, and a runny duck egg. The scorching hot bowl sears the fish and transforms the rice kernels into a toothsome amber crust. Parachute's unique ideology continues through to desert when black sesame cake arrives crowned with blueberry sorbet and powdered browned butter.

# Parson's Chicken & Fish

✕

**2952 W. Armitage Ave. (at Humboldt Blvd.)**

| | | |
|---|---|---|
| **Phone:** | 773-384-3333 | Lunch & dinner daily |
| **Web:** | www.parsonschickenandfish.com | |
| **Prices:** | **$$** | California (Blue) |

If the cherry-red 1977 El Camino emblazoned with a crossed fish-bone-and-drumstick logo doesn't pique your curiosity, the young, cool kids waiting to stuff their faces with tricked-out junk food makes Parson's impossible to miss. It's no surprise that this throwback chicken shack is the brainchild of the Longman & Eagle team.

Slurp a neon Negroni slushy while waiting for an open booth or communal table and peruse the menu, which draws inspiration from coastal, comfort, soul, and street food. Cold chickpea salad with grilled octopus and *chermoula* or hush puppies with chopped scallion should be a new picnic standard; as should the expertly seasoned, crunchy fried chicken with hot sauces. For sweet? Funnel cake with green peppercorn brittle, of course.

# The Radler

German

2375 N. Milwaukee Ave. (at Fullerton Ave.)

**Phone:** 773-276-0270  
**Web:** www.dasradler.com  
**Prices:** $$

Lunch & dinner daily

 California (Blue)

With around 20 suds on tap and more than 95 bottles to sample, The Radler is everything you want a beer hall to be. Though the space is new, it has an old soul: communal benches hearken back to the days of classic Bavarian *biergartens*, and the enormous Bohemian Export beer mural that commands guests' attention is indigenous to the building—a happy discovery during demolition.

A stack of small plates on each table sends the message that everything on the menu is meant for sharing. German onion pie arrives straight from the oven, topped with shaved asparagus and made-to-order Pilsner soubise. Four types of wurst are available by the link like Thüringer—served over a bed of spring green peas with authentic marinated cucumber salad and traditional mustard.

# Semiramis

Lebanese ✗✗

4639 N. Kedzie Ave. (bet. Eastwood & Leland Aves.)

**Phone:** 773-279-8900  
**Web:** www.semiramisrestaurant.com  
**Prices:** ⌾⌾

Lunch & dinner daily

 Kedzie (Brown)

Heed the advice advertised on the staff's T-shirts and "take it easy, Lebaneasy" at the pleasantly casual Semiramis. Set in the heart of Middle Eastern-mobbed Kedzie Ave., this **BYO** Lebanese café sees a diverse crowd fill their simple tables set atop tiled floors and lit softly through stained glass window shades. A separate counter and lounge caters to the stream of takeout regulars grabbing the popular $9 rotisserie chicken for tonight's dinner.

Fresh, flavorful fixings make classics like tabbouleh, crispy falafel, and flaky baklava shine. *Ful* is a warm fava bean-and-garlic stew tinged with zingy lemon juice and mint; while steak fries dusted with piquant sumac and whipped garlic mousse for dipping are best paired with the chicken shawarma special.

# Shokran Moroccan Grill

✕

## 4027 W. Irving Park Rd. (bet. Keystone Ave. & Pulaski Rd.)

Phone: 773-427-9130                     Dinner Wed – Mon
Web:    www.shokranchicago.com
Prices: ⊖⊜                              🚇 Irving Park (Blue)

Judging by the ordinary façade, commercial surroundings, and hovering highway, you may be tempted to pass right by. But, oh, the delights that would be missed! Arabic for "thank you," Shokran is a scrumptious spot for homemade Moroccan, where rich silk fabrics billow from the ceiling; framed mother-of-pearl artifacts hang on burnt sienna walls; and hookah pipes and copper chargers bedeck the room.

Brace yourself for the couscous royale—melt-in-your mouth braised lamb; juicy merguez (spicy sausage stuffed with ground lamb and beef); tender zucchini, rutabaga, carrots, and chickpeas snuggled into fluffy couscous. Satiate the sweet tooth with handmade cookies—from almond pastries to *fekkas*, each morsel is fresh and irresistible. Thank you, Shokran.

# Smoque BBQ 😀

✕

## 3800 N. Pulaski Rd. (at Grace St.)

Phone: 773-545-7427                     Lunch & dinner Tue – Sun
Web:    www.smoquebbq.com
Prices: ⊖⊜                              🚇 Irving Park (Blue)

At this unassuming barbecue joint set upon a dull corner in Irving Park, the focus is more on food than ambience. This may be a take-a-number counter service, but after one forkful of meltingly tender brisket, smoked for 15 hours, you won't be giving a second thought to your surroundings.

Beyond brisket, the meats—by the pound, on platters, or in sandwiches—are the main draw. Pulled pork, smoked chicken, saucy-slick ribs, and peppery Texas sausage weigh down platters, accompanied by piles of sides like cider vinegar slaw, crispy fresh-cut fries, or creamy macaroni and cheese. There's only one dessert option and it's peach cobbler. But, place your trust with the geniuses in the kitchen, and it's all one needs to end a meal here.

# Sol de Mexico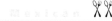

XX

**A3**

Mexican

**3018 N. Cicero Ave. (bet. Wellington Ave. & Nelson St.)**

**Phone:** 773-282-4119
**Web:** www.soldemexicochicago.com
**Prices:** $$

Lunch & dinner Wed – Mon

Thanks to this hugely skilled kitchen, dishes are bold and authentic, tortillas are made on the spot, and *moles* are the renowned house specialty. Mexican paintings, carved masks and colorful artifacts hang on bright orange walls and splashes of cobalt blue pop against white linens.

Start with freshly made guacamole, then explore the roster of exciting and interesting fare, such as the *chambandongo*, layering fresh tortillas, shredded pork, almonds, pecans, and raisins in deeply flavored *Teloloapense* red *mole*. The *camarones en mole verde* is a delightfully classic sauce combining herbs, tomatillos, pumpkin seeds, and epazote over juicy grilled shrimp, and served with grilled vegetables and rice. Feeling adventurous? Try the five-course chef's choice menu.

# Table, Donkey and Stick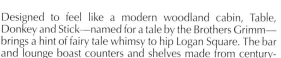

XX

**C4**

Austrian

**2728 W. Armitage Ave. (bet. California Ave. & North Point St.)**

**Phone:** 773-486-8525
**Web:** www.tabledonkeystick.com
**Prices:** $$

Lunch Sat – Sun
Dinner Wed – Mon
Western (Blue)

Designed to feel like a modern woodland cabin, Table, Donkey and Stick—named for a tale by the Brothers Grimm—brings a hint of fairy tale whimsy to hip Logan Square. The bar and lounge boast counters and shelves made from century-old Illinois barn wood, and a patio fire pit cozies up chilly evenings.

The popular restaurant menu and wine list focus on the traditional fare of the Alps, presenting elegantly composed versions of tavern-friendly comfort food. A sweet-and-salty punch of candied kalamata olives offsets the crisp richness of a braised, then fried chicken leg, and woodsy accompaniments of pickled ramps and celery root pair with roasted rabbit in a *ballotine*. For dessert, caramelized *chicharrónes* garnish homemade pineapple-fennel ice cream.

# Yusho

**2853 N. Kedzie Ave. (bet. Diversey Pkwy & George St.)**

| | |
|---|---|
| **Phone:** 773-904-8558 | Lunch Sun |
| **Web:** www.yusho-chicago.com | Dinner Wed – Mon |
| **Prices:** $$ | Logan Square |

Just off the beaten (and quickly gentrifying) path from its Logan Square brethren, Yusho quietly draws a crowd. A narrow façade hides a deceptively expansive room done up in a rustic-chic mix of weathered wood planks, cement floors, plaid-upholstered booths, and Danish midcentury chairs.

Diners show up in droves for a rotating selection of steamed buns, crispy chicken bits, and slurpable noodle bowls. "Logan Poser Ramen" showcases Chef/owner Matthias Merges' house-made noodles, a swirl of thick, al dente strands in spicy tonkatsu broth. A poached hen egg and crispy pig's tail croquette take it over the top. Vegetarians delight in an elegant pickled gobo root salad with translucent Asian pear and black plum slices and silky tofu-*tobanjan* dressing.

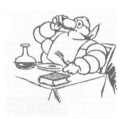

Look for our symbol ஃ
spotlighting restaurants
with a notable wine list.

# Lakeview & Wrigleyville

## ROSCOE VILLAGE

Lakeview is the blanket term for the area north of Lincoln Park, including Roscoe Village and Wrigleyville (named after its iconic ball field). On that note, enjoy a boisterous game with maximum conveniences at a Wrigley Field rooftop like **Murphy's Bleachers**, where hot dogs and hamburgers are washed down with many pints of beer. When the beloved Cubs finish their season each October, don't despair as these American summertime classics continue to shape the neighborhood's cuisine. Thanks to a large Eastern European population, an impressive array of sausages and wursts can be found in a number of casual eateries and markets, including **Paulina**—a local institution where expected items like corned beef and lamb are offered beside novel items like ground venison and loin chops. It's also a hot spot for local Swedish families, who come for time-tested faves like pickled Christmas hams and cardamom-infused sausages. Other Swedes may sojourn to **Ann Sather**, a sweet brunch spot branded for its baseball glove-sized cinnamon buns.

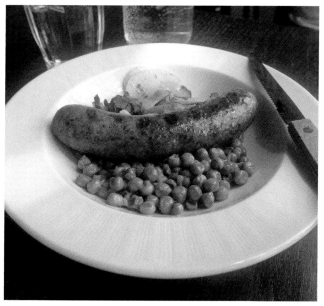

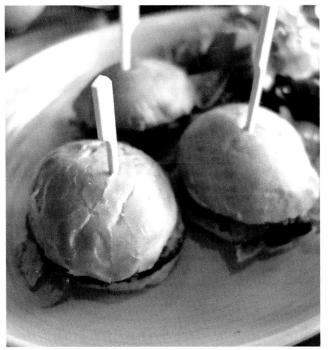

## CLASSIC CHICAGO

Diners are all the craze in this quarter, starting with **Glenn's** whose menu reads like a seafaring expedition with over 16 varieties of fresh fish on offer. Additionally, between its kitchen's savory egg specialties, 30 types of cereal, and a blackboard menu that makes Egyptian tombs look brief, this is a veritable Seinfeld kind of spot and flaunts something for everyone. Similarly, the Windy City's passion for the humble hot dog is something to bark home about, and Lakeview offers plenty of proof. Case in point—the dogs and burgers at **Murphy's Red Hots**, which may be relatively simple in presentation, but are entirely delicious in taste. Note that the location near Wrigley only has outdoor picnic tables and no inside seating.

## BAKING IN BAVARIA

Even Chicagoans can't survive on hot dogs alone. Thankfully, Lakeview has an antidote for practically every craving under the sun. Should you have a hankering for Bavarian baked goods, for example, **Dinkel's Bakery** is right around the corner. Originally opened by a master baker from Bavaria in 1922, this family-run business (in its current locale since 1932) is renowned for traditional renditions of strudels, *butterkuchen*, and stollen. Their big breakfast sandwich, Dinkel's Burglaur, is less traditional but just as tasty, as are their decadent donuts. Items can, of course, be

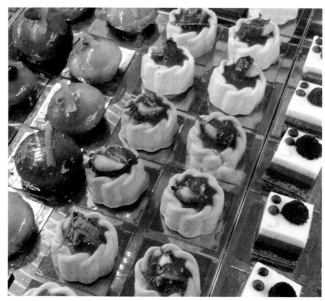

purchased fresh, but are also available frozen for shipping to lucky out-of-town fans.

## FASCINATING FOOD FINDS

For a different type of sugar high, stop by **Mayana Chocolates** to indulge in globally influenced flavors that run the gamut—from accessible (cookies n' cream or lime and raspberry?) to more exotic flavors like Sumatra coffee or coriander praline. Connoisseurs of quality-baked goods will want to pop into **Bittersweet Pastry Shop**, where Chef/owner Judy Contino has been whipping up decadent desserts for almost two decades. It's a one-stop shop for everything from breads, pastries, and cupcakes, to exquisitely sculpted wedding confections. Those seeking a classic American experience should proceed to **Fritz Pastry** for a faithful breakfast spread that includes

bakery specials like banana bread, cinnamon rolls, hand pies, and macarons. Another laudation (even if it comes in buttery and sugary packages) to Chicago's neighborhoods is **City Caramels**, home to a plethora of lip-smacking treats. Settle in and make your way through Bucktown (think coffee-inspired caramels with chocolate-covered espresso beans); Lincoln Square (toasted hazelnuts anybody?), and Pilsen (Mexican drinking chocolate with ancho chili) with their respective caramel and candy cuts. If savory dessert is more your style, make a beeline for **Pastoral**, which is hailed as one of the country's top spots for cheese. Their classic and farmstead varietals—as well as fresh breads and olives—are local favorites, not unlike their intermittently scheduled tastings. An offbeat yet quirky vibe is part and parcel of Lakeview's fabric and testament to this fact is **The Flower Flat**, boasting a comforting breakfast or brunch affair in an actual flower shop. Meanwhile, **Uncommon Ground** is as much a restaurant serving three meals a day as it is a coffee shop revered for its musical acts. During the months between June and September, stop by at any time to admire their certified organic sidewalk garden before tasting its bounty on your plate inside. And around the corner, aspiring young chefs with big dreams proudly present a wholesome grab-n-go restaurant called **Real Kitchen**. On the menu, a home-style dish like baked Amish chicken is paired with a unique and crusty pork belly BLT.

Everyone loves a rollicking street fair, and this nabe's **Guinness Oyster Festival**, with its diverse music, epic beer selection, and slurp-worthy guests of honor (a certain mollusk believed to have aphrodisiac qualities) doesn't disappoint. Homesick New Yorkers and transplants take note: Roscoe Village is also home to **Apart Pizza**, Chicago's very own homage to the thin-crust pie. (Just remember, you're in deep-dish land, so you might want to refrain from admitting how much you enjoyed it!) And because pizza is never complete without gelato, you'll want to make your way to **Black Dog** whose creamy concoctions count renowned local chefs among their fans.

Chicago ▶ Lakeview & Wrigleyville

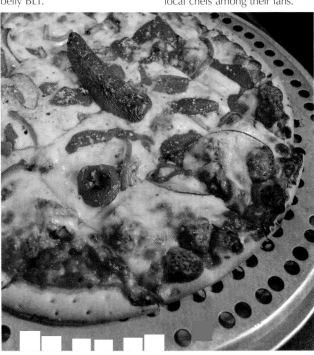

119

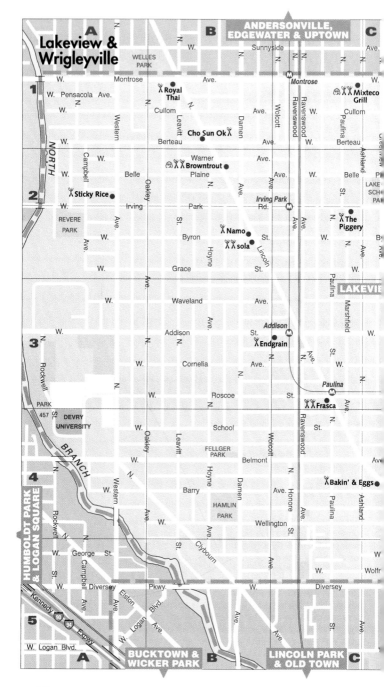

# Lakeview & Wrigleyville

WELLES
PARK

Montrose

W. Pensacola Ave.

Royal Thai

Sunnyside

Montrose

Mixteco Grill

Cullom

Cullom

Berteau

Cho Sun Ok

Berteau

Warner

Browntrout

Belle

Plaine

Sticky Rice

LAKE
SCH
PA

Irving Park

REVERE
PARK

Irving

Park

The Piggery

Namo

Byron

sola

Grace

LAKEVIE

Waveland

Addison

Addison

Endgrain

Cornelia

Roscoe

Frasca

DEVRY
UNIVERSITY

School

FELLGER
PARK

Belmont

Bakin' & Eggs

Barry

HAMLIN
PARK

Wellington

HUMBOLDT PARK
& LOGAN SQUARE

George St.

Diversey

Pkwy.

Diversey

Wolfr

Kennedy
Expwy.

W. Logan Blvd.

A     BUCKTOWN &
WICKER PARK     B     LINCOLN PARK
& OLD TOWN     C

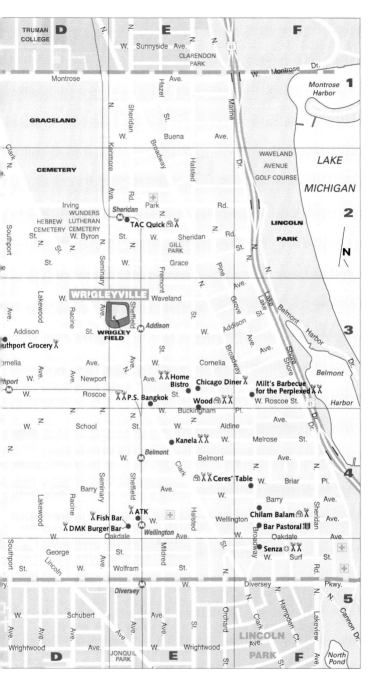

TRUMAN COLLEGE **D**

**E**

**F**

W. Sunnyside Ave.
CLARENDON PARK

W. Montrose Dr.

Montrose Ave.

**1**

Montrose Harbor

**GRACELAND**

Sheridan St.

W. Buena Ave.

Hazel

Broadway

Halsted

Marine Dr.

WAVELAND AVENUE GOLF COURSE

**LAKE**

Clark N.

**CEMETERY**

Kenmore Ave.

Southport

HEBREW CEMETERY

WUNDERS LUTHERAN CEMETERY

St.

Irving Park Rd.

*Sheridan* ⓜ●

W. Byron St.

St.

St.

Seminary

W. Sheridan Rd.

W. Grace

Fremont

GILL PARK

Pine

N.

Rd.

St.

**MICHIGAN**

**2**

**N**

**LINCOLN**

**PARK**

*TAC Quick* ✄ ✗

**WRIGLEYVILLE**

Lakewood Ave.

Racine Ave.

Sheffield Ave.

W. Waveland

*Addison* ●

St.

Grove Ave.

Lake St.

Belmont Harbor

Lake Shore Dr.

**3**

Addison

**ST. WRIGLEY FIELD**

W. Addison Ave.

ornelia

Southport Grocery ✗

Lakewood Ave.

Ave.

W. Newport Ave.

Racine Ave.

St.

Sheffield Ave.

Ave.

W. Cornelia

Broadway

Belmont

**Belmont**

*Belmont*

Ave.

Belmont

W. Roscoe St.

✗ ✗ *Home Bistro*

*Chicago Diner* ✗

*Milt's Barbecue for the Perplexed* ✗ ✗

Harbor

✗ ✗ *P.S. Bangkok*

*Wood* ✄ ✗ ✗

W. Buckingham Pl.

W. Aldine

Pl.

Ave.

**4**

W. School

St.

● *Kanela* ✗ ✗ W. Melrose St.

N.

Seminary Ave.

Sheffield Ave.

*Belmont* ⓜ

Barry Ave.

Clark Ave.

Belmont

Ave.

Z.

W. Briar Pl.

Barry Ave.

Sheridan Rd.

⓪ ✗ ✗ *Ceres' Table* W.

Lakewood

Racine Ave.

✗ *Fish Bar*

✗ *ATK*

Halsted

Wellington

W.

*Chilam Balam* ⓪ ✗

N.

✗ *DMK Burger Bar*

*Wellington* ⓜ Ave.

Mildred St.

St.

Broadway

*Bar Pastoral* ⓘ

W. Oakdale Ave.

Rd.

Southport

George

Lincoln

Ave.

Oakdale

St.

St.

W. Wolfram St.

*Senza* ⓪ ✗ ✗
W. Surf St.

ry.

*Diversey* ⓜ

W.

Diversey Pkwy.

N.

**5**

W. Schubert Ave.

Ave.

St.

Orchard

Clark Ave.

Hampden Ct.

Lakeview Ave.

Cannon Dr.

Ave.

Ave.

Ave.

Ave.

W. Wrightwood

**LINCOLN PARK**

N.

Wrightwood Ave.

JONQUIL PARK

**D**

**E**

St.

**F**

North Pond

# ATK

Thai 🍴

**E4**

### 946 W. Wellington Ave. (at Sheffield Ave.)

**Phone:** 773-549-7821                                          Lunch & dinner daily
**Web:** www.andysthaikitchen.com
**Prices:** $$                                                    🚇 Wellington

💲

BYO

Chef Andy Aroonrasameruang's Thai kitchen has earned numerous accolades and a devout following in its brief existence. Bring friends and settle in to the slender, spotless room arranged with ebony-finished tables and accent walls painted with hues evocative of turmeric and purple onion.

Cooked-to-order creations are spicy, sour, crunchy, and aromatic; as in the snappy Isaan-style sausage sided by a mouthwatering dipping sauce. The *kao soy* features thin egg noodles in a rich golden-yellow curry stocked with pounded chicken, bean sprouts, raw cabbage, and pickled mustard greens—all topped by a nest of crunchy fried noodles. The duck in red curry is chili-revved, redolent of five-spice, and balanced by the sweetness of diced pineapple, grapes, and tomato.

# Bakin' & Eggs

American 🍴

**C4**

### 3120 N. Lincoln Ave. (bet. Barry & Belmont Aves.)

**Phone:** 773-525-7005                                          Lunch daily
**Web:** www.bakinandeggschicago.com
**Prices:** 🪙🪙                                                   🚇 Paulina

♿

BYO

A pastry case chockablock with cupcakes, cookies, and brownies entices passersby into this relaxed Lincoln Ave. breakfast and lunch hangout. Whitewashed repurposed church pews provide ample seating for both big families and solo hipsters. Intelligentsia coffee is on hand for a pick-me-up; alcohol is best for boozy weekend brunches.

As the sibling of Wicker Park's Lovely Bake Shop, it's no wonder the moist, generously frosted cupcakes take the cake. Flavors like pumpkin spice, peanut butter and jelly, and red velvet make it hard to pick a favorite. Latin influences on the savory menu mean carb-loaded and dense *chilaquiles* with avocado and tomatillos. A kids' menu offers mini breakfast burritos or buttermilk pancakes with whipped cream smiles.

# Bar Pastoral

**F4**      International

### 2947 N. Broadway (bet. Oakdale & Wellington Aves.)

**Phone:** 773-472-4781      Lunch Sat – Sun
**Web:** www.barpastoral.com      Dinner nightly
**Prices:** $$       Wellington

When Wrigleyville denizens want to say cheese, they head to Bar Pastoral, the rustic bistro companion to an artisan cheese and wine shop. Subtly styled like a cave for aging, the restaurant's barrel-vaulted ceilings and exposed brick walls evoke intimacy. A glossy half-moon bar, marble-topped cheese counter, and rustic tables inlaid with wine crate ends let guests gather and sample.

As expected, many dishes feature cheese, though shareable plates run from house-made charcuterie to bone-in pork chops. Thick slices of bacon-wrapped country pâté are generously studded with pistachios. A succinct wine list offers a number of by-the-glass selections for pairing with cheese—such as the raw cow's milk Kentucky Rose served with caramelized onion chutney.

# Browntrout

**B2**      American

### 4111 N. Lincoln Ave. (bet. Belle Plaine & Warner Aves.)

**Phone:** 773-472-4111      Lunch Sun
**Web:** www.browntroutchicago.com      Dinner Wed – Sun
**Prices:** $$       Irving Park (Brown)

The natural beauty of a fish caught by Chef Sean Sanders during his New Zealand honeymoon inspired this pleasant neighborhood spot. Front windows swing wide open in warmer months and bring a breeze to the mocha-hued dining room. The neatly sketched chalkboard displays nightly specials and a list of their favorite (often organic) farmers—sources used in addition to their own rooftop garden.

The menu is broken down into "Smalls" like the whitefish brandade or smoked crappie and "Bigs" like Texas Bandera quail with almond, pineapple, and sage *pistou*. Brunch is a hit with the likes of blueberry beignets and cured salmon with a soft-cooked duck egg.

Kids eat free before 7:00 P.M. and Wednesdays allow you to create your own three-course bargain menu for $35.

# Ceres' Table

Chicago ▲ Lakeview & Wrigleyville

Italian ✗✗

**F4**

### 3124 N. Broadway (bet. Barry Ave. & Briar Pl.)

**Phone:** 773-922-4020
**Web:** www.cerestable.com
**Prices:** $$

Lun Sun
Dinner Mon – Sat
🚇 Belmont (Brown/Red)

Though Ceres' Table has moved from Uptown into an expanded Lakeview space, its menu of superbly prepared Italian specialties hasn't skipped a beat. The new digs keep things casual but contemporary: stylish gray loveseats sub for the usual wall banquettes, and an open kitchen showcases the addition of a wood-burning oven.

Each of the Sicilian- and Roman-inspired dishes finds a match on the all-Italian wine list. *Bucatini* with sardines and sweet raisins gets an extra-verdant twist: the pasta is perfumed with fennel-infused water, boosting the creamy anise flavor. Two juicy slabs of rosemary and garlic-roasted pork exemplify the platonic ideal of porchetta. An Oreo crumble on salted caramel budino lends a whimsical touch to a refined dessert.

# Chicago Diner

Vegetarian ✗

**E3**

### 3411 N. Halsted St. (at Roscoe St.)

**Phone:** 773-935-6696
**Web:** www.veggiediner.com
**Prices:** ⊜⊛

Lunch & dinner daily

🚇 Addison (Red)

"Meat free since '83" is the slogan at Chicago Diner, where servers have been slinging creative, healthy fare to grateful vegetarians and vegans for decades. The ambience evokes a neighborhood diner with fire engine-red tables trimmed in chrome, shiny black vinyl chairs, and raised booths. And the food? It looks and tastes the part.

Convincingly crispy seitan buffalo wings cool down the spice factor with vegan ranch dressing; while *flautas* filled with mashed potato, faux cheese, and jalapeños are served with tons of flavorful fixings so that the meat is not missed at all. With a popular brunch menu, numerous gluten-free choices, and a stronghold on the local vegan scene, waits can be long. So, get there early or hope for good Karma—and a seat.

# Chilam Balam

**F4**

Mexican ✗

### 3023 N. Broadway (bet. Barry & Wellington Aves.)

**Phone:** 773-296-6901
**Web:** www.chilambalamchicago.com
**Prices:** $$

Lunch Sat – Sun
Dinner Tue – Sat

🚇 Wellington

**BYO**

Duck into Chilam Balam's subterranean dining room, where low ceilings and a perpetually full house keep conversation levels high. Servers weave through a tight mosaic of tables with pitchers of virgin sangria and limeade from the tiny bar (consider bringing a mini-bottle of tequila to spike your own). Creative, shareable Mexican dishes pair seasonal ingredients in surprising combinations, and arrive at the table just as unpredictably. Grilled pork loin atop blue corn waffles and creamy chorizo gravy balances richness with the refreshing tang of thin zucchini pickles. Chocolate-chili mousse with toasted marshmallow sauce echoes the nostalgic taste of s'mores, but its goat cheese center turns the dessert into a pleasantly grown-up treat.

# Cho Sun Ok

**B1**

Korean ✗

### 4200 N. Lincoln Ave. (at Berteau Ave.)

**Phone:** 773-549-5555
**Web:** www.chosunokrestaurant.com
**Prices:** 🍲🍲

Lunch & dinner daily

🚇 Irving Park (Brown)

**BYO**

Service with a smile may not be the motto here, but satisfaction with the food is a near-guarantee at this small but beloved Korean barbecue spot. Booths and tables with central cooktop grills crowd the cozy, wood-paneled room, ensuring that even if the staff is gruff, the atmosphere remains very warm.

Large portions are the norm, making it easy for groups to sample and share the flavorful entrées. Complimentary *banchan* including pickled goodies and kimchi are copious enough to be a meal, but don't fill up on the snacks. Save room to sample authentic Korean food like thin, tender *chadul-goi* and marinated *bulgogi* for grilling at the table; pork belly tossed with spicy kimchi; or eggy shrimp-and-octopus pancakes with a scallion-soy dipping sauce.

# DMK Burger Bar

American

**E4**

### 2954 N. Sheffield Ave. (at Wellington Ave.)

**Phone:** 773-360-8686
**Web:** www.dmkburgerbar.com
**Prices:**

Lunch & dinner daily

 Wellington

Want a stellar burger? Hit DMK Burger Bar, brainchild of David Morton (of steakhouse fame) and Michael Kornick (mk). Grab a seat at the lengthy bar or cop a squat on an old church pew and admire concrete floors, exposed pale brick, and weathered wood borders contrasting the chocolaty-purple pressed-tin ceilings. What this place lacks in comfort, it makes up for in comfort food.

Follow the locals, and order by number. Perhaps #11: a dolled-up gyro featuring sheep's milk feta, olive tapenade, and *tzatziki* atop a grass-fed lamb patty; or go for #3: beef topped with pastrami, Gruyère, sauerkraut, and rémoulade. Cross over to the bad side and pair your sammie with hand-cut gourmet fries. And for a fine finale, slurp up a cold brew or homemade soda.

# Endgrain

American

**C3**

### 1851 W. Addison St. (at Wolcott Ave.)

**Phone:** 773-687-8191
**Web:** www.endgrainrestaurant.com
**Prices:**

Lunch Fri – Sun
Dinner Tue – Sat
 Addison (Brown)

For those moments when you just want a bite of breakfast or snack on-the-go, Endgrain is happy to meet your needs. In an appropriately carpentry-themed room featuring a rustic wood counter lined with shop stools and cupboards shelved with stacks of planks, Roscoe Villagers stop here as part of their routine—for a cup of coffee with a blackberry-peppercorn or butterscotch-bacon donut. The treats arrive courtesy of pastry wunderkind and Chef/owner Enoch Simpson.

While the menu leans toward breakfast—with emphasis on baked and fried pastry items—savory dishes also abound. Gravy-smothered biscuits topped with *harissa*-tinged fried eggs and crispy onion rings are very hearty. A pulled pork hand pie balances rich meatiness with tangy soybean sprout kimchi.

# Fish Bar

Seafood

**E4**

### 2956 N. Sheffield Ave. (at Wellington Ave.)

**Phone:** 773-687-8177        Lunch & dinner daily
**Web:** www.fishbarchicago.com
**Prices:** $$       Wellington

Chicago may not be known for local seafood, but Fish Bar makes sure to handpick the best from both the Atlantic and Pacific coasts to fill its chilled coffers. A blackboard above the semi-open kitchen lists the fresh daily fish and oyster offerings, ready to be shucked, steamed, fried, and grilled for guests lining up at the wood bar snaking around the room.

The casual menu pays homage to classic coastal fish shacks, yet throws in a few gussied-up items like tartare and octopus *à la plancha*. Bowls of gumbo stick to the classic recipe with zippy andouille sausage, okra, and chunks of blue crab. The Satchmo po'boy is a mouthful, combining fried rock shrimp and crawfish tails along with slaw and sweet pickles in a traditional, buttery split-top roll.

# Frasca

Italian

**C3**

### 3358 N. Paulina St. (at Roscoe St. )

**Phone:** 773-248-5222       Lunch Sat – Sun
**Web:** www.frascapizzeria.com       Dinner nightly
**Prices:** $$       Paulina

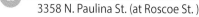

Like stepping into a warm, aromatic wine barrel, Frasca embraces its name (Italian for "branch") with a wraparound wooden bar flanking the wood-fired pizza oven, tables fashioned from tree trunks, planked walls, and forest-motif wallpaper.

As denoted by the brick oven, Frasca's pizzas with fresh, flavorful toppings (perhaps the *rustica* with fennel sausage?) are the heart of the operation, though seasonal pastas and entrées are also available. An "Old World Farmer's Table" menu lets diners check off items from a list of *bruschette*, cheeses with homemade jams, and cured meats for a choose-your-own antipasto adventure. Sharing plates is encouraged, down to the list of wines by the glass that allows for mixing and matching with other menu components.

# Home Bistro

**E3**

### 3404 N. Halsted St. (at Roscoe St.)

**Phone:** 773-661-0299

**Web:** www.homebistrochicago.com

**Prices:** $$

Lun Sun

Dinner Tue – Sun

🚇 Belmont (Brown/Red)

Home Bistro dishes up loads of quirk and charm with a healthy dash of humor in the heart of Boystown. Its radiant yellow-hued walls, lined with quotes from Miss Piggy, Beethoven, and other luminaries, inspire contemplative chuckles from first-timers. As if that weren't enough, the friendly servers and cooks always put a smile on the face of locals and regulars alike.

Comfort food by way of France and the Netherlands translates to a roundup of satisfying plates like Amsterdam-style mussels with beer broth and truffle fries; or artichoke and Edam fritters with roasted garlic aïoli. Almond butter and raspberry-jalapeño *gastrique* perk up tender house-smoked chicken thighs; while homemade Belgian chocolate candy bars are almost too good to save for the end.

# Kanela

**E4**

### 3231 N. Clark St. (bet. Belmont Ave. & School St.)

**Phone:** 773-248-1622

**Web:** www.kanelabreakfastclub.com

**Prices:** 💰💰

Lunch daily

🚇 Belmont (Brown/Red)

A comfortable, lived-in setting makes this breakfast club more like a home away from home for many Lakeview residents. The cozy chocolate-brown dining room packs in hungry brunchers on weekends, but the flung-open front windows, efficient kitchen (and a Bloody Mary or two) keep everyone happy.

Since Kanela is Greek for "cinnamon," the signature pastry is appropriately loaded with spiced sugar, vanilla frosting, and blueberries. A flight of four kinds of French toast sweetens the deal for indecisive types. But savory brunchers have a host of options too, including the Lorraine scramble with Gruyère, peppered bacon, and sprightly scallions. Brunch cocktails, fresh-squeezed juices and smoothies, and Julius Meinl coffee cover all the beverage bases.

# Milt's Barbecue for the Perplexed

B a r b e c u e   ✗✗

**3411 N. Broadway (bet. Hawthorne Pl. & Roscoe St.)**

| | |
|---|---|
| **Phone:** 773-661-6384 | Lunch Sun – Fri |
| **Web:** www.miltsbbq.com | Dinner Sun – Thu |
| **Prices:** | 🚇 Addison (Red) |

The full name of this kosher spot is Milt's Barbecue for the Perplexed, and those who wander in looking for baby back ribs or pulled pork may initially be confused. But even without these treats (or dairy), the catalog of smoky barbecue and Jewish deli delights are bound to appease one and all. Additionally, 100% of their profits go to charity, so get in here and get your craving on.

Tender chopped brisket on a toasted hamburger bun arrives with a trio of barbecue sauces—mustardy Carolina, smoky Memphis, and sweet Kansas City—and fries in a wire fryer basket; while pulled smoked chicken makes its way into the homemade soup. Don't expect to take your Friday night date here as Milt closes at sundown out of respect for the Sabbath.

# Mixteco Grill

M e x i c a n   ✗✗

**1601 W. Montrose Ave. (at Ashland Ave.)**

| | |
|---|---|
| **Phone:** 773-868-1601 | Lunch Sat – Sun |
| **Web:** www.mixtecogrill.com | Dinner Tue – Sun |
| **Prices:** | 🚇 Montrose (Brown) |

Floor-to-ceiling windows that wraparound the corner of Montrose and Ashland are flanked by cheery orange curtains that reflect the fiery and flavorful Mexican cuisine inside Mixteco Grill. A large open kitchen splits the dining room, giving the front room's hungry patrons a first-hand look at the mesquite-fired grill action.

As Mixteco is a region in culinarily diverse Oaxaca, Chef Raul Arreola has room to play with a variety of meats, seafood, *moles*, and salsas. Standouts in his menu include *chiles rellenos* stuffed with sweet bay shrimp, scallops, and crab in a creamy chipotle sauce; and crispy *taquitos* with an *escabeche*-spiked sauce that's only for the bold, not the bashful. *Flan de mamey* adds a sweet potato accent to the traditional custard.

# Namo

Thai

**B2**

### 3900 N. Lincoln Ave. (at W Byron St.)

**Phone:** 773-327-8818
**Web:** www.namothaicuisine.com
**Prices:** ✿✿

Lunch daily
Dinner Mon – Fri
Irving Park (Brown)

BYO

Namo tweaks traditional Thai food with deliciously contemporary touches in a mod space that matches its culinary philosophy. Woven baskets and fish traps double as pop art-style ceiling installations and lighting fixtures in this restrained dining room; wooden banquettes and tables in dark tones counterbalance the whitewashed brick.

Authentic flavors come in novel packages throughout the menu. "Sea bags" are actually crispy, deep-fried dumplings filled with spicy scallops, shrimp, and glass noodles; and "mozza crab sticks" replace cream cheese with mozzarella for a chewier version of crab Rangoon. A neatly constructed egg net covers an entire lobster tail in a luxurious take on lobster pad Thai.

Lunch and dinner prix-fixes are a splendid steal.

# The Piggery

American

**C2**

### 1625 W. Irving Park Rd. (at Marshfield Ave.)

**Phone:** 773-281-7447
**Web:** www.thepiggerychicago.com
**Prices:** $$

Lunch & dinner daily

Irving Park (Brown)

The bacon is back—as well as the ham, the shoulder, and the rest of the pig too. This Lakeview sports bar and shrine to all things porcine pays homage to its whimsical ways by way of kitschy pig paraphernalia that shares shelf and wall space with flat-screens tuned to Cubs and Sox games, naturally.

The menu may be hell for vegans, but it's a pork lover's paradise: cuts from every part of the animal find their way into nearly each dish, from hearty ham-stuffed burgers to the signature bacon-wrapped jalapeño poppers. Gently charred slabs of ribs basted with the Piggery's own heady barbecue sauce are teeth-sinkingly tender. Even salads may give you the meat sweats, with pulled pork or buffalo chicken—and bacon, of course—offered as toppings.

# P.S. Bangkok

  **E3**

T h a i

### 3345 N. Clark St. (bet. Buckingham Pl. & Roscoe St.)

**Phone:** 773-871-7777        Lunch & dinner Tue – Sun
**Web:** www.psbangkok.com
**Prices:** 💰💰        🚇 Belmont (Brown/Red)

Even first-timers are part of the family at P.S. Bangkok, a charming Lakeview retreat run by a trio of sisters. Wind chimes ring softly as Sue, who runs the front of the house, graciously welcomes each guest. Linen-draped tables, wooden arches, and bamboo accents lend subtle elegance to the space.

Diners do double takes at intriguingly titled dishes that depart from the usual Thai menu. "Love me tender" duck is a sweetheart of a meal, featuring fanned duck breast slices with crackling, sugary skin in a citrus-tinged sauce. "Beef paradise" is marinated in garlic and spices, and served with Thai barbecue dipping sauce. Stir-fried entrées named for flavor profiles like pungent, tangy, or peppery let guests cater to their own taste buds.

# Royal Thai

**B1**

T h a i

### 2209 W. Montrose Ave. (bet. Bell Ave. & Leavitt St.)

**Phone:** 773-509-0007        Lunch & dinner Wed – Mon
**Web:** www.royalthaichicago.com
**Prices:** 💰💰        🚇 Western (Brown)

 Stately elephants march down the silk runners on each linen-draped table at this age-old Lakeview Thai spot, adding a regal air to the already-polished dining room. Glossy bamboo floors, dark wood high-backed chairs, and ceiling fans atop light walls hung with mirrors make the space look larger than it is.

What this minuscule spot lacks in size, it makes up for in big and bold flavors. Be mindful of your spice tolerance, as the kitchen is known to turn up the heat. They're not fooling around so don't plan on kissing anyone after sucking on plump Royal Thai prawns topped with a potent mix of minced, fresh garlic, dried red chillies, and fragrant cilantro. Ask for a second bowl of rice to sop up the homemade peanut curry in spicy *rama* chicken.

Chicago ▲ Lakeview & Wrigleyville

# Senza ✿

Contemporary ✕✕

**2873 N. Broadway (bet. Oakdale Ave. & Surf St.)**

**Phone:** 773-770-3527      Dinner Tue – Sat
**Web:** www.senzachicago.com
**Prices:** $$$$      🚇 Wellington

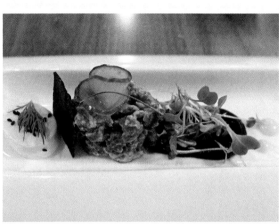

There may be no more fitting place for young foodies on date-night. In contrast to the serious nature of Senza's cuisine, the dining room feels distinctly laid-back both in look and spirit. Modern art, bare tables, and throw pillows help bridge the worlds of casual and fine dining. The décor mixes disparate pieces like colored chalk renderings of a fantastical mushroom forest, and eclectic terrariums filled with plastic dinosaurs, mini-gnomes, and succulents. This is a restaurant that knows how to run on all cylinders—except for the one that uses gluten. (And you'll never miss it. Promise.)

Begin with diced lamb tartare with crème fraîche, chives, and a pickle, accompanied by young mustard greens, caraway cracker, and a delicate mustard flan. That dish is even more harmonious if you ignore the waiter's comment that it was inspired by a Burger King Whopper. Move onto a velvety-sweet parsnip soup poured over kisses of pungent horseradish mousse, crisp *guanciale*, chunks of poached lobster tail, dried cherries, and micro-arugula sprouts.

Finish with a beautifully composed cheese course, such as creamy raclette resting beneath powdered pancetta and a tiny *membrillo*-filled éclair.

# sola

Contemporary ✗✗

**B2**

### 3868 N. Lincoln Ave. (at Byron St.)

**Phone:** 773-327-3868  
**Web:** www.sola-restaurant.com  
**Prices:** $$

Lunch Sat – Sun  
Dinner nightly  
Irving Park (Brown)

California transplant and Chef/owner Carol Wallack brings her love of sun, sand, and surf to the eclectic cuisine of sola. The discreet Byron Street entrance leads to a lively dining room with a lengthy bar, where creative cocktails are shaken from brunch through dinner. Warm tones on high-backed striped banquettes glow in the light of modern hanging lanterns.

The adventurous menu has a distinctly tropical feel, featuring Pacific-inspired entrées like ginger-glazed salmon over truffle-teriyaki sauce with edamame purée. Brunch offers ham and cheese French toast, a savory-sweet update of the Monte Cristo sandwich with whole-grain mustard and plum-ginger preserves on brioche. *Togarashi* hash browns tingle with a subtle hint of Japanese rice seasoning.

# Southport Grocery

American ✗

**D3**

### 3552 N. Southport Ave. (bet. Addison St. & Cornelia Ave.)

**Phone:** 773-665-0100  
**Web:** www.southportgrocery.com  
**Prices:** ⊙⊙

Lunch daily

Southport

Whether breakfast or lunch is your bag, you'll find a plate to suit your style at this hopping local hangout that's both a café and (of course) a grocery. Browse the racks of locally made specialty ingredients or peruse the counter stacked with made-from-scratch baked goods while you wait for a spot at the wooden communal table.

Bread pudding pancakes or a "grown-up" pop tart filled with local preserves, mascarpone, and roasted vanilla-tinged walnuts send sweet lovers into seventh heaven. On the savory end of the spectrum, the Southport Cuban, layered with ham and house-smoked brisket, giardiniera, and Swiss on freshly grilled challah, gets even better with a side of creamy mashed Red Bliss potatoes. An ancho chile Bloody Mary is sure to end any hangover.

# Sticky Rice

Thai ✕

**A2**

**4018 N. Western Ave. (at Cuyler Ave.)**

| | |
|---|---|
| **Phone:** 773-588-0133 | Lunch & dinner daily |
| **Web:** www.stickyricethai.com | |
| **Prices:** 💰 | 🚇 Irving Park (Blue) |

**BYO**

Yes, there's no dearth of Thai joints in this neighborhood, but Sticky Rice stands out not only for its focus on Northern Thai specials, but for the quality and abundance of dishes made to order. Step inside the sunny lemon- and tangerine-hued space with teak wood carvings, but step away from the satay and pad Thai. In fact, move outside your comfort zone and find a new favorite craving from their extensive menu.

*Gang hung lay* exemplifies the dark, chili-rich, and Northern-style curry with chunks of pork, garlic, and julienned ginger. Banana blossom salad, one among nearly thirty on the menu, mixes sour, floral, and spicy flavors in a vinegar-rich shrimp chili paste. Feeling truly bold? More exotic dishes include jellyfish salad and fried bamboo worms.

# TAC Quick

Thai ✕

**E2**

**3930 N. Sheridan Rd. (at Dakin St.)**

| | |
|---|---|
| **Phone:** 773-327-5253 | Lunch & dinner Wed – Mon |
| **Web:** www.tacquick.net | |
| **Prices:** 💰 | 🚇 Sheridan |

Only a short jaunt from Wrigley Field, this modest, modern corner spot hides a secret behind its windowed façade: some of the most authentic Thai cooking in Chicagoland. Loyal followers fill every seat in the minimal dining room framed by tall windows. They are here to slurp up curries, chow down on mouthfuls of noodles, and snap up spicy stir-fries.

Though there is a so-called secret menu, TAC Quick happily posts it everywhere, much to the relief of diners looking for such genuine dishes as sour curry with *cha om*-flecked omelette. Even familiar plates like pork *prik king* or *yum woon sen*, a spicy, refreshing cold mélange of glass noodles, shrimp, and chicken tossed with lime, cilantro, and chilies, superbly mix crisp textures with aromatic flavors.

# Wood

**Contemporary** ✗✗

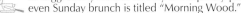

### 3335 N. Halsted St. (at Buckingham Pl.)

**Phone:** 773-935-9663
**Web:** www.woodchicago.com
**Prices:** $$

Lunch Sun
Dinner nightly
🚇 Belmont (Brown/Red)

The décor at this Boystown spot might be all grown-up with rich wood tones set against pale tufted booths and a glossy cream bar, but witty winks to the gay community pop up throughout the menu. Cocktails like a "manhandled sour" are as suggestively named as they are superbly prepared. Heck, even Sunday brunch is titled "Morning Wood."

That said, the menu is incredibly refined. Choose from seasonal American food like roasted venison with creamed spinach as well as homemade sausage and spaetzle. Or opt for the country ham flatbread topped with creamy raclette and charred black kale, presented in squares for easy sharing. The bar continues to pour long after the kitchen closes, so night owls sample from the "Backwoods" menu of Belgian frites and sauces.

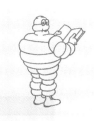

Red=Particularly Pleasant.
Look for the red ✗ symbols!

# Lincoln Park & Old Town

The congregation of history, commerce, and nature is what makes Lincoln Park and Old Town one of Chicago's most iconic districts. Scenically situated along Lake Michigan's shore, the eponymous park offers winter-weary Chicagoans an excuse to get out. As if that isn't enticing enough, the park also keeps its patrons happy with a spectacular array of cafés, restaurants ranging from quick bites to the city's most exclusive reservations, and takeout spots rife with picnic-perfect products. Populated by college grads, young families, and wealthy upstarts, as well as home to more than a handful of historic districts, museums, shopping, music venues, and the famous (not to mention, free) zoo, Lincoln Park remains a hugely sought-after destination year-round.

## DELICIOUS DINING

Wallet-happy locals and well-heeled gourmands make reservations to come here and dine at some of the most exclusive restaurants in town. But beyond just glorious, white-glove restaurants, there's more delicious dining to be had here. During the weekend, these streets are jumping thanks to a combination of the theater, bar scene, and scores of high-rises catering to affluent and boisterous yuppies. On Wednesdays and Saturdays during the **Green City Market**, the south end of the park is transformed into hipster-chef-foodie central. With the aim to increase availability of top-notch produce and to improve the link between farmers and local producers with restaurants and food organizations, this

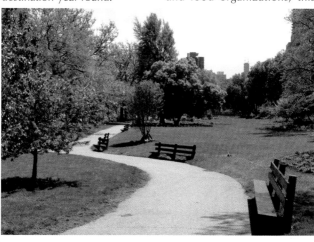

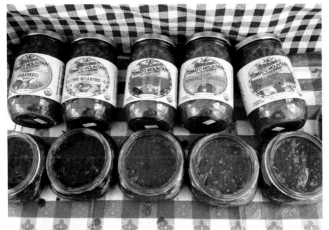

market works to educate the Windy City's masses about high-quality food sourcing. (In winter it is held across the street inside the Peggy Notebaert Nature Museum).

## BEST IN BITES

Lincoln Park's outpost of **Floriole Café & Bakery** brought about much jubilation, and along with it, a regular lunch lineup. In fact, the aromas wafting from freshly baked breads, pastries, and cookies never fail to tempt onlookers. For more savory goodness, try the heartwarming **Meatloaf Bakery**, where meatloaf and mashed potatoes are crafted into all manner of dishes. Leaving aside their quirky titles ("loaf-a-roma" or "no buns about it burger loaf"), this may just be some of the best baked goods in town. Like many foods (Juicy Fruit, Cracker Jack, and Shredded Wheat, for example), it is said that the Chicago-style dog may have originated at the Chicago World's Fair and Columbian Exhibition in 1893. Others credit the Great Depression for its birth. Regardless of its source, one thing is for certain: chef-driven **Franks 'n' Dawgs** is Chicago's most desirable hot dog destination, by virtue of employing only fresh, locally sourced ingredients for their hand-crafted creations. Similarly, **The Wieners Circle** is as known and loved for its late hours (as late as 5:00 A.M.) and intentionally rude service, as for its repertoire of delicious dogs and fries. Carnivores may choose to carry on the party at **Butcher & the Burger** as they do their part to stay at the helm of the burger game. Meanwhile the ocean's bounty can be relished in all its glory at **Half Shell**—whose cash-only policy has done nothing to deter crowds from consuming fresh crab legs and briny oysters.

## BOOZE CRUISE

Wash down these salty treats with cool sips from a choice selection at **Goose Island Brewery**, makers of the city's favorite local beers.

Continue the alcohol-fueled fun at **Barrelhouse Flat**, which is always hip and happening thanks to their litany of hand-crafted punches, before winding up in time—for brunch perhaps?—at **The Drinking Bird**. From sweet and stirring sake punch to spicy house sausages, their carte du jour is nothing short of crowning.

Lincoln Park is one of the dog-friendliest areas around, but then what else would you expect from a neighborhood named after a huge expanse of grass? Big bellies and bold palates with Fido in tow are forever devouring savory spreads, followed by decadent desserts prevalent throughout this 'hood. Finally, find them walking off the calories at **Ginkgo Organic Garden**, where most visitors feel good about the fact that their exquisite yield of vegetables, fruit, and flowers is ultimately donated to non-profit organizations. If that doesn't put a smile on your face, those deep-friend oreos at **Racine Plumbing** or decadent popcorn from **Berco's** boutique will certainly do the trick. It's a whole different ballgame at **Karyn's Fresh Corner and Raw Café** where a full vegan menu keeps vegetarians raving and gratified year-round. Just adjacent, **Fresh Corner Market** keeps the raw movement in fine fettle by selling meals-to-go. These may include "meatballs" made from lentils, and soy protein "sloppy Joes."

## OLD TOWN

The Old Town quarter has a few quaint cobblestoned streets that house the Second City comedy scene (now with a Zanies, too, for even more laughs). Also housed here is June's annual must-see (and must-shop) Old Town Art Fair; the Wells Street Art Fair; as well as places to rest with beers and a groovy jukebox like the **Old Town Ale House**. Wells Street is the neighborhood's main drag, and is really where browsing should begin. Any epicurean shopping trip should also include **The Spice House** for its exotic spice blends, many named after local landmarks; or **Old Town Oil** for hostess gifts like infused oils and aged vinegars. Prefer a sweeter vice? **The Fudge Pot** tempts with windows of toffee, fudge, and other chocolate-y decadence. Lastly, you may not be a smoker, but the Up Down Cigar is worth a peek for its real cigar store Indian carving.

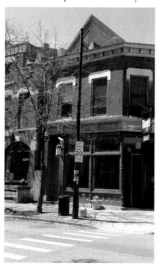

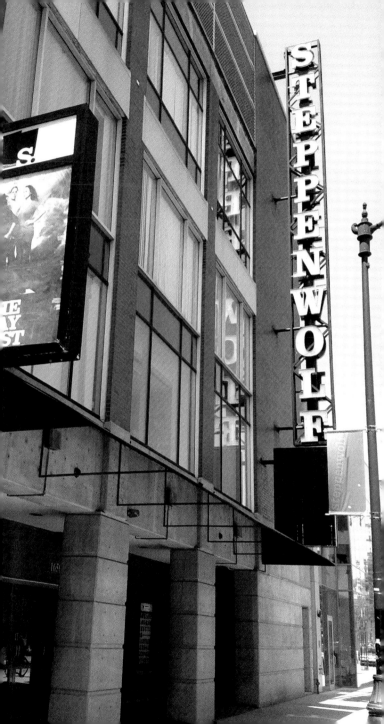

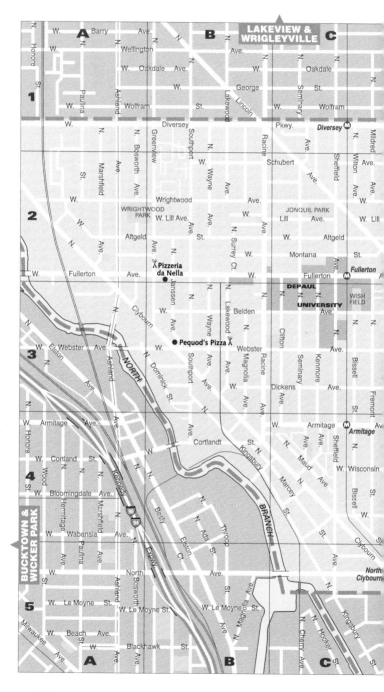

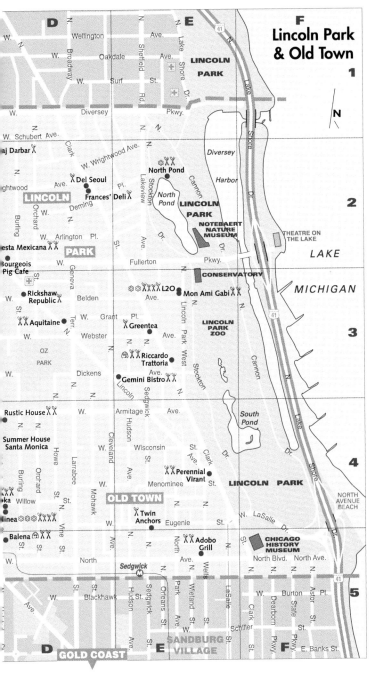

# Lincoln Park & Old Town

**D**  **E**  **F**

**1**

**2**

**3**

**4**

**5**

N

W. Wellington Ave.

W. Oakdale Ave.

Broadway

Sheffield

Lake Shore Dr.

W. Surf St.

LINCOLN PARK

W. Diversey Pkwy.

W. Schubert Ave.

aj Darbar

W. Wrightwood Ave.

Clark

Del Seoul

Frances' Deli

North Pond

Diversey

Harbor

LINCOLN PARK

NOTEBAERT NATURE MUSEUM

THEATRE ON THE LAKE

LAKE

ghtwood Ave.

LINCOLN

Orchard

Burling

Deming

Lakeview

Stockton

North Pond

W. Arlington Pl.

esta Mexicana

PARK

W. Fullerton Pkwy.

CONSERVATORY

MICHIGAN

Bourgeois Pig Cafe

Geneva

Rickshaw Republic

Belden Ave.

L2O

Mon Ami Gabi

Aquitaine

W. Grant Pl.

Greentea

Lincoln Park West

LINCOLN PARK ZOO

OZ PARK

Webster Ave.

Dickens

Riccardo Trattoria

Gemini Bistro

Lincoln

Sedgwick

Stockton

South Pond

Rustic House

Armitage Ave.

Cleveland

Hudson

Clark

Ave.

Dr.

Summer House Santa Monica

Wisconsin St.

Howe

Larrabee

Mohawk

W. Menominee St.

Perennial Virant

LINCOLN PARK

NORTH AVENUE BEACH

Burling

Orchard

Willow St.

ka

OLD TOWN

inea

Twin Anchors

Eugenie St.

Balena

Vine St.

North

North Ave.

Adobo Grill

Wells

CHICAGO HISTORY MUSEUM

North Blvd. North Ave.

Sedgwick

Blackhawk

Hudson

Sedgwick

Orleans St.

Park

Wieland

LaSalle

Burton Pl.

Clark

Dearborn

State

Astor

Pkwy.

GOLD COAST

SANDBURG VILLAGE

Schiller St.

E. Banks St.

# Adobo Grill

### 1610 N. Wells St. (bet. Eugenie St. & North Ave.)

**Phone:** 312-266-7999
**Web:** www.adobogrill.com
**Prices:** $$

Lunch Sat – Sun
Dinner nightly
 Sedgwick

Fun, festive, and flavorful, Adobo Grill is celebrated as a longtime Old Town crowd-pleaser. Housed within a meandering building, it is at once cozy and lively with everyone from local denizens and families to solo diners at the bar.

First, order a lip-smacking margarita with fresh lime, then flag down one of the roving guacamole carts for a wildly popular tableside rendition. The solid Mexican bill of fare offers something for everyone, like little tostadas with achiote-marinated chicken, pickled onions, black beans, and sour cream; and *arrachera adobado*—grilled flank steak with a rich adobo, smoky *frijoles puercos*, grilled tomatoes, onions, and their unique house-made tortillas.

Brunch brings signature starters, small plates, and *huevos rancheros*.

# Aquitaine

### 2221 N. Lincoln Ave. (bet. Belden & Webster Aves.)

**Phone:** 773-698-8456
**Web:** www.aquitainerestaurant.com
**Prices:** $$

Lunch Sun
Dinner nightly
 Fullerton

Eleanor of Aquitaine wasn't a restaurateur as far as we know, but Chef/partner Holly Willoughby channels her regal, refined spirit at this romantic Lincoln Avenue mainstay. Dark brocade wallpaper, polished wood floors, and red leather banquettes face a long, welcoming bar, while French doors swing open when the weather cooperates.

The seasonally changing menu complements the casually elegant space. Duck finds its way into many of the French-influenced entrées such as juicy roasted duck breast with crushed celery root and Sauternes-apricot jam; or duck crêpes with maple-shallot brown butter. The signature amber cake, reminiscent of a French opera cake, pairs caramel *fleur de sel* cream, lemon madeleines, and crisp streusel for multi-layered bliss.

# Alinea ✿ ✿ ✿

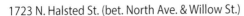

**1723 N. Halsted St. (bet. North Ave. & Willow St.)**

Phone: 312-867-0110
Web: www.alinea-restaurant.com
Prices: $$$$

Dinner Wed – Sun

North/Clybourn

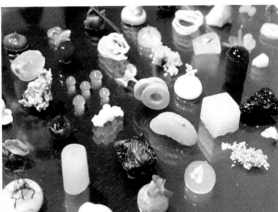

Who needs a meal followed by a show when you can have both together? That's because eating at Alinea, which involves around 20 courses over about three hours, is more than simply dinner—it's culinary theater. Perhaps it could qualify for a Tony Award along with its Michelin stars, because you're even invited backstage afterwards to meet the talented protagonists in the kitchen. Alinea provides such a vivid, visceral experience, that you'll even forget about the somewhat painful and entirely inhospitable booking procedure.

Neophytes have nothing to fear here as there's a veritable army of charming, clued-up helpers and servers to guide you effortlessly through each and every dish. And guidance is certainly needed because the only menu you'll see is the one presented to you like an award certificate as you leave.

The cooking is strikingly original and very clever. It can surprise but it can also challenge; at times dishes can be playful or even whimsical. But underpinning all those clever techniques and all those dazzling arrangements and quite striking presentations is an inherent understanding of flavor—and this is what gives the cooking such great depth.

# Balena

**D5**

### 1633 N. Halsted St. (bet. North Ave. & Willow St.)

**Phone:** 312-867-3888
**Web:** www.balenachicago.com
**Prices:** $$

Dinner nightly

🚉 North/Clybourn

Since it's a mere stone's throw from the Steppenwolf and Royal George theaters, Balena is always popular among the pre-show crowds. Those who can linger and disregard the giant clock hanging from the back wall should go for lucky seats at the chef's counter for a little dinner theater of their own.

Italian techniques and flavors inspire the menu, but your *nonna* wouldn't recognize many of these dishes at first glance. Modern interpretations include house-made *orecchiette* tossed in a lemony cream sauce, hearty Tuscan kale salad dressed with a Caesar-like riff on classic *tonnato* sauce, or pizza with cauliflower, burrata, and *anchoïade*. Splurge on the bread basket for seasonal surprises like heirloom beet crostini or orange and anise *grissini*.

# Bourgeois Pig Cafe

**D2**

### 738 W. Fullerton Pkwy. (at Burling St.)

**Phone:** 773-883-5282
**Web:** www.bpigcafe.com
**Prices:** 

Lunch & dinner daily

🚉 Fullerton

Scholarly types from nearby DePaul University adore this bookish café on a quiet block of Fullerton. Choose from a litany of salads, sandwiches, and drinks from oversized chalkboard menus behind the counter, then stake out one of the premium second-floor tables. Upstairs, chandeliers, cozy couches, and scattered antiques (not to mention frequent study groups guzzling caffeine and homemade cookies) lend character.

Many sandwiches take names from literary works, like *The Old Man and the Sea* (tuna salad) or *Catcher in the Rye* (reuben). The muffuletta is a lightly pressed panini rendition of the New Orleans standard, stacking a deli's worth of ham, salami, mortadella, provolone, and mild giardiniera in fresh focaccia for a hearty yet delicate sandwich.

# Boka

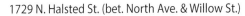

XXX

**1729 N. Halsted St. (bet. North Ave. & Willow St.)**

**Phone:** 312-337-6070                              Dinner nightly
**Web:** www.bokachicago.com
**Prices:** $$$                                      North/Clybourn

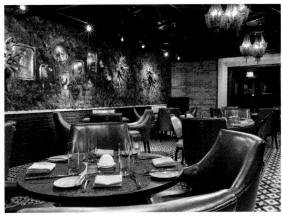

The changes here may be massive, but all are for the better. A complete remodel has done away with the billowing white sails of fabric to reinvent this sultry dining room. The new look exudes class with a bit of romance and occasional quirk (note the escutcheon-covered doorway and whimsical paintings). Against dark pebbled walls, find oversized horseshoe booths, long banquettes, and mirrored lightbulbs casting funky shadows. The semi-outdoor solarium has a living wall of moss and ferns. Servers are friendly and genuine without a hint of pretense.

This is the kind of place where one can sink into and not care to leave.

Chef Lee Wolen's menu may be modern, but it is widely appealing with a Mediterranean edge. Begin with Spanish octopus that is tender with a bit of pleasant chew from the grill, served with a harmonious hodgepodge of Japanese eggplant coins, fingerling potatoes, cubes of compressed Granny Smith apple, and shredded pork finished with pork broth and shiso leaves. Thin and finely crafted ravioli may be filled with chopped salt cod and tossed with fresh favas, wilted arugula, and near-melting artichokes in velvety velouté sauce. The salty-sweet chocolate cake is not to be missed.

# Del Seoul

Korean 🍴

**D2**

**2568-2570 N. Clark St. (bet. Deming Pl. & Wrightwood Ave.)**

**Phone:** 773-248-4227                                   Lunch & dinner daily
**Web:** www.delseoul.com
**Prices:** 😋                                              🚇 Diversey

Korean street food makes its way from the trendy trucks to a fast-casual space that gives the people what they crave. All the intoxicating flavors of Korean cuisine are here in finger food form, perfect for sharing or creating your own personal buffet. Choose from the video screens above the counter, take a number, and grab a seat.

Bite-sized barbecue tacos are the star of the menu, filled with a variety of meats including *kalbi*-style braised beef short ribs or panko-breaded sesame-chili shrimp. Both get a topping of bright cilantro-onion slaw on grilled white corn tortillas. Canadian poutine crosses a number of borders when topped with more of those tender short ribs, house-made kimchi, pickled red onions, and a melted trio of cheddar, jack, and *crema*.

# Fiesta Mexicana

Mexican 🍴🍴

**D2**

**2423 N. Lincoln Ave. (bet. Fullerton Ave. & Halsted St.)**

**Phone:** 773-348-4144                                   Lunch & dinner daily
**Web:** www.fiestamexicanachicago.com
**Prices:** 😋                                              🚇 Fullerton

Cheerful and bright, Fiesta Mexicana is truly a party for the eyes and tastebuds. High-ceilinged rooms are lined with colorful murals of small-town Mexican life, and wide-open front windows invite in warm evening breezes. Live mariachi bands turn up the heat on weekends.

Creative Mexican fare begins with the usual suspects like tacos *al pastor* and piquant, spunky house-made salsa, but unique dishes broaden the offerings. Here, a bowl of *fundido* is a Latin cousin to spinach and artichoke dip, with a blend of tangy cheeses and plenty of roasted poblanos for extra warmth. Pan-fried pork tenderloin medallions come smothered in tomatillo sauce alongside drunken beans, bacon-wrapped shrimp, and a side of smashed red potatoes with oozing *Chihuahua* cheese.

# Frances' Deli

**2552 N. Clark St. (bet. Deming Pl. & Wrightwood Ave.)**

**Phone:** 773-248-4580                                    Lunch daily
**Web:** www.francesdeli.com
**Prices:**

Frances' Deli is the type of quaint, lived-in diner everyone dreams of having just around the corner from home. Lucky Lincoln Park residents get that wish fulfilled at this authentic pre-war haunt packed with American antiques and memorabilia, where weekend waits are the norm as half the neighborhood vies for a place at one of the closely spaced tables.

As with any good diner, breakfast, lunch, and dinner all know how to hit the spot. The deli roasts its own meats and does Jewish-American staples right, from flavorful, crisp-tender potato pancakes to oversized pastrami and brisket sandwiches with all the fixings (slaw, fries, and potato salad). As long as you're going for the full nostalgia trip, slurp down a made-to-order milkshake or malt.

# Gemini Bistro

**2075 N. Lincoln Ave. (at Dickens Ave.)**

**Phone:** 773-525-2522                                    Lunch Sun
**Web:** www.geminibistrochicago.com                    Dinner Tue – Sun
**Prices:** $$                                     Armitage

Opposites attract at this delightful neighborhood bistro that offers the best of both worlds: a chic, upscale setting with a casual, approachable attitude. Dark Venetian blinds and awnings remove outside distractions, letting guests focus their attention on the white marble bar and the lychee martinis shaken there. Most street parking in the area is permit only, so consider the valet.

Seasonal American fare pulls inspiration from the Mediterranean in dishes like plump double-boned pork chop Lyonnaise, cooked to a juicy medium, draped in herbed demi-glace, and nestled with *cipollini* onions and roasted fingerling potatoes. Smaller bites like a trio of seared scallops are paired with the timeless flavors of brown butter, capers, and lemon zest.

# L20

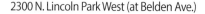

Seafood XXXX

**E3**

## 2300 N. Lincoln Park West (at Belden Ave.)

**Phone:** 773-868-0002
**Web:** www.l2orestaurant.com
**Prices:** $$$$

Dinner Thu – Mon

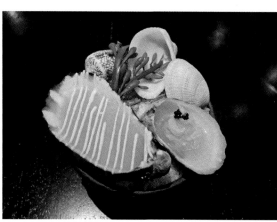

The lobby of the magnificent Belden Stratford building offers few clues that you're in the right place, but pass through the door on the right and you'll find yourself instantly transported into this most ethereal of restaurants. The room boasts a timeless grace and elegance thanks largely to the warm, natural tones provided by dark and light wood. Clever room dividers ensure it manages the trick of feeling intimate yet open at the same time, and the young service team play their part by being unfailingly cheerful, attentive, and informative, which in turn keeps the atmosphere buoyant.

Seafood and shellfish of unimpeachable quality and in all its forms are celebrated here, from caviar, oysters, and abalone, to cusk, trout, and *daurade*. The style of cooking is intricate and exact, with the dishes displaying a delicacy and precision that certainly leaves an impression. The presentation is remarkable but is matched by the intriguing and well-thought through textural contrasts and the wonderful balance of flavors.

While a wine pairing is offered here, better luck will be had on the impressive list.

# Greentea

✗

**2206 N. Clark St. (bet. Belden & Webster Aves.)**

**Phone:** 773-883-8812
**Web:** N/A
**Prices:** $$

Lunch Tue – Sat
Dinner Tue – Sun

 **BYO**

Regulars would rather your eyes glaze past Greentea's nondescript storefront so they can keep this secret to themselves. The bento box-sized room isn't glitzy, so the scene is limited to a few lucky cat sculptures and plants to punctuate the seafoam green walls. Otherwise, the focus is kept on the *itamae* in colorful chef's coats and the pristinely fresh seafood they're preparing.

Purists love the well-priced nigiri, sashimi, and manageably sized rolls showcasing silky hamachi or glistening uni with a touch of minerality. Tiger Eyes salad is a visual showstopper: squid stuffed with smoked salmon, julienned cucumber, and marinated carrots sliced into thin rounds create a clever and flavorful resemblance to an orange-pupiled eye.

# Mon Ami Gabi

✗✗

**2300 N. Lincoln Park West (at Belden Ave.)**

**Phone:** 773-348-8886
**Web:** www.monamigabi.com
**Prices:** $$

Dinner nightly

Within the historic Belden-Stratford hotel, Mon Ami Gabi offers an instant trip to Lyon by way of Lincoln Park. This appealing brasserie stays lively with the cozy ambience of a French bistro straight from central casting. Leather banquettes, dusky yellow walls, and wooden wine racks set the scene, while old-world, tuxedo-clad servers play the part, perfectly.

Gabino Sotelino (the "ami" referenced in the restaurant's name) and team turn out faithful renditions of classic brasserie food such as an anchovy-rich Caesar salad with shards of baguette croutons, dusted with black pepper ground at the table; plump and on-point medium-rare filet mignon with a healthy dab of butter and béarnaise; or French onion soup capped with gooey Gruyère.

# North Pond ✿

**E2**

### 2610 N. Cannon Dr.

**Phone:** 773-477-5845
**Web:** www.northpondrestaurant.com
**Prices:** $$$

Lunch Sun
Dinner Tue – Sun

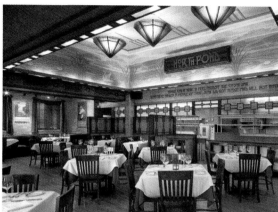

A pleasant stroll through the neighborhood's namesake park leads you to North Pond. This former ice-skaters' warming house has been reincarnated as a cozy but elegant cottage with carefully considered Craftsman-era detail. With the Chicago skyline reflected in the rippling water and the verdant landscape framed by the windows, the scene is the very dictionary definition of "picturesque."

Inside, the gracious space is filled with sophisticated arts and crafts accents like patterned friezes and room dividers, as well as nature-inspired details and a recessed ceiling mural that echoes the view outside.

Chef Bruce Sherman presents surprisingly complex and modern seasonal dishes instead of straightforward farm-to-table fare, though his tremendous creativity can lead to competing flavors. Composed salads feature roasted Chioggia beets interspersed with cured Arctic char cubes as well as both smoked and fresh salmon caviars. Main courses can be decadently tender and rich as in pork medallions with cherry gelée, or rabbit served three ways: buttermilk-braised, bacon-wrapped saddle, and a "truffle" of nut-coated liver with rhubarb jam. Architecturally impressive desserts are an equal delight.

# Pequod's Pizza

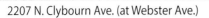

**2207 N. Clybourn Ave. (at Webster Ave.)**

Phone: 773-327-1512

Web: www.pequodspizza.com

Prices: $$

Lunch & dinner daily

🚇 Armitage

Ditch your diet, grab your fellow Blackhawk fans, and head to this Lincoln Park stalwart for some of the best pies in town. Christened for Captain Ahab's whaling ship, Pequod's menu promises smooth sailing, featuring bar food apps, hearty sandwiches (try the tender Italian beef with melted cheese and hot peppers), and fantastic pizzas.

Crusts range from thin to deep-dish, but the specialty is the pan pizza, with its cake-like crust and halo of caramelized cheese that sticks to the sides of the pan. Toppings like spicy sausage and pepperoni are heaped on with abandon, as if the pizza makers are whipping up a pie to take home for themselves. Pequod's stays open till 2:00 A.M. most nights, so stop by for a late-night nosh and ponder the great white whale.

# Perennial Virant

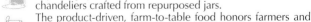

**1800 N. Lincoln Ave. (at Clark St.)**

Phone: 312-981-7070

Web: www.perennialchicago.com

Prices: $$

Lunch Sat – Sun
Dinner nightly

Housed in this upmarket quarter and packed with patrons to match, this Paul Virant operation is a perennial hit. Book in advance and take the time to truly appreciate the philosophy followed here—local, sustainable cuisine combined with an appealing, pared down décor, featuring earthy shades and chandeliers crafted from repurposed jars.

The product-driven, farm-to-table food honors farmers and seasonality. Start with fermented veggies and rustic boards arranged with charcuterie and cheese. Pickled items star in nearly every plate, including a fluffy three-egg skillet with salsa, corn relish, and smoky cheddar. Black Earth bacon is crunchy, delicious, and perfect. End with a freshly baked turnover highlighting semi-crisp pastry and sweet rhubarb filling.

# Pizzeria da Nella

Lincoln Park & Old Town ▶ Chicago

Italian

B2

**1443 W. Fullerton Ave. (bet. Greenview & Janssen Aves.)**

**Phone:** 773-281-6600 Lunch & dinner daily
**Web:** www.pizzeriadanella.com
**Prices:** $$ Fullerton

Though it calls itself a pizzeria, this cheerful and vast Italian hang near DePaul University is so much more. A mosaic-tiled wood-burning oven gleams from the rear of the dimly lit space, brightened by sunny yellow and Mediterranean blue walls. Craft beer nerds should take a seat at the bar for a sampling from the varied list of artisanal Italian beers.

Authentic Neapolitan pizzas share menu space with modern stuffed "bomba" pies like the Ciotta Ciotta, which mounds a deli case's worth of salumi and cheeses between two pizza dough rounds. Pasta selections are equally sprawling, and include fresh combinations like pappardelle with plump mussels, black truffles, and pecorino. Limoncello-soaked strawberries over homemade sponge cake keep the finale light.

# Raj Darbar

Indian

D2

**2660 N. Halsted St. (bet. Schubert & Wrightwood Aves.)**

**Phone:** 773-348-1010 Dinner nightly
**Web:** www.rajdarbar.com
**Prices:** $$ Diversey

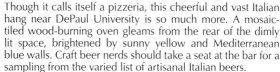

Though discreetly set a few steps below street level, Raj Darbar feels roomy and bright, thanks to a warm color scheme, mirrored accents, and wide windows looking out onto Halsted Street. This large cavern is a favorite among Indians for family gatherings and celebrations, though locals and regulars pop in routinely for takeout and filling dinners.

The expansive menu covers all bases with a host of standards, pleasantly prepared with aromatic spices. Large half-moons of naan arrive fluffy and blistered from the tandoor, and are a perfect vessel for the spicy yogurt sauce in lamb *rogan josh* or richly balanced and velvety chicken *makhani*. Vegetable samosas, crispy on the outside and stuffed with spiced peas and potatoes, are impossible to put down.

# Riccardo Trattoria

XX

## 23

### 2119 N. Clark St. (bet. Dickens & Webster Aves.)

**Phone:** 773-549-0038 Dinner nightly
**Web:** www.riccardotrattoria.com
**Prices:** $$

The understated wood-and-cream décor doesn't look anything like an Italian *nonna*'s kitchen. But, the soulful personality of Chef/owner Riccardo Michi and his cache of family recipes make his eponymous restaurant a second home to half the city, it seems—a go-to spot equally suited to flirty date-nights and big, boisterous dinners.

As intimated by the word "trattoria," authentic rustic Italian cooking presides over the menu. One baseball-sized *arancino* would suffice for a hearty appetizer, but in the spirit of *abbondanza*, you get two. Veal roulades, pounded thin, stuffed with sausage and pistachios, and paired with Tuscan fries are standouts among the *secondi*; while a light, fluffy version of tiramisu makes even those who beg off dessert take a second bite.

# Rickshaw Republic

X

## D3

### 2312 N. Lincoln Ave. (bet. Belden Ave. & Childrens Plz.)

**Phone:** 773-697-4750 Lunch Tue – Sun
**Web:** www.rickshawrepublic.com Dinner Tue – Sat
**Prices:** ⊜⊜ ▦ Fullerton

The fire engine-red façade of the Adler & Sullivan building grabs your attention, but the smells and tastes of the Southeast Asian street food at this fresh family-run spot keep you glued to your seat. The colorful handmade marionettes and inverted parasols hanging from the ceiling next to batik-patterned wood carvings and handcrafted Indonesian masks are eye-catching, too.

Specials are listed as "whatever mommy feels like making," and it's wise to trust Mom when it comes to dishes like crispy, sweet, and sticky chicken wings; *mie goreng* noodles with crunchy puffed shrimp chips; or fried *pastel* dumplings stuffed with ground chicken. The house-made *sambal*, red as the building's exterior with an equally fiery finish, goes with everything.

# Rustic House

American

### 1967 N. Halsted St. (bet. Armitage Ave. & Willow St.)

**Phone:** 312-929-3227          Dinner Tue – Sun
**Web:** www.rustichousechicago.com
**Prices:** $$         Armitage

Lincoln Park denizens who aren't at Gemini Bistro are usually here at Rustic House, where wagon-wheel chandeliers and burlap walls add just the right touch of country. Cocktails and snacks like honey-peppered bacon or Marcona almonds fried in duck fat make the bar a destination in its own right.

At the rear of the dining room, the glass-front rotisserie displays juicy, organic chickens in constant rotation, often joined by Kurobuta pork or whole ducks. Pair a rotisserie meat with sweet corn brûlée and garlicky, smooth mashed potatoes; or slice into a prime aged steak from the wood-burning grill. Arrive before 6:30 P.M. to take advantage of the $35 prix-fixe, with the option of Scotch whiskey or dessert as a third course.

# Summer House Santa Monica

American

### 1954 N. Halsted St.(bet. Armitage Ave. & Willow St.)

**Phone:** 773-634-4100        Lunch Fri – Sun
**Web:** www.summerhousesm.com       Dinner nightly
**Prices:** $$       Armitage

Sunny days and southern California come to Lincoln Park in the form of this bright and breezy restaurant that resembles a beach house, albeit an enormous one with lots of house guests. It's the perfect choice for a summer's day—and not a bad one in the colder months either if you're having a quick bite before the theater or want to shake off those winter blues for a while. There's even a countdown showing the number of days till summer.

The menu proves a good fit for the surroundings by keeping things easy. There are sandwiches, tacos, and salads, but it's the meat and fish from the wood-fired oven that stand out. For dessert, choose a big cookie from the counter by the entrance. There's also a pizza restaurant and bar attached.

# Twin Anchors

 Barbecue  %

### 1655 N. Sedgwick St. (at Eugenie St.)

| | | |
|---|---|---|
| **Phone:** | 312-266-1616 | Lunch Sat – Sun |
| **Web:** | www.twinanchorsribs.com | Dinner nightly |
| **Prices:** | **$$** | Sedgwick |

Within the brick walls that have housed Twin Anchors since 1932, generations have made their way across the checkerboard linoleum floor to throw a quarter in the jukebox and get saucy with a slab of their legendary ribs in one of the curved booths. Though the bar is wall-to-wall on weekends, most weekdays are low-key, with families and groups ready for a casual night out.

Fall-off-the-bone baby back ribs are the real deal, made with sweet and spicy rub, served with their own "zesty" sauce or the newer Prohibition version, with brown sugar and a hint of ghost-pepper heat. Classic sides like onion rings, baked beans, or hearty chili round out the meal. If there's a wait at this no-reservations spot, try the beer of the month while cooling your heels.

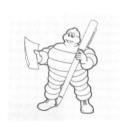

Chicago ▲ Lincoln Park & Old Town

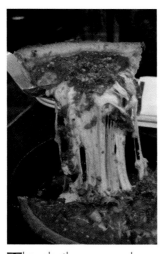

foodies and visitors can contact the Chicago Cultural Center's "culinary concierges" with any food tourism-related queries.

## SENSATIONAL SPREADS

The relentless pace and race of Chicago's main business district is named after the "El" tracks that make a "loop" around the area. Their cacophony may be an intrinsic part of the soundtrack of the Windy City, but that isn't to say that this neighborhood doesn't have a culinary resonance as well. In fact, it is one that is perpetually evolving with the region. It wasn't that long ago that the Loop turned into a no-man's land once the business crowd headed home for the evening. However thanks to a revitalized Theater District, new residential high-rises, hotels, and student dorms, the tumbleweeds have been replaced with a renewed dining scene, wine boutiques, and gourmet grocery stores that stay open well past dusk. In fact, as a testament to the times, local

Start your voyage here by exploring **Block 37**, one of the city's original 58 blocks. It took decades of hard work and several political dynasties, but the block now cradles a five-story atrium with shopping, restaurants, and entrances to public transportation. Next up: **Haute Sausage**, a food truck-turned-storefront that boasts numerous creations infused with Middle Eastern and South African elements. Top off these savory spreads with a bit of sweet at the Chicago outpost of New York City hot spot **Magnolia Bakery**, where folks wait in line for such treasures as banana pudding and melt-in-your-mouth cupcakes. For those watching their waistline, probiotic **Starfruit Café**—with a spectrum of delicious frozen yogurts—is heaven on earth. Catering to the hordes of office lunchers in the Loop are several fast food options on the Pedway level (a system of tunnels that links crucial downtown buildings underground, which is essential during those cruel Chicago winters.) For a quick grab-and-go lunch, **Hannah's Bretzel** is top notch. Lauded as "über sandwich makers," their version of the namesake, crafted from freshly baked German bread, features ultra-tasty fillings (think of a grass-fed sirloin spread with nutty Gruyère, vine tomatoes, and spicy horseradish aïoli). While summer brings a mélange of musical performances to Millennium Park, Grant Park, and the Petrillo Music Shell that's just begging for a picnic *en plein air*, winter evenings are best spent at **The Walnut Room**. Besides fantastic people-watching, a family-friendly vibe, and stunning Christmas décor, this Marshall Fields favorite also warms the soul with delicious comfort food like Mrs. Hewing's Original Chicken Pot Pie—the recipe for which dates back to 1890. Local foodies can also be found feasting at **Park Grill**, a full-service restaurant flanked by an ice rink in the winter. Finally, no trip to Chicago, much less the Loop, would be complete without munching on Italian specialties from **Vivere**, a long-lived, local institution mixing formality with spirited charm in a handsome and curvaceous wood-toned space.

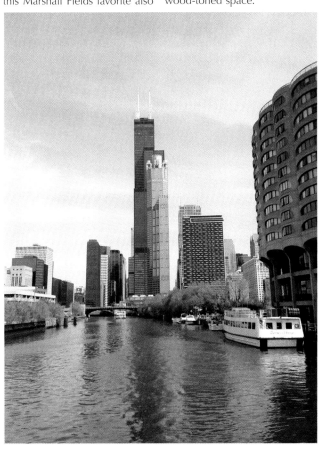

## TOURING & CAROUSING

Calling all sweet tooths: throughout the week, **Valerie's Original Chicago Chocolate Tours** gives two-plus hour guided walking tours of the downtown area's hottest chocolate shops, bakeries, and cafés. If dessert isn't your thing, stops on **Tastebud Tours'** Loop route include hot dogs, pizza, and **The Berghoff**, the city's oldest restaurant known for its enormous steins of beer. And since no tour of the Second City would be complete without pizza, the popular **Chicago Pizza Tour** is also headquartered here. From visiting restaurant kitchens, getting schooled on top ingredients, ovens, the physics of pizza-making, and, of course, digging into some deep-dish pies, this expedition is designed to showcase the essence behind Chicago's most notable food. During warmer months, several farmers' markets cater to the downtown crowd, including the ones at Federal Plaza on Tuesdays and Daley Plaza on Thursdays. Though concession carts dot the streets in nearby Millennium Park, true foodies are in for a treat at **Mariano's Fresh Market**. This gourmet grocery store offers everything from gluten-free lemon bars for stiletto-clad socialites, to holiday gift ensembles popular among local businesses. Moving from food to wine, **Printers Row Wine Shop's** carefully curated, all-embracing wine selection, and weekly wine tastings (every Friday at 5:00 PM.) make it the district's go-to wine spot, intent on equipping real folks with the right amount of relevant information. The city also sees its fair share of coffee connoisseurs and those weary from sightseeing should be sure to get a pick-me-up at **Intelligentsia Coffee**—a local coffee chain with an emphasis on direct trade. Locations can be found all over town, but the **Millennium Park Coffeebar** is especially convenient and delicious.

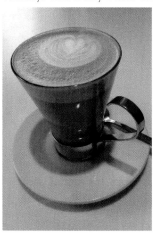

## TASTE OF CHICAGO

One of the Windy City's biggest events (and the second largest attraction in the state), **Taste of Chicago** is a five-day summer extravaganza in Grant Park. For the last 30 years, the festival's never-ending maze of real food booths and live music has attracted hordes of hungry diners and gourmands from all over the world. It may be hot and crowded, but that's just part of the fun—or torture.

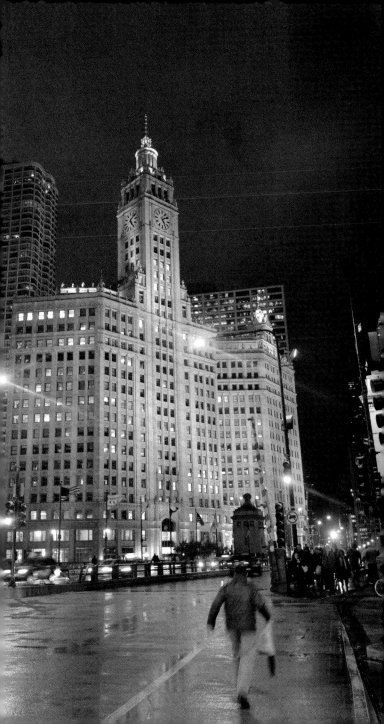

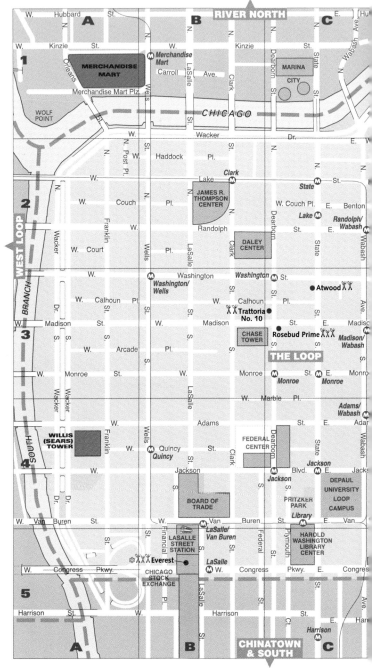

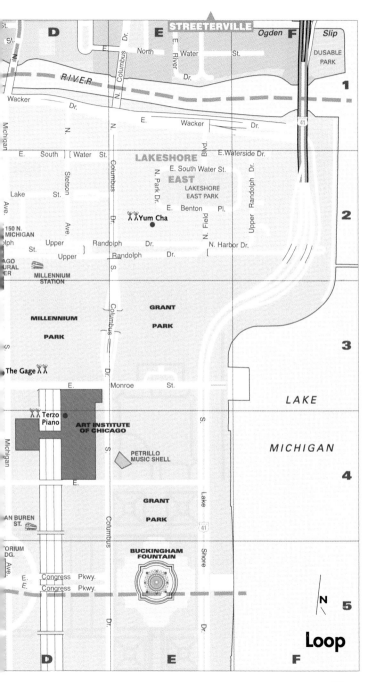

# Atwood

Contemporary ✗✗

**C3**

### 1 W. Washington St. (at State St.)

| | | |
|---|---|---|
| **Phone:** | 312-368-1900 | Lunch & dinner daily |
| **Web:** | www.atwoodrestaurant.com | |
| **Prices:** | $$ | 🚇 Washington |

Set beside Hotel Burnham, this N'Orleans-cum-Parisienne bijou is bold, bright, and fun. A perfect mix of comfort and polish make the compact space snug for some, while soaring ceilings, wood-framed windows, and gorgeous chandeliers make it a supreme choice among handsome hotel guests, suits on the run, and lunching ladies.

Even if the kitchen is located below, every dish turned out of it is top-notch. Service is on-point with minor blemishes that are bound to be forgotten when served piping-hot poutine tater tots dipped in delicious pork gravy. Beer-battered cod is perfectly fried and very tasty when teamed with crispy potato chips and creamy sauce *gribiche*, whereas a red-apple strudel infused with cinnamon is divine on its own and all alone.

# The Gage

Gastropub ✗✗

**D3**

### 24 S. Michigan Ave. (bet. Madison & Monroe Sts.)

| | | |
|---|---|---|
| **Phone:** | 312-372-4243 | Lunch & dinner daily |
| **Web:** | www.thegagechicago.com | |
| **Prices:** | $$ | 🚇 Madison |

Set across from Millennium Park, this expansive gastropub is used to accommodating crowds. And yet, its buzzy, collegial vibe never feels overwhelming. Handsome banquette booths and columns wrapped in glazed celadon tiles lend a clubby allure. A sidewalk patio and bar stretching half the length of the restaurant gets its fair share of happy-hour crowds, so walk to the rear dining rooms for a more sedate setting.

Pub classics with flair stand out on the menu. House poutine is a delicious deviation from tradition, smothering fries with smoked wild boar ragout, cheese curds, and pickled red onions. The mushroom sandwich is simply named but deeply flavorful, layering roasted earthy varieties with pecorino, arugula, and truffle oil on a crusty baguette.

162

# Everest

 French

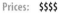 **B5**

## 440 S. LaSalle St. (bet. Congress Pkwy. & Van Buren St.)

**Phone:** 312-663-8920                          Dinner Tue – Sat
**Web:** www.everestrestaurant.com
**Prices:** $$$$                           LaSalle/Van Buren

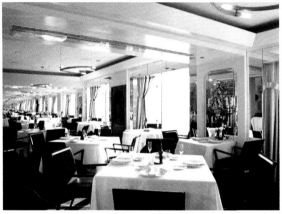

Reservations are essential here. When a restaurant is perched atop the Chicago Stock Exchange, you'll need one just to get through security. (Remember to change elevators on the 39th floor!)

Upon entering this restaurant, prepare to be swept away by panoramic views comparable to those seen from an airplane, especially on a clear, summer night. The interior is a gallery of sorts, with abstract paintings, tabletop sculptures, and plenty of mirrors to exaggerate the dominating views. Everyone who dines here is dressed to the nines, celebrating a special occasion, and making an over-the-top effort. The feeling is a bit dated, but nonetheless lovely.

Chef Jean Joho's French menu is wonderfully old-school, with plenty of Alsatian accents. Each dish is sure to be beautifully executed, as in the cold-pressed lobster tail enrobed in blanched leek served with *brandade*-potato terrine, celeriac remoulade, and tears of crème fraîche dotted with Herruga caviar. Expect meat courses inspired by the tables of kings, like Louis XIV's *lièvre à la royale* stuffed with pheasant, duck, and foie gras in a deep brown sauce with buttery noodles, roasted squash, and turnip purée. Chocolaty chestnut beignets for dessert ooze with decadence.

# Rosebud Prime

Steakhouse

## 1 S. Dearborn St. (at Madison St.)

**Phone:** 312-384-1900
**Web:** www.rosebudrestaurants.com
**Prices:** $$$

Lunch Mon – Fri
Dinner nightly
 Monroe

Though it's only been part of the Rosebud empire since 2007, this Loop darling plays the part of a throwback American steakhouse to the hilt. Crimson-hued faux-alligator chairs and banquettes punctuate a sprawling wood-paneled dining room, where tuxedoed servers weave expertly among suited bankers. A winding staircase leads to a lofty mezzanine.

Bread baskets filled with soft pretzels and ciabatta start the parade of steakhouse staples. Rounding out the beef, tender Berkshire pork chops are sautéed with red cherry bomb peppers and spiced with a pinch of chili for surprising heat with every bite. Keep the mashed potatoes a secret from your cardiologist: already decadent and buttery, they're studded with bacon and topped with broiled cheddar.

# Terzo Piano

Italian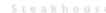

## 159 E. Monroe St. (in the Art Institute of Chicago)

**Phone:** 312-443-8650
**Web:** www.terzopianochicago.com
**Prices:** $$$

Lunch daily
Dinner Thu
 Monroe

With a stunning architectural backdrop of the Chicago skyline and Millennium Park, oohs and aahs come with the territory at this hot spot in the Art Institute of Chicago. As such, Terzo Piano allows itself to be a blank canvas for the surrounding view—and the artistry of food and drink on each table. Walls of windows flood the room with natural light that's further amplified by white tables and chairs.

Many elements of the restaurant's menu are made in-house, including tea blends and sodas. Dishes span the globe, like smoky chicken skewers over charred eggplant purée and couscous studded with apricots and almonds. Earthy but surprisingly delicate Nebrodini mushroom sauce bathes springy hand-cut pappardelle and gets a peppery bite from wilted arugula.

# Trattoria No. 10

Italian

### 10 N. Dearborn St. (bet. Madison & Washington Sts.)

**Phone:** 312-984-1718
**Web:** www.trattoriaten.com
**Prices:** $$

Lunch Mon – Fri
Dinner Mon – Sat
 Washington

Don't be deceived by its small entrance next to Sopraffina Marketcaffè—Trattoria No. 10's cavernous, subterranean rooms seem to spread out for miles under the Loop. Lunch reservations are necessary to secure a spot here among the legal and financial power lunchers scarfing up rustic Italian specialties, alongside a selection of beer lovers perusing the craft varietals.

Seasonality is the driving force behind many of their items including the justly famous ravioli, filled one day with squash blossoms and pancetta, and another day with the always in-demand spicy sausage. Other fresh pasta creations may include fluffy spinach *gnudi* with fennel pollen in a creamy heirloom tomato sauce; or miniature orecchiette tossed with chopped rapini and fontina.

# Yum Cha

Chinese

### 333 E. Randolph St. (bet. Columbus Dr. & Field Blvd.)

**Phone:** 312-946-8885
**Web:** www.yumchachicago.com
**Prices:** $$

Lunch & dinner daily

 Randolph

This dim sum parlor may be a new kid on the block, but don't be fooled by its modern, angular structure as it's the ideal place to shoot the breeze over authentic steamed treats. Inside, grab a perch up front or settle into a seat in the attractive rear dining area overlooking the park. Alcoves with padded banquettes and dark fittings feel cozy and intimate—not unlike the warm staff who are always eager to please.

Plump pouches of *har gow* followed by octopus rings sautéed with tofu, garlic, and spicy Sichuan chilies are always a hot choice. Bamboo steamers of chicken-and-mushroom *siu mai* or vegetable rolls filled with glass noodles are inherently satisfying, and mango pudding with tapioca cream makes for a rich finale.

# Pilsen, University Village & Bridgeport

This cluster of neighborhoods packs a perfect punch, both in terms of food and sheer vitality. It lives up to every expectation and reputation, so get ready for a tour packed with literal, acoustic, and visual flavor. The Little Italy moniker applies to a stretch of Taylor Street that abuts the University (of Illinois at Chicago) Village neighborhood, and it's bigger and more authentically Italian than it first appears. The streets are as stuffed with epicurean shops as an Italian beef sandwich is with meat. On that note, bring an appetite and try a prime example of the iconic (and messy) Chicago treat at **Al's No. 1 Italian Beef**. After combing through the wares at **Conte Di Savoia**, an Italian grocery and popular takeout counter, stop for lunch at **Fontano Foods** (locally famous for their hearty subs) or old-school **Bacchanalia**.

Then, save room for dessert at **Mario's Italian Lemonade**, where you can wash down your meal with a frozen fruit slush. Later, consider popping into **Scafuri Bakery** for a sugar refill, some biscotti, or a *sfogliatelle*. This charming sanctum has been delivering traditional Italian sweets to the community since opening its doors in 1904. Well-loved for fresh breads, pastries, and cookies, wedding cakes and pies are now also part of their ever-evolving repertoire.

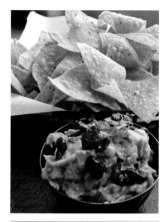

## UNIVERSITY VILLAGE

Like any self-respecting college "town," University Village is home to a range of warm and toasty coffee shops. Add to that the mélange of doctors, medical students, nurses, and others working in the neighborhood hospital, and you've got a perpetually bustling vibe with great people-watching potential. Take a break from the hustle to quench your thirst at **Lush Wine & Spirits** showcasing the expected varietals, or sate a salt craving at local obsession, **Salted Caramel**, noted for their popcorn, especially the bacon-bourbon caramel. On Sundays, follow the local crowd to Chicago's legendary **Maxwell Street Market**. Having relocated to Desplaines Street in 2008, this sprawling bazaar welcomes over 500 vendors selling fresh produce, Mexican street eats, and non-food miscellanea.

Watch celebrity chef, Rick Bayless as he scours these stalls for locally grown tomatoes and tomatillos; while lesser Gods can be seen rummaging around for tonight's dinner essentials.

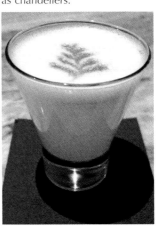
## PILSEN & BRIDGEPORT

Chicagoland's massive Mexican population (more than 500,000 according to the latest U.S. Census count) has built a patchwork of regional specialties, many of which are found in the south side's residential Pilsen and Little Village neighborhoods. Pilsen is also home to the free National Museum of Mexican Art, the only Latino museum accredited by the American Alliance of Museums, as well as countless authentic taquerias and bakeries. **Birrieria Reyes de Ocotlan** is one such model whose main attraction is tender, delicious, and flavorful goat meat folded into juicy tacos. If goat sounds too gamey, then **Pollo Express** oozing with the tantalizing aroma of whole chargrilled chickens, is always reliable. Join their endless queue for Styrofoam containers filled with fresh guacamole, spicy adobo-rubbed chicken, and individually wrapped sweet empanadas.

Everyone goes all out for Mexican Independence Day in September, including more than 25 participating area restaurants, while the Little Village Arts Festival packs 'em in every October. Just as **the Pilsen Community Market** held every Sunday in the Chicago Community Bank, with its assortment of fruit and vegetables, does much to replenish the soul; carb addicts get their fill of freshly made tortillas and crispy corn chips at **Sabinas Food Products**. Meanwhile, carnivores can be found gushing over **Carnitas Uruapan's** plates of slow-cooked pork carnitas paired with salty, fatty, and crispy *chicharrónes*. Since 1950, **El Milagro** has been proffering a unique taste with its cafeteria-style restaurant complete with a tamale-centric menu, as well as a store bursting with burritos and handmade tortillas. Finally, lovers of all things "green" cannot resist the siren call of **Simone's Bar**. This certified eco-friendly joint is not just hip and happening, but also an ideal spot for sipping on beers and cocktails while savoring an array of well-prepared food. Over in Bridgeport, **Maria's Packaged Goods & Community Bar** has been a neighborhood institution in one form or another since 1939. Here, antique collectible beer cans line the space, and leftover clusters of beer bottles are being constantly repurposed as chandeliers.

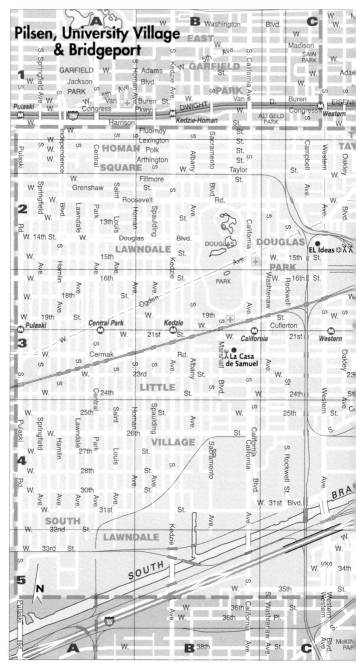

# Pilsen, University Village & Bridgeport

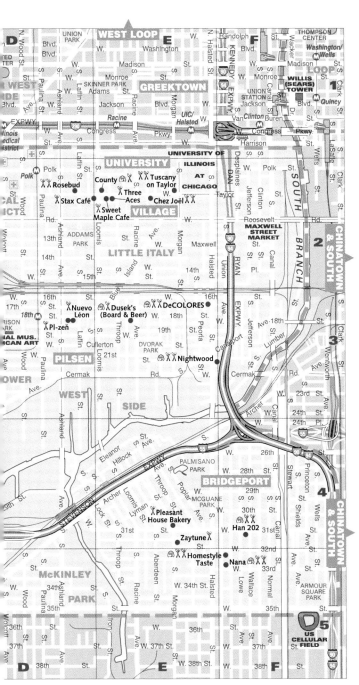

# Chez Joël

French

**1119 W. Taylor St. (bet. Aberdeen & May Sts.)**

**Phone:** 312-226-6479
**Web:** www.chezjoelbistro.com
**Prices:** $$

Lunch Fri – Sun
Dinner Tue – Sun

With tables covered in archetypal butcher's paper, butter-yellow walls, and red velvet window dressings, Chez Joël adds a touch of *je ne sais quoi* to Little Italy. The cozy, romantic setting is filled with expats and locals reliving memories of their trips to the City of Light. Taxidermied pheasants keep watch over the room from their high perches, like a Deyrolle curiosity.

The kitchen gives classic French cuisine a soupçon of international embellishment. Three plump scallops spooned with basil pesto are set over a pool of tomato coulis for a Franco-Italian take on *coquilles St. Jacques.* Simple Caesar salad benefits from fresh ingredients like tender grilled chicken and crisp romaine lettuce in a garlicky dressing. Tasty pastas round out the menu.

# County

Barbecue

**1352 W. Taylor St. (bet. Ada & Loomis Sts.)**

**Phone:** 312-929-2528
**Web:** www.dmkcountybarbeque.com
**Prices:** ⊜⊜

Lunch & dinner daily

🚇 Polk

Go ahead; guess which building on this block of Taylor belongs to County. If you chose the one done up in gingham, you're on the money. Chef Michael Kornick's barbecue-focused outpost exudes pure Americana, and is dressed in deep mahogany-tinted walls and the heavenly aroma of smoking meats.

The same cheeky 'tude that gave us County's technicolor façade appears in creative starters like the bacon-and-barbecue parfait: a shot glass layered with charred brisket and white cheddar grits, topped with a crisp bacon strip. Covering swaths of regional barbecue styles, other riches include St. Louis ribs smoked for five hours; moist, lacquered chicken; and spicy grilled hot links. Sides, like cheesy potato casserole with pickled jalapeños, are fun and filling.

# DeCOLORES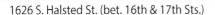

🕽🕽

**1626 S. Halsted St. (bet. 16th & 17th Sts.)**

**Phone:** 312-226-9886
**Web:** www.decolor.us
**Prices:** $$

Lunch Thu – Sun
Dinner Tue – Sun

This family-owned Mexican restaurant in Pilsen's art district appropriately doubles as a gallery, with locals' works rotating frequently on the coffee-colored walls. If the pieces for sale don't strike a chord, just admire the bar's halting design of stylized metal branches snaking between shelves of colorful sugar skulls and paper flags.

Recipes passed down through generations highlight fresh vegetables and healthy fare. The salsa with house-made corn chips as a starter changes every day, but each variety is a pleasure. A smattering of raw shaved cabbage, radish, and red onion in pozole offers a fresh take on traditional hominy stew with roast pork and cucumber salsa. Boneless *guajillo*-marinated pork loin chops gain sweetness from grilled pineapple.

# Dusek's (Board & Beer)

🕽

**1227 W. 18th St. (at Allport St.)**

**Phone:** 312-526-3851
**Web:** www.dusekschicago.com
**Prices:** $$

Lunch Sat – Sun
Dinner nightly
🚇 18th

Housed in Thalia Hall, a former theater and public hall, Dusek's has room to be a triple threat. The dining room is on the main floor, while the upstairs is a live music venue with a subterranean bar pouring a strong selection of classic and contemporary cocktails. "Re-established" in 2013 by the team behind Longman & Eagle, it's got the same cool factor with a comfy neighborhood vibe.

The soulful American menu changes daily, so don't get too hung up on favorites. Recent hits include partially deboned quail—"Kentucky fried" for crunch and paired with a plank of foie gras cornbread and pickled okra to cut the richness. Deviled pigtail rillettes arrive as crisp panko-coated cylinders atop paprika-cured soft egg yolk dotted with celery foam and sweet relish.

# EL Ideas ঞ্চ

XX

**2419 W. 14th St.** (at Western Ave.)

Phone: 312-226-8144
Web: www.elideas.com
Prices: $$$$

Dinner Tue – Sat

🚇 Western (Pink)

BYO

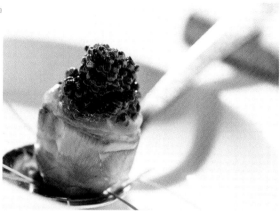

Free your mind, keep your expectations high, and ignore the hand-made sign and desolate locale that make this undeniably edgy restaurant seem like a David Lynch movie.

No one comes here for high-end pampering; rather, the interior is an amalgam of heavy wood timber, zinc ductwork, abstract art, and a homespun curtain made of wine corks. The open kitchen and its team of freewheeling anti-heroes lend a dinner-party vibe, with guests bringing bottles of bourbon as gifts for the chefs and others getting up to mingle.

Those who prefer some sort of ice-breaker before jumping into the spirited conversation over the 14-course prix-fixe may rest assured that the first dish must be licked directly off the plate. That fresh uni arrives on a bed of smoked shiitake mushrooms with trout roe to cut the richness, colorful nasturtium leaves, and citrusy yuzu jelly. A supremely smooth potato soup has tremendous depth of flavor, topped with crisped potato cubes, and finished with nitrogen frozen vanilla granité. Beguiling simplicity is at the heart of a stunning slice of fine-grained, pink, and delicate antelope served in a light jus with chewy sautéed ramps, mixed baby vegetables, and pickled rhubarb.

# Han 202

🍴🍴

605 W. 31st St. (bet. Lowe Ave. & Wallace St.)

**Phone:** 312-949-1314                                Dinner Tue – Sun
**Web:** www.han202.com
**Prices:** $$

BYO

In a neighborhood dominated by sports bars and Irish pubs, Han 202 stands apart as a sophisticated pan-Asian alternative for White Sox watchers. Bare wood tables and high-backed coffee-and-cream leather seats convey polish—an attitude reinforced by the skilled chefs and servers. Dramatic driftwood sculpture and framed art play against pale walls.

The $35 four-course prix-fixe menu is a true bargain, with each course punctuated by precisely cut fresh bites of sushi. Jeju Island *hirame* is lightly brushed with mirin and kissed with wasabi. Lobster tail arrives warm and buttery with a dollop of fresh ricotta and tender red beet halves, drizzled with olive oil. Seared duck breast adds juicy flavor to standard steamed vegetables in fermented bean sauce.

# Homestyle Taste 🍢

🍴🍴

3205 S. Halsted St. (bet. 32nd & 33rd Sts.)

**Phone:** 312-949-9328                                Lunch & dinner daily
**Web:** N/A
**Prices:** 🍜

BYO

When the winter winds start whipping, step into this family-run restaurant, where the name says it all. Homestyle Taste is authentic, chili-heavy Chinese food that will warm even the most bone-chilled Chicagoan. The dining room's dangling red fabric strands of chilies are harbingers of what is to come. Even the freshly brewed tea verges on scalding, though the hot and sour soup is perfectly balanced with vinegar, white pepper, and full-bodied flavors. Just don't forget to try the ethereally light, "hand pancake" and pull it apart, shred by shred. Chopped spicy chicken is served cold on the bone, bathed in scarlet chili oil that's at once searingly hot, salty, and sweet. Garlicky fried string beans are perfect for those who can't take the heat.

# La Casa De Samuel

B3

Mexican ✕

**2834 W. Cermak Rd. (bet. California Ave. & Marshall Blvd.)**

**Phone:** 773-376-7474

**Web:** www.lacasadesamuel.com

**Prices:** 🍝🍝

Lunch & dinner daily

🚇 California (Pink)

Though the sign over the awning reads "Cocina Internacional," make no mistake: this Mexican restaurant has been bringing tacos and *queso fundido* to Pilsen since 1989. Exposed wood beams, brick walls, and bright oil paintings add a true-blue vibe; while a tortilla station where an *abuelita* works masa into thin discs gets the appetite going. Multi-generational families return time and again to share spicy *molcajete*-crushed salsa.

Along with the freshly made tortillas that arrive swaddled and warm from the grill, the bustling kitchen turns out solid standards like fajitas as well as unusual wild game options like grilled wild boar, rabbit, or alligator. Wash down baby eels sizzling with garlic and chile with an icy lime-infused margarita.

# Nana

F5

Latin American ✕✕

**3267 S. Halsted St. (at 33rd St.)**

**Phone:** 312-929-2486

**Web:** www.nanaorganic.com

**Prices:** $$

Lunch daily
Dinner Wed – Sun

While Nana Solis is the matriarch of this family-run Bridgeport favorite, her children (who were raised just upstairs) keep the kitchen and dining room humming. A devoted breakfast crowd takes up residence at the coffee bar and butcher block tables each day, often perusing the colorful modern artwork for sale on the walls.

Locally sourced and organic are the guiding principles behind every ingredient here; many dishes also get a little Latin flavor. Soft avocado wedges are tossed in panko, then flash-fried for a crispy exterior and creamy center. "Nanadicts" give a Southwestern accent to eggs Benedict by adding chorizo, corn *pupusas*, and poblano cream. Sunday nights feature family-style fried chicken dinners fit for large groups with larger appetites.

# Nightwood

XX

**2119 S. Halsted St. (at 21st St.)**

Phone: 312-526-3385
Web: www.nightwoodrestaurant.com
Prices: $$

Lunch Sun
Dinner Mon – Sat

An oasis of stylish simplicity on an otherwise bland stretch of Halsted, Nightwood gleams like a beacon with its enchanting courtyard and welcoming entrance. Solo diners love the chef's counter with its view into the bustling kitchen. Dark wood and brick accents throughout make the dining room casually romantic.

Speaking of which, get your palate going with a whiskey cocktail or seasonal non-alcoholic bevy like a concord fizz. Rustic inflections like spit-roasted chicken and hand-shaped pasta complement elegant touches that show the kitchen's finesse. A purse of soft scrambled eggs opens to reveal creamy quail egg yolks and steelhead roe; and caramelized pigs' ears take on the texture of peanut brittle when paired with maple-habanero butter.

# Nuevo Léon

**1515 W. 18th St. (bet. Ashland Ave. & Laflin St.)**

Phone: 312-421-1517
Web: N/A
Prices: ☺☺

Lunch & dinner daily

 18th

Nuevo Leon's colorful trompe l'oeil exterior is almost as loud as the din inside this family favorite in the heart of Pilsen. A jukebox competes with the chatter as it blasts Mexican tunes throughout multiple dining rooms, bouncing off clay tile floors and rattling the hand-painted plates on festive yellow walls.

The crowds come for large portions of straightforward Mexican fare like slabs of carne asada with warm corn tortillas to wrap the lightly seasoned meat and beans. Munch on a complimentary beef-and-potato soft taco while poring over the extensive menu. Sizzling platters arrive in a heartbeat once the order's been placed. Just add summery tomato salsa or taqueria-style pickled carrots and jalapeños to give each bite a bit more zing.

# Pleasant House Bakery

**E4**

### 964 W. 31st St. (bet. Farrell St. & Lituanica Ave.)

**Phone:** 773-523-7437 — Lunch & dinner daily
**Web:** www.pleasanthousebakery.com
**Prices:**

A lucky horseshoe tucked under Pleasant House's shingled yellow eaves might be nothing but insurance, as this tiny shop specializing in British meat pies has a rabid cult following. UK expats are thrilled to taste authentic renditions of their favorite foods without a trip through customs, and locals appreciate the simple artisanal fare.

**BYO**

Owners Art and Chelsea Jackson fill buttery crusts with savory and seductively curried chicken *balti*. Scotch eggs faithfully follow the classic recipe: hard-boiled, then encased in sausage and breading before taking a dip in the fryer. You may have to BYOB, but the bakery has a symbiotic relationship with Maria's Packaged Goods next door, so feel free to take your pies to the bar or bring a bottle into the café.

# Pl-zeň

**D3**

### 1519 W. 18th St. (bet. Ashland Ave. & Laflin St.)

**Phone:** 312-733-0248 — Lunch Sat – Sun
**Web:** www.pl-zen.com — Dinner Tue – Sun
**Prices:** $$ —  18th

The beckoning tentacles of an enormous octopus painted on a brownstone point the way to this quirky subterranean spot. More murals lead diners down a brick-lined alley and into the dining room, where the dim space is lightened by blonde wood barstools and a hospitable vibe from the cool young staff.

Though *chilaquiles* and sesame-crusted tilapia tacos find their way to the menu, Pl-zeň offers a full slate of gastropub fare that steps away from the traditional Mexican bent of the neighborhood. Raisin- and pignoli-studded boar meatballs are simmered in tomato sauce and finished with ricotta and caramelized onions. A poached egg adds richness to crispy pig ear salad with Fresno aïoli. Cinnamon-sugar beignets deserve a dip in luscious strawberry-pinot grigio sauce.

# Rosebud

**1500 W. Taylor St. (at Laflin St.)**

Phone: 312-942-1117
Web: www.rosebudrestaurants.com
Prices: $$

Lunch & dinner daily

 Polk

Handsomely appointed and sultry even at lunch, Rosebud evokes those Italian red-sauce joints where deals are brokered by wise guys in hushed voices over the likes of a fat pork chop Calabrese. This is the original location that launched a mini-chain of Rosebuds throughout Chicago, and its nostalgic charm still retains its character—as well as the characters who've been coming here for more than 30 years. Live out your Godfather fantasy in a seat by the leaded glass windows, watched over by a painting of the Chairman of the Board, while slurping down *pasta e fagioli*, sausage and peppers, or chicken Vesuvio. And since we're reliving this fantastical classic, leave the gun, as they say, and take the crispy cannoli garnished with pistachios and strawberries.

# Stax Café

**1401 W. Taylor St. (at Loomis St.)**

Phone: 312-733-9871
Web: www.staxcafe.com
Prices:

Lunch daily

"We're Breakfast Geeks. We take this stuff way too seriously" reads one of the server's T-shirts at Stax Café, and UIC students and staff are grateful for their dedication to heart-warming wake-up fare. From the coffee and fresh juice bar for on-the-go types, to flat-screen TVs for those dying to catch up on sports, this corner restaurant aims to get everyone's day started right.

Breakfast items with tasty twists abound, like ricotta pancakes with strawberry-rhubarb compote; or the Spanish Harlem omelet served frittata-style with chorizo, roasted tomatoes, and poblano peppers. Can't choose? Get a side of mini waffles dusted with powdered sugar alongside your main dish, and don't forget to check out the chalkboards for specials—perhaps breakfast tacos?

# Sweet Maple Cafe

**1339 W. Taylor St. (bet. Loomis St. & Racine Ave.)**

Phone: 312-243-8908                                    Lunch daily
Web:   www.sweetmaplecafe.com
Prices:

Sweet Maple piles on the country charm for the loyal crowd of regulars who know that its register of made-from-scratch breakfast plates (with a few lunch items too) is worth getting up for each morning. Checkered oilcloth tablecloths, scuffed wood floors, and rustic dowel furniture give this Taylor Street spot a lived-in look, while fresh flowers on each table brighten the mood.

Whatever your choice, make sure to include a homemade sweet milk or cornmeal biscuit with your order—whether as part of a sandwich with freshly scrambled eggs and cheese, or on the side of a rotating special like the *chorissimo* taco. Corned beef hash with expertly poached eggs and firm, flavorful bits of corned beef is an eye-opener for those who've avoided lesser versions.

# Three Aces

**1321 W. Taylor St. (bet. Loomis & Throop Sts.)**

Phone: 312-243-1577                            Lunch & dinner daily
Web:   www.threeaceschicago.com
Prices: **$$**                                     Racine

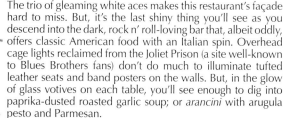

The trio of gleaming white aces makes this restaurant's façade hard to miss. But, it's the last shiny thing you'll see as you descend into the dark, rock n' roll-loving bar that, albeit oddly, offers classic American food with an Italian spin. Overhead cage lights reclaimed from the Joliet Prison (a site well-known to Blues Brothers fans) don't do much to illuminate tufted leather seats and band posters on the walls. But, in the glow of glass votives on each table, you'll see enough to dig into paprika-dusted roasted garlic soup; or *arancini* with arugula pesto and Parmesan.

A cracker-thin *pizzetta* with seasonal toppings like homemade merguez and crumbled *ricotta salata* is an all-time fave; whereas big appetites go for the famously towering Ace burger.

# Tuscany on Taylor

## 1014 W. Taylor St. (bet. Miller & Morgan Sts.)

**Phone:** 312-829-1990
**Web:** www.tuscanychicago.com
**Prices:** $$

Lunch Mon – Fri
Dinner nightly
UIC-Halsted

Italian and Chicago accents co-mingle at Tuscany on Taylor, where the classic cuisine and service are perfectly old-school (no pun intended—the university is a few blocks away). The formal staff tends to diners at white linen-topped tables in the terra cotta-tiled dining room. Chefs in puffy toques man the open kitchen amid shelves of polished copper pans.

A wide-ranging menu of modern Italian interpretations takes guests on a whirlwind tour of the boot. Tiny ravioli stuffed with roasted pears are set in a densely flavorful mascarpone cream sauce with toasted pine nuts and strips of sundried tomatoes. Simple caprese salad arrives as three stacks of thickly sliced heirloom tomatoes, buffalo mozzarella, and basil pesto drizzled with balsamic reduction.

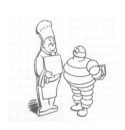

Look for the symbol for a brilliant breakfast to start your day off right.

179

# River North

Urban, picture-perfect, and always-happening River North not only edges the Magnificent Mile, but is also set north of the Chicago River, just across the bridge from the Loop. Once packed with factories and warehouses, today this capital of commercialization is the ultimate landing-place for art galleries, well-known restaurants, swanky shopping, and a hopping nightlife. Thanks to such versatility, the area attracts literally everybody—from lunching ladies and entrepreneurs, to tour bus-style crowds. Visitors are sure to drop by, if only to admire how even mammoth chain restaurants ooze a particular charm here. Among them is **Rock 'n' Roll McDonald's**, a block-long, music-themed outpost of the ubiquitous burger chain. This is one of the world's busiest **MickeyD's** with an expanded menu, music memorabilia, and bragging rights to the first two-lane drive-through. Speaking of drive-throughs, River North is also home to the original **Portillo's**, a hot dog, burger, and beer favorite, whose giant exterior belies its efficient service and better-than-expected food. When it comes to size, few buildings can rival **Merchandise Mart** (so large it has its own ZIP code), known for its retail stores, drool-worthy kitchen showrooms, and two great food shops—at **Artisan Cellar**, in addition to boutique wines and cheeses, you can also purchase Katherine Anne Confections' fresh cream caramels. Locals also adore **The Chopping Block** for

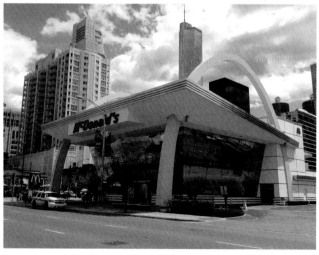

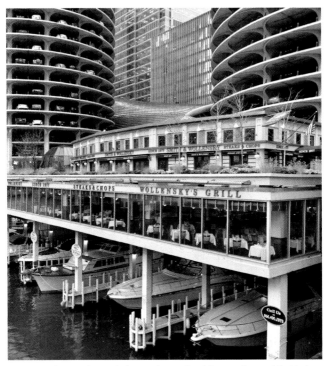

its expertly taught and themed cooking courses, updated, well-edited wine selections, and sparkling knife lines.

From trends to legends, **Carson's** is a barbecue institution. This squat brick box has no windows, but is just the kind of spot where wise guys like to do business, with a bib on of course! This old-school treasure features framed pictures of every local celebrity, who can also be seen gracing the walls at seafood superstar, **Shaw's Crab House**. Their nostalgic bar and dining den is dotted with stainless steel bowls to collect the shells from the multitude of bottom-dwellers on offer. Crab is always available of course, but selections spin with the season. For those who aren't down with seafood in any form, this kitchen turns out a few prime steaks as well. Combat the bitter-cold winters and warm the soul with hearty food and easy elegance at **Lawry's Prime Rib**, housed in the 1890's McCormick Mansion. Inside, the opulent dining room covers all bases from prime rib dinners to seafood signatures. But, true carnivores that like their meat and potatoes done in grand style will find deep comfort in **Smith & Wollensky's** elaborate affair. Another nationwide chain, **Fleming's Prime Steakhouse & Wine Bar** is as well-regarded and recognizable as the aromas wafting from **Blommer Chocolate Outlet Store**, beckoning city dwellers to its Willy Wonka-esque confines. Further indulge

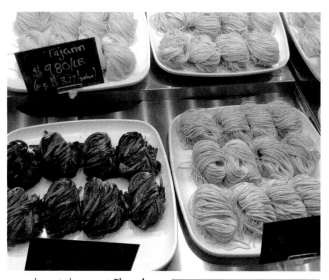

your dessert dreams at **Firecakes Donuts** where moist, coconut cream-filled buns are chased down by delicious, piping-hot chocolate bobbing with soft marshmallows. The Windy City's recent doughnut craze carries on at **Doughnut Vault**, brought to you by restaurateur Brendan Sodikoff, who appears to have the Midas touch with this morning-fried dough. Formerly the location for the infamous Cabrini-Green government housing, today **Chicago Lights: Urban Farm** showcases organic produce, nutritional education, and workforce training, thereby elevating the level of economic opportunities available to this vibrant community. On the other hand, **Eataly** is a huge Italian ode to food, employing a massive workforce. This gourmet paradise may present the same delicacies as its NYC flagship, but the Nutella (corner) with the likes of muffin con Nutella is sure to keep folks infatuated.

## DEEP-DISH DELIGHTS

Thanks to its diverse community, River North is also an excellent destination for various food genres including the local phenomenon of deep-dish pizza. With a doughy crust holding abundant cheese, flavorful sauce, and other toppings some may say this is closer to a casserole or "hot dish" than an Italian-style pizza. Either way, these pies take a while to craft—so be prepared to wait wherever you go. **Pizzeria Uno** (or sister **Pizzeria Due**), and **Giordano's** are some of the best-known pie makers in town. If a little indigestion isn't a concern, chase these down with another local specialty: the Italian beef sandwich. At **Mr. Beef's**, these "parcels" resemble a messy, yet tasty French dip, wrapping thinly sliced and well-seasoned beef with hot or sweet peppers on a hoagie. If you order it "wet," both the meat and bread will be dipped in pan juices. You could also add cheese, but hey, this isn't

Philly! Distinguished by day, River North pumps up the volume at night with sleek cocktail lounges, night clubs, and authentic Irish bars. Slip into **Three Dots and a Dash**, a retro, tiki-inspired bar featuring some of the city's most well-regarded mixologists. For a more rootin'-tootin' good time, stop by the electric **Underground Wonder Bar** whose dangerously tenacious punchbowls and succinct pan-Asian menu make it a favorite for private parties. Meanwhile, happy hour is always hopping at **Green Door Tavern**, which gets its name from the fact that its colored front told Prohibition-era customers where to enter for a drink. To appreciate what all the fuss is about, order their "famous sandwich" or "Green Door Burger."

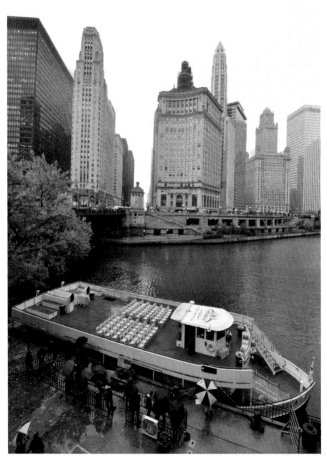

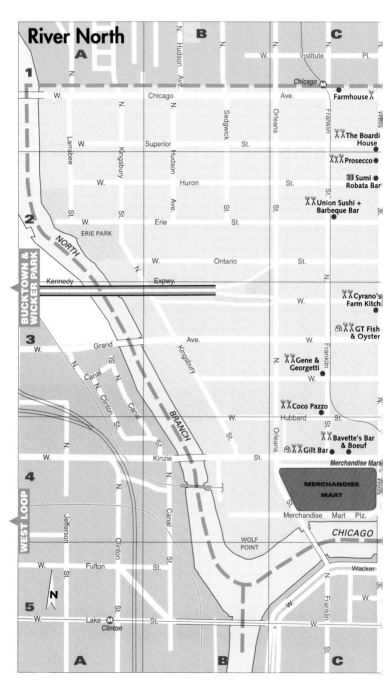

# River North

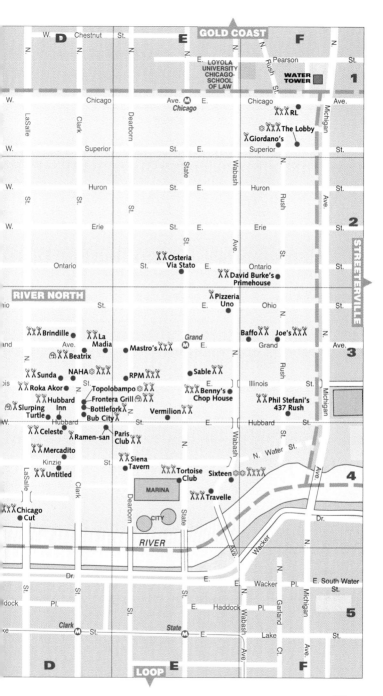

185

# Baffo

 **F3**

### 44 E. Grand Ave. (bet. Rush St. & Wabash Ave.)

| | |
|---|---|
| **Phone:** 312-521-8700 | Lunch Fri – Sun |
| **Web:** www.eataly.com/baffo | Dinner nightly |
| **Prices:** $$$ |  Grand (Red) |

The handlebar pins adorning servers' ties give away the name of the game at Baffo, a visual reminder that the restaurant is named after the Italian word for mustache. As Eataly's fine-dining option, the kitchen makes the most of its 63,000 square-foot pantry upstairs. In typical Mario Batali fashion, a rocking soundtrack bounces off the intricately tiled floor and long marble entry bar.

Though presented in classic Italian fashion from antipasti to *contorni*, modern touches abound in each dish. Finely diced Calabrese salami turns up the heat on al dente squid ink fettuccine tossed with tender lobster chunks, while *vitello tonnato* combines veal carpaccio, tuna aïoli, and *bottarga*-style shaved dried tuna loin for an umami-packed rendition of the classic.

# Bavette's Bar & Boeuf

 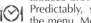

**C4**

### 218 W. Kinzie St. (bet. Franklin & Wells Sts.)

| | |
|---|---|
| **Phone:** 312-624-8154 | Dinner nightly |
| **Web:** www.bavetteschicago.com | |
| **Prices:** $$$ |  Merchandise Mart |

Restaurateur Brendan Sokoloff (also of Maude's Liquor Bar and Au Cheval) breathes new life into the tried and true steakhouse concept with this swanky destination. The vibe inside may be dark and loud, but that only adds to the bonhomie of the chic and cavernous den, outfitted with exposed brick walls, mismatched dangling light fixtures, and tobacco-brown Chesterfield-style sofas.

Predictably, steakhouse and raw bar standards dominate the menu. Most steaks are wet-aged, and though some may prefer more funk, the cuts are expertly broiled. The kitchen deserves praise for unexpected options like creamy short rib stroganoff featuring hand-cut pasta; buttermilk fried chicken; and sides such as *elote*-style corn in a rich cheese sauce sparked with lime.

# Beatrix

**D3**                                     International    ✗✗

### 519 N. Clark St. (at Grand Ave.)

| | | |
|---|---|---|
| **Phone:** | 312-284-1377 | Lunch & dinner daily |
| **Web:** | www.beatrixchicago.com | |
| **Prices:** | **$$** | 🚇 Grand (Red) |

From a spartan façade to an industrial décor, Beatrix is the epitome of cool. Then consider its many meal options, popular tunes, and trendy scene rife with hotel guests from adjacent Aloft, and know why it's jamming. Servers don stylish hairdos and tattoos to match the vibe while attending to the giant room scattered with seats and a coffee bar dispensing excellent local brews.

Meanwhile, the menu veers from creative to quirky with pleasing results. A spring pea soup highlights aroma, flavor, and texture when shot with mint, ricotta, and croutons. Salads may headline, but mains like roasted chili- and chocolate-glazed salmon are a smoky surprise. End with the apple strudel flavored with caramelized brown sugar—it's big in size and faultless in flavor.

# Benny's Chop House

**E3**                                     Steakhouse    ✗✗✗

### 444 N. Wabash Ave. (bet. Hubbard & Illinois Sts.)

| | | |
|---|---|---|
| **Phone:** | 312-626-2444 | Lunch & dinner daily |
| **Web:** | www.bennyschophouse.com | |
| **Prices:** | **$$$** | 🚇 Grand (Red) |

Old-school service meets modern elegance at Benny's Chop House. A far cry from the clubby, masculine steakhouses of yesteryear and just a stone's throw away from the Magnificent Mile, this expansive but welcoming space goes for understated glamour, with tasteful inlaid wood and burgundy columns offset by natural stone walls, white birch branches, and a marble bar.

Though Benny's steaks are the draw, those prime cuts of filet mignon and ribeye are matched by fresh seafood like simply roasted bone-in halibut fillet and classic raw bar towers, along with a variety of pastas and salads. A trio of sliders featuring mini portions of Benny's burger, crab cake, and sliced filet with horseradish cream elevate the idea of bar snacks to new heights.

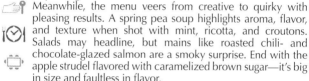

Chicago ► River North

# The Boarding House

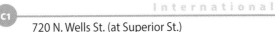

International 🍴🍴

**C1**

## 720 N. Wells St. (at Superior St.)

**Phone:** 312-280-0720
**Web:** www.boardinghousechicago.com
**Prices:** $$

Dinner nightly

🔲 Chicago (Red)

The long-awaited passion project from Chicago master sommelier Alpana Singh, The Boarding House has thrown its doors open to four floors of grandeur. The impressively shimmering wine glass clusters dangling in the first floor bar lead way to the upper dining room, which pulls out all the stops by virtue of its arched, mullioned windows and an installation made from more than 4,000 green wine bottles. Small and larger plates make sharing an appealing proposition. House-made *tagliolini* ribbons tossed with fresh peas, mint, and pickled ramps are bright and zesty. Garlic lovers use crispy chicken thighs to sop up every last bit of aromatic green-garlic pistou. Scoops of sour cherry gelée and merlot-chocolate chip ice cream crown rich brownies for dessert.

# Bottlefork

Contemporary 🍴

**D3**

## 441 N. Clark St. (bet. Hubbard & Illinois Sts.)

**Phone:** 312-955-1900
**Web:** www.bottlefork.com
**Prices:** $$

Lunch daily
Dinner Mon – Sat
🔲 Grand (Red)

Bottlefork, Forkbottle—yup, we get it, it's a "bar & kitchen" but, in this case, a very good one. The narrow room is dominated by a 40-foot bar which morphs into an open kitchen. The lights are turned down and the music is turned up—and unless they know Big Audio Dynamite it's not music for kids. When it comes to the food, "locally sourced and globally inspired" is their USP with the chef, a Four Seasons alumnus, making much of his largely European peregrinations. Expect punchy flavors, teasing combinations, clever twists, and everything from *salumi* and tuna crudo in a jar to "popcorn" sweetbreads, pastas, and Moroccan stews. The terrific cocktail and drinks list covers all bases too. And who isn't tempted to take dessert in liquid form?

# Brindille

French

 D3

**534 N. Clark St. (bet. Grand Ave. & Ohio St.)**

**Phone:** 312-595-1616                                  Dinner Mon – Sat
**Web:** www.brindille-chicago.com
**Prices:** $$$$                                           Grand (Red)

Old-world sophistication mingles with modern artistry at Brindille, the posh and intimate spot from cousins Carrie and Michael Nahabedian (of NAHA). Leather and weathered wood as well as neutral tones give the sumptuous space a hushed feel, though a mosaic wall depicting delicate branches and a glass-enclosed host stand offer a hint of sparkle.

Luxe ingredients in French-inspired dishes are highlighted by eye-catching presentations. Caraway-tinged onion crème soup contains a wealth of surprises: crisp Brussels sprout leaves, Bartlett pear rounds, and semi-melted chunks of blue cheese in the bottom of the bowl. Equally decadent is the Paris-Brest filled with *fromage blanc*, caramelized hazelnuts, and topped with hibiscus granita and spun sugar.

# Bub City

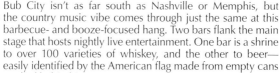

Barbecue

 D3

**435 N. Clark St. (bet. Hubbard & Illinois Sts.)**

**Phone:** 312-610-4200                                  Lunch & dinner daily
**Web:** www.bubcitychicago.com
**Prices:** $$                                             Grand (Red)

 Bub City isn't as far south as Nashville or Memphis, but the country music vibe comes through just the same at this barbecue- and booze-focused hang. Two bars flank the main stage that hosts nightly live entertainment. One bar is a shrine to over 100 varieties of whiskey, and the other to beer—easily identified by the American flag made from empty cans stacked behind its counter.

 Along with the extensive lineup of traditional smoked brisket, ribs, and fried chicken, a raw bar brings chilled seafood refreshment before spicy cheese-stuffed Texas Torpedoes and  loaded hot link sandwiches. A bowl of Smokie's chili arrives with a kick from sliced jalapeño, but the caddy of barbecue and hot sauces on each table lets heat fiends intensify the seasoning.

# Celeste

**111 W. Hubbard St. (bet. Clark & LaSalle Sts.)**

**Phone:** 312-828-9000                                    Dinner Mon – Sat
**Web:** www.celestechicago.com
**Prices:** $$$                                            Grand (Red)

Celeste celebrates the city's close relationship with that great American institution—the bar. It is a veritable fun palace evoking the great drinking establishments of the last century and is spread over three floors. On the first floor is a bar with an abbreviated menu. On the second floor is the narrow and nominally named Deco Room where the marble-topped tables face another bar; and upstairs is reserved for private parties.

The food is certainly more than a mere addendum to the terrific cocktail list and the kitchen is clearly a skilled one. Dishes are quite elaborate in their construction—order lamb and you may find it includes the loin, belly and sweetbreads— and they are as flavorsome as they are attractive.

# Chicago Cut

**300 N. LaSalle St. (at Wacker Dr.)**

**Phone:** 312-329-1800                                    Lunch & dinner daily
**Web:** www.chicagocutsteakhouse.com
**Prices:** $$$                                            Merchandise Mart

Chicago Cut is a steakhouse perfectly suited for the City of the Big Shoulders. The finely tailored locale bustles day and night, thanks to being wrapped in windows along the riverfront, sumptuous red leather furnishings, warm wood trim, and a crackerjack service team cementing its steakhouse vibe.

Non-meat entrées include cedar-planked salmon with a *sriracha*-honey glaze, but make no mistake: beef is boss here. Prime steaks, butchered and dry-aged in-house for 35 days, get just the right amount of time under the flame, as is the case with the perfectly cooked-to-order Porterhouse—pre-sliced and plated for each guest. Sides are a must and should include the dome of hashbrowns, creamed spinach redolent of nutmeg, or tender stalks of grilled asparagus.

# Coco Pazzo

✕✕

 **C3**

**300 W. Hubbard St. (at Franklin St.)**

**Phone:** 312-836-0900
**Web:** www.cocopazzochicago.com
**Prices:** $$

Lunch Mon – Fri
Dinner nightly
Merchandise Mart

Vibrant blue-and-orange awnings help Coco Pazzo make its mark among the area's stellar restaurants, though their reputation for seasonal Tuscan cuisine has been going strong since 1992. Navy velvet curtains hung in the wide, welcoming, high-ceilinged room may dampen the din, but not the enthusiasm from regulars ready for serious *abbondanza* and a bottle from the all-Italian wine list.

Business types fill every seat for the $18 *piatti unici*, a chef-chosen lunch special that changes daily but is always made with expert care. Selections may include Rushing Rivers trout over lentils and spinach paired with speck- and mushroom-studded Carnaroli risotto. Dinner options like pancetta-wrapped quail with taleggio fondue showcase the kitchen's ambitious side.

# Cyrano's Farm Kitchen

 **C3**

✕✕

**546 N. Wells St. (bet. Grand Ave. & Ohio St.)**

**Phone:** 312-467-0546
**Web:** www.cyranosfarmkitchen.com
**Prices:** $$

Dinner Tue – Sat
 Grand (Red)

 Cheerful cherry-red marks the façade of Cyrano's Farm Kitchen on Wells Street. A rustic wood-and-brick dining room continues the haute barnyard theme, complete with decorative pitchforks, roosters, and a portrait of Chef Didier Durand tending to a pot of moules that hangs above glowing crimson banquettes.

The menu strives for a nostalgic tone with French onion soup, steak frites, and other classics. Duck rillettes are picnic perfect, accompanied by crusty country bread and julienned apple coleslaw to balance the richness. Individual Staub casseroles are fragrant with comforting servings of stewed ratatouille. Though Cyrano's serves dinner only, their Cafe On The River offers lunch—and ice cream on the riverwalk in warm months.

# David Burke's Primehouse

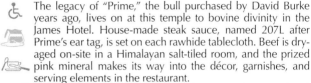

**F2**

**616 N. Rush St. (bet. Ohio & Ontario Sts.)**

**Phone:** 312-660-6000                                    Lunch & dinner daily
**Web:** www.davidburkesprimehouse.com
**Prices:** $$$                                            Grand (Red)

The legacy of "Prime," the bull purchased by David Burke years ago, lives on at this temple to bovine divinity in the James Hotel. House-made steak sauce, named 207L after Prime's ear tag, is set on each rawhide tablecloth. Beef is dry-aged on-site in a Himalayan salt-tiled room, and the prized pink mineral makes its way into the décor, garnishes, and serving elements in the restaurant.

Thin slices of crimson Wagyu sashimi coated in powdered black truffle are fanned on a brick of Himalayan salt for additional seasoning, and a 55-day aged bone-in ribeye gains a deep meaty flavor thanks to its hang time. For those overwhelmed by the menu's savory richness, a salad of young and sprouting arugula with truffle-smoked tomatoes is a refreshing accompaniment.

# Farmhouse

**C1**

**228 W. Chicago Ave. (bet. Franklin & Wells Sts.)**

**Phone:** 312-280-4960                                    Lunch & dinner daily
**Web:** www.farmhousechicago.com
**Prices:** $$                                             Chicago (Brown)

Like shaking the hand of your local farmer, grab the pitchfork door handles of Farmhouse and you'll be almost as close to the source of your food. Much of the décor is salvaged and much of the menu is procured right from the Midwest. From Indiana chicken to Michigan wine, local is more than a buzzword. Exposed brick, rough-hewn wood, and wire-encased filament bulbs make it the quintessential modern tavern.

Highlights of the harvest headline each course. Whole-grain mustard dresses up a vibrant (and requisite) beet salad. Nueske's bacon is the star in a rustic BLT, accompanied by Klug Farms peaches tossed with balsamic dressing. Cream cheese-frosted carrot-bread pudding is fragrant from autumn spices, layered with golden raisin purée and nutmeg crunch.

# Frontera Grill

 **D3**

Mexican ✗✗

### 445 N. Clark St. (bet. Hubbard & Illinois Sts.)

**Phone:** 312-661-1434     Lunch & dinner Tue – Sat
**Web:** www.fronterakitchens.com
**Prices:** $$      Grand (Red)

It may be the casual sibling to Topolobampo next door, but Frontera Grill is a cornerstone of Rick Bayless' empire. Tourists and locals alike line up for this famed dining room, as colorful as a kaleidoscope and peppered with Mexican masks, paintings, and artifacts. Those in-the-know hang at the bar with a margarita in hand until a table is ready, tapping their toes to peppy Latin music.

Despite Bayless' worldwide recognition, everyone is here for the food. The regularly changing menu focuses on regional dishes made with quality ingredients, such as smoky guacamole folded with crispy bacon, toasted chiles, and smoked tomato. Also sample grilled lamb in red peanut *mole* tucked with wintery squash and heirloom runner beans into fresh tortillas.

# Gene & Georgetti

 **C3**

Steakhouse ✗✗

### 500 N. Franklin St. (at Illinois St.)

**Phone:** 312-527-3718     Lunch & dinner Mon – Sat
**Web:** www.geneandgeorgetti.com
**Prices:** $$$$      Merchandise Mart

No, it's not a Hollywood set. This Italian-American steak joint is the real thing, and those wiseguys at the bar have been clinking their ice cubes in this wood-paneled room for decades. This historic spot, founded in 1941, is boisterous downstairs with the aforementioned regulars and guys grabbing a bite; upstairs is more refined for local politico lunches and a bit of old-school romance at dinner.

Gene & Georgetti is a steakhouse with an Italian bloodline, prominently displayed in the heaping helping of fried *peperoncini* and bell peppers with the signature "chicken alla Joe." The cottage fries (oversized potato planks that come with most entrées) might necessitate a doggie bag, but all the better to leave room for a slice of classic carrot cake.

# Gilt Bar

 Gastropub ✗✗

**C4**

**230 W. Kinzie St. (at Franklin St.)**

**Phone:** 312-464-9544
**Web:** www.giltbarchicago.com
**Prices:** $$

Dinner nightly

🔲 Merchandise Mart

In the shadow of Merchandise Mart, it's not easy to miss the revolving door entrance to Gilt Bar, a moody and imposing River North favorite. The bar up front mixes cocktails to a metronomic rhythm, while the back is more intimate with brick walls, studded leather banquettes, and nostalgic lighting.

However make no mistake: this is no Bugsy Malone speakeasy, but a grown-up version for bar-flies with astute palates. Snack on creamy burrata and shaved ham finished with a swig of extra virgin olive oil before savoring tender, flavorful pork meatballs on a bed of wilted kale with romesco and almond *gremolata*. In the end, gorge on an unctuous brown butter-apple cake with salted caramel and vanilla ice cream—perhaps to the dulcet tunes of Bob Dylan. Bliss.

# Giordano's

Pizza ✗

**F1**

**730 N. Rush St. (at Superior St.)**

**Phone:** 312-951-0747
**Web:** www.giordanos.com
**Prices:**

Lunch & dinner daily

🔲 Chicago (Red)

Value, friendly service, and delicious deep-dish pizza make Giordano's a crowd sweetheart. With several locations dotting the city and suburbs, this restaurant has been gratifying locals with comforting Italian-American fare for years. Come during the week—service picks up especially at dinner—to avoid the cacophony.

Giordano's menu includes your typical salads, pastas, et al., but you'd do well to save room for the real star: the deep-dish. Bring backup because this pie could feed a small country. The spinach pie arrives on a buttery pastry crust, filled with spreads of sautéed (or steamed) spinach and tomato sauce, and topped with mozzarella and Parmesan cheese. For those cold, windy nights, opt for delivery—their website sketches a detailed menu.

# GT Fish & Oyster

Seafood XX

**C3**

### 531 N. Wells St. (at Grand Ave.)

**Phone:** 312-929-3501
**Web:** www.gtoyster.com
**Prices:** $$

Lunch & dinner daily

 Grand (Red)

Quaint seaside shacks have nothing on this urban spot that exudes nautical chic. A boomerang-shaped communal table by the raw bar makes a perfect oyster-slurping perch. Lead fishing weights keep napkins in place on nautically styled, brass-edged tables, lined up under an enormous chalkboard-style mural of a jaunty swordfish skeleton.

Pescatarians savor the numerous seafood dishes meant for sharing, but those who forego fish are limited to three meat options. Rectangular crab cakes, stuffed to the gills with sweet meat, get a crunchy sear on all sides. *Salade* Niçoise spotlights pristine slices of fresh tuna and snappy green beans in a cider-mustard dressing. Key lime pie, a traditional meal-ender, is transformed into light layers of curd and cake in a glass jar.

# Hubbard Inn

Mediterranean XX

**D3**

### 110 W. Hubbard St. (bet. Clark & LaSalle Sts.)

**Phone:** 312-222-1331
**Web:** www.hubbardinn.com
**Prices:** $$

Lunch & dinner daily

 Grand (Red)

Handsome from head-to-toe, the Hubbard Inn takes the idea of a classic tavern and dresses it to the nines. Brass-clad globe lights glow above lacquered plank tables in the front bar room, leading to tufted leather couches and fireplaces in the book-lined and Hogwarts-worthy library. The second floor is low-slung and loungy. A wall-sized chalkboard behind the marble bar whets whistles with descriptions of house cocktails.

Shareable farm-to-table dishes appeal to nearly every appetite. Kale salad, that ubiquitous menu staple, gets a new twist when tossed with pickled blackberries, candied walnuts, and grated *ricotta salata*. A quartet of juicy, beautifully cooked lamb chops over rustic chickpea purée is brightened by a handful of chopped olives and mint.

# Joe's

**60 E. Grand Ave. (at Rush St.)**

**Phone:** 312-379-5637
**Web:** www.joes.net
**Prices:** **$$$$**

Lunch & dinner daily

Grand (Red)

Despite the ample neighborhood competition, this outpost of the original Miami seafood, steak, and stone crab palace does just fine up north. Clubby, masculine décor fashions a classic scene, while business diners and lively martini-toasting groups keep the leather booths full from lunch through dinner.

Stone crab claws accompanied by signature mustard sauce are shared by nearly every table, followed by decadent dishes like a bone-in filet with their simple yet delicious coriander-spiked seasoning. Americana sides like Jennie's fontina and asiago mashed potatoes, or grilled tomatoes topped with cheesy spinach pesto, are ample enough to share. Joe's Key lime pie is rightly famous, but other retro sweets like coconut cream are worth a forkful.

# La Madia

**59 W. Grand Ave. (bet. Clark & Dearborn Sts.)**

**Phone:** 312-329-0400
**Web:** www.dinelamadia.com
**Prices:** **$$**

Lunch & dinner daily

Grand (Red)

Those corner slice joints have nothing on this hip, contemporary Italian spot on Grand, where the see-and-be-seen crowd takes over the colorful striped booths and the marble dining counter surrounding the wood-fired pizza oven. A floor-to-ceiling wine wall telegraphs La Madia's upscale selection, but keeps it tasting-friendly with 4- or 7-oz. pours.

Pizza and salads are the draw for the club-happy crowd, though well-sourced ingredients like fresh butter lettuce and hearts of palm with a lemon-chili dressing ensure flavors are more "hey there!" than ho-hum. Neapolitan-style pies get sparing but flavorful toppings like homemade lamb sausage, pesto, and truffle oil. A pizza fondue featuring cheese-laced tomato sauce is perfect for the after-party.

# The Lobby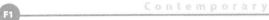

Contemporary ✕✕✕

### 108 E. Superior St. (at Michigan Ave.)

**Phone:** 312-573-6760
**Web:** www.peninsula.com
**Prices:** $$$

Lunch & dinner daily

🚇 Chicago (Red)

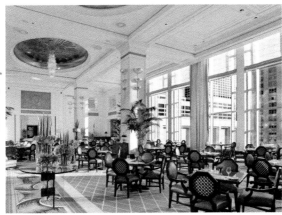

You can't say you weren't warned. The Peninsula people sensibly realized that honesty was best when naming this vast space which looks remarkably like…a lobby. Let's face it; intimate it ain't and no amount of anodyne musical accompaniment emanating from a gallery in the gods is going to make it so. At least the friendly and not overly formal service manages to wrestle back some control, and you know your conversation won't be overheard by tables near you— because there aren't any tables near you.

So why the recommendation? Because the food is very good. The lunch menu doesn't really get past lobster rolls and chicken legs, but at night the kitchen's innate skill is very much in evidence, with the high standard maintained through a 2014 change in chef. Dishes are good-looking, but also have depth and ingredients are of irreproachable quality. Flavors marry well and there are intriguing touches of originality but never at the expense of the overall balance of the dish.

In any big city there should be room for all sorts and styles of restaurant. And that includes restaurants that resemble lobbies.

# Mastro's

Steakhouse

### 520 N. Dearborn St. (at Grand Ave.)

**Phone:** 312-521-5100                 Dinner nightly
**Web:** www.mastrosrestaurants.com
**Prices:** $$$$                  Grand (Red)

Mastro's may be relatively young on the Windy City's steakhouse scene, but it shows up with the swagger of an old pro. Black SUVs unload VIPs in front of the revolving door, which leads to a gleaming wall of bottles at the gilded bar. Live lounge music may take the level of conversation up a notch, but sip on a shaken martini to blank out the surrounding din.

Steaks on screaming hot platters come unadorned unless otherwise listed, and servers will happily rattle off recommendations for toppings, sauces, and crusts. Salads like Mastro's house version, a local favorite stocked with chopped jumbo shrimp and a giant steamed prawn, are hearty (read: oversized), but smaller portions are on offer so you can leave room for the renowned butter cake.

# Mercadito

Mexican

### 108 W. Kinzie St. (bet. Clark & LaSalle Sts.)

**Phone:** 312-329-9555                 Lunch & dinner daily
**Web:** www.mercaditorestaurants.com
**Prices:** $$                  Merchandise Mart

If the Mayans turned their design skills toward modernism, they'd end up with a temple like Mercadito. Commissioned work from graffiti artist Ernie Valdez adorns the lively spot with its white terrazzo tabletops and weathered metal façade. Clubby music keeps friendly servers bouncing between tables, while margaritas keep hungry guests reaching for more.

The menu is built for mixing and matching: orders of small tacos filled with rosemary-marinated steak or Michoacàn-style pork carnitas pair with a half-dozen guacamole varieties and snappy ceviche. A torta Baja stuffed with beer-battered mahi mahi and coleslaw is big enough to satisfy on its own. Some may balk at shelling out for chips and salsa, though the smoky chipotle heat makes a convincing case.

# NAHA

American ✕✕✕

**500 N. Clark St. (at Illinois St.)**

**Phone:** 312-321-6242
**Web:** www.naha-chicago.com
**Prices:** $$$

Lunch Mon – Fri
Dinner Mon – Sat
Grand (Red)

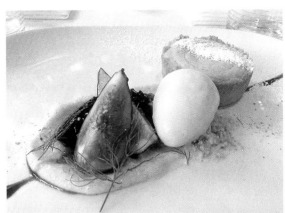

Upon entering this *très* sophisticated venue, it's apparent that the cadres of servers take hospitality seriously. The art of the welcome is alive and well as guests are soothingly greeted and even thanked for choosing to dine at this window-wrapped Clark Street corner. Fine service continues to play out as lovely meals unfold against a warm, refined backdrop of bold abstract artwork, concrete and wood accents, and vibrant greenery.

Like its understated scene, the menu doesn't have to shout to prove its worth. Mediterranean notes pepper Chef Carrie Nahabedian's seasonally driven cuisine, which is exemplified by the risotto starter. The creamy bowlful of organic *carnaroli* rice was riddled with shredded suckling pig and studded with seasonal treats including diced pumpkin, caramelized garlic cloves, and slivered leeks. Finely grated *Parmigiano Reggiano* and a drizzle of flavorful pork jus rounded out this stellar composition.

Entrée options are numerous, but pan-seared skate was skillfully rendered. The excellent quality fish was presented with myriad embellishments including plump nuggets of poached blue crab, beluga lentils, and a novel finishing touch of pickled lemon *beurre noisette*.

# Osteria Via Stato

**E2**

### 620 N. State St. (at Ontario St.)

**Phone:** 312-642-8450

**Web:** www.osteriaviastato.com

**Prices:** $$

Dinner nightly

Grand (Red)

Though it is adjacent to the Embassy Suites, this pitch-perfect cozy *enoteca* complete with stone walls and barrel-vaulted archways is a local standby for its across-the-board value in a neighborhood of pricey plates. The all-Italian wine list sparkles with well-priced gems, but those who can't decide can simply ask for the "just bring me wine" feature—a tasting flight of three different wines.

Order à la carte or bring a group for the *molto* popular "Italian dinner party" that lets diners choose their own entrée and share antipasti, pastas, and sides, family-style. With hearty portions of mini meatballs in marinara sauce; braised lamb shank with cipollini onions and rosemary; or ravioli stuffed with tender short rib, no one leaves hungry.

# Paris Club

**D4**

### 59 W. Hubbard St. (bet. Clark & Dearborn Sts.)

**Phone:** 312-595-0800

**Web:** www.parisclubbistroandbar.com

**Prices:** $$

Dinner nightly

Grand (Red)

Big changes in 2014 resulted in a smaller Paris Club, as some of its space was commandeered to create a ramen restaurant next door. In return for this munificence, it got a full makeover—which was executed so well you'd think it's looked like this for years.

With its red leather seats, wood panelling and globe lighting, it perfectly captures the look of a traditional Parisian brasserie. The only thing missing is insouciant service and someone with a dog on their lap. The menu is unapologetically Gallic, "Le Prime Steakburger" notwithstanding, and all the classics are present: from *fruits de mer* to steak frites and *baba au rhum*. The pommes purée is so wonderfully buttery you'll need a defibrillator on standby. The wine list is all French too.

# Phil Stefani's 437 Rush

Italian  🗡🗡

**437 N. Rush St. (bet. Hubbard & Illinois Sts.)**

| | | |
|---|---|---|
| **Phone:** | 312-222-0101 | Lunch Mon – Fri |
| **Web:** | www.stefanirestaurants.com | Dinner Mon – Sat |
| **Prices:** | $$$ | 🚇 Grand (Red) |

Two classic styles of Chicago restaurant—steakhouse and Italian—converge at 437 Rush St. The tasteful room recently received a refresh and now employs a neutral palette throughout, commissioned photography on the walls, and the newly installed Salumeria Bar, making this a standout contender among the many stylish steakhouses thriving in the city.

Elegant, unfussy Italian dishes complement the primo selection of well-prepared steaks, chops, and seafood platters. *Tonno con caponata Siciliana* arrives as seared slices of sashimi-grade tuna fanned over artichoke hearts, pine nuts, and eggplant caponata. Grilled Atlantic salmon with silky organic fava bean purée showcases the restaurant's commitment to sustainability without skimping on flavor.

# Pizzeria Uno

Pizza 🗡

**29 E. Ohio St. (at Wabash Ave.)**

| | | |
|---|---|---|
| **Phone:** | 312-321-1000 | Lunch & dinner daily |
| **Web:** | www.unos.com | |
| **Prices:** | 💰💰 | 🚇 Grand (Red) |

Since 1943, this establishment has been laying claim to the (somewhat disputed) title of creating the original Chicago-style pizza. Its tiny booths and wood tables wear their years of graffiti etchings like a badge of honor. Nonetheless, an intricate pressed-tin ceiling reflects the cheerful atmosphere as everyone counts down the 40 or so minutes it takes for these deep-dish delights to bake.

Of course, the main attraction here is, was, and always will be the flaky, buttery crust generously layered with mozzarella, other toppings, and tangy tomato sauce that comprise this belly-busting pizza. The menu also includes a selection of good basic bar food like Buffalo wings and a simple salad, but most just save the room for an extra slice.

# Prosecco

Italian

**710 N. Wells St. (bet. Huron & Superior Sts.)**

**Phone:** 312-951-9500
**Web:** www.prosecco.us.com
**Prices:** $$

Lunch Mon – Fri
Dinner Mon – Sat
Chicago (Brown)

No matter the hour, it's always time for bubbly at Prosecco, where a complimentary flute of the namesake Italian sparkler starts each meal. This fizzy wine inspires the restaurant's elegant décor, from creamy pale walls and damask drapes to travertine floors. Sit at the long wooden bar or in one of the well-appointed dining rooms for a second glass chosen from the long list of *frizzante* and *spumante* wines.

Hearty dishes spanning the many regions of Italy cut through the heady bubbles. Carpaccio selections include the classic air-dried *bresaola* as well as whisper-thin seared rare duck breast. *Saltimbocca di vitello* marries tender veal medallions with crispy *Prosciutto di Parma* and creamy mozzarella, with hints of sage in the tomato-brandy sauce.

# Ramen-san

Asian

**59 W. Hubbard St. (bet. Clark & Dearborn Sts.)**

**Phone:** 312-377-9950
**Web:** www.ramensan.com
**Prices:** 😊😊

Lunch Mon – Sat
Dinner nightly
Grand (Red)

Lettuce Entertain You brings you bowlfuls of ingredient-driven noodle soups served up right next door to the restaurant group's Paris Club. The menu at this Asian concept revolves around a handful of tastefully crafted broths dancing with thin, wavy noodles produced by Sun Noodle. The *tonkotsu* ramen is a traditional pleasure afloat with sweet slices of *chasu*, *wakame*, and molten egg. Meanwhile, the smoked brisket ramen is a novel departure defined by a black garlic-enriched chicken broth and slices of Bub City's 18-hour brisket.

Ramen-san's loyal following is comprised of hipsters and suits alike, and they all seem to dig the salvaged look and booming playlist. Night owls take note: Japanese whiskies rule the bar and fried rice is served late into the night.

# RL

 American XXX

115 E. Chicago Ave. (bet. Michigan Ave. & Rush St.)

**Phone:** 312-475-1100
**Web:** www.rlrestaurant.com
**Prices:** $$$

Lunch & dinner daily

 Chicago (Red)

If you swoon for tartan and pine for the posh life Ralph Lauren represents, head for the boîte attached to the flagship Michigan Avenue store. Like a stylish private club but without the centuries of stuffiness, RL offers options for a quick solo lunch, cocktail at the mahogany bar, or full dinner. The odd Blackhawks jersey here and there doesn't detract from the overall aura.

The menu is as classically American as the name, featuring bistro favorites like Waldorf salad and raw bar offerings alongside well-prepared dishes like sweet and plump pan-seared scallops with white balsamic-crème fraîche. The thin, flaky crust of a goat cheese- and caramelized onion-tart nearly steals the show from the rich atmosphere of the wood-paneled dining room.

# Roka Akor

 Asian XX

456 N. Clark St. (at Illinois St.)

**Phone:** 312-477-7652
**Web:** www.rokaakor.com
**Prices:** $$$

Lunch Mon – Fri
Dinner nightly
 Grand (Red)

There's no shortage of flash at Roka Akor, the local offshoot of a London-based-via-Scottsdale Japanese steakhouse and sushi temple. The massive LED-illuminated glass hood of the showstopping *robata* station grabs attention in the center of the vast space, with a brigade of black-clad line cooks working the flames. For a front row seat of the action, sit at the surrounding counter topped with charred *shou-sugi-ban* wood.

With such a prominent display, guests would be remiss not to try choices from the *robata*. Lightly blackened lamb chops in a sweet-and-spicy glaze are tender, smoky, and ready for dipping in crimson Korean chili sauce. A starter of plump Wagyu and kimchi dumplings nearly bursting with spicy, rich beef expertly toe the line between crispy and moist.

# RPM

**E3**

Italian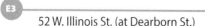

### 52 W. Illinois St. (at Dearborn St.)

**Phone:** 312-222-1888
**Web:** www.rpmitalian.com
**Prices:** $$

Lun Sun
Dinner nightly
Grand (Red)

You'll want to bust out the Dolce & Gabbana for a sultry night at RPM. This see-and-be-seen scene starts at the wraparound Carrara marble bar and works its way to the mod black-and-white dining room, where sexy white leather chairs and booths don't detract from the pretty people on display. Even servers get into the spirit with white coats and skinny black ties.

If you can tune out the diversions, the poster-sized menu of modern Italian antipasti, snacks, and family-style plates won't disappoint. Classically prepared peppered beef carpaccio and shaved Parmesan is garnished with crispy mushrooms, while a hearty entrée of gnocchi is tossed with mild Italian sausage and rapini. Save room to share a plate of freshly fried *bomboloni* oozing with Nutella.

# Sable

**E3**

American

### 505 N. State St. (at Illinois St.)

**Phone:** 312-755-9704
**Web:** www.sablechicago.com
**Prices:** $$

Lunch & dinner daily

Grand (Red)

Set beside Hotel Palomar, this handsome gastro-lounge is adorned in shades of brown, bronze, and pewter. Between banquette-lined tables, free-standing seats, and an elevated dining room, everyone from chic hotel guests to stylish regulars is comfortably accommodated.

Sable lives in a league of its own thanks to a bar pouring notable cocktails and a lively kitchen preparing excellent eats. Shelves of vials may resemble a lab, but the food is truly heartwarming: rich lobster salad slathered between buttery brioche, or well-seasoned buttermilk fried chicken and crunchy waffles kissed with maple syrup. Portions are small, so order a lot and share—unless it's a bowl of thick Greek yogurt with berries and granola. You'll want that for yourself!

# Siena Tavern

Italian ✕✕

**E4**

## 51 W. Kinzie St. (at Dearborn Pkwy.)

**Phone:** 312-595-1322
**Web:** www.sienatavern.com
**Prices:** $$

Lunch & dinner daily

 Merchandise Mart

Chef Fabio Viviani's TV-ready Italian charisma extends to every corner of this huge, lively restaurant. A mixture of funky décor elements—like cascading plants "growing" from filing cabinets on walls—somehow manage to work in incongruous harmony with sexy black marble and stainless steel throughout the multilevel space.

Various bars offer pizza, crudo, fresh mozzarella, and house-made pasta, though even globally influenced dishes have a Mediterranean touch. The Tavern burger accompanied by Parmesan-dusted fries is stacked with melted Taleggio, crispy speck, and garlic aïoli. Order the lush, creamy tiramisu for dessert, which gets a crunch from chopped nuts and crisp homemade meringues, and you'll be tempted to lick the bottom of the zinc tin.

# Slurping Turtle

Japanese ✕

**D3**

## 116 W. Hubbard St. (bet. Clark & LaSalle Sts.)

**Phone:** 312-464-0466
**Web:** www.slurpingturtle.com
**Prices:** $$

Lunch & dinner daily

 Merchandise Mart

Both turtles and noodles symbolize longevity, so a meal at Slurping Turtle should add a few years to your life (and warmth to your belly). Inside the minimalist bento box of a space, diners sit elbow-to-elbow at sleek white communal tables. Boutique Japanese beverages like Hitachino Nest beer and Ramuné bubble-gum soda bring smiles to patrons in the know.

Along with deep, steaming bowls of ramen and udon, the lengthy menu serves small plates, sushi, and other Japanese comfort food for snacking and sharing. Tender ribeye and chicken skewers arrive moist and glistening, straight from the *bincho* charcoal grill. Deep-fried Brussels sprouts are crispy outside and tender inside without a hint of grease, topped with sliced scallions and fried shallots.

# Sixteen

Contemporary    XXXX

**401 N. Wabash Ave. (bet. Hubbard St. & the Chicago River)**

**Phone:** 312-588-8030

Lunch & dinner daily

**Web:** www.trumpchicagohotel.com

**Prices:** $$$$

State/Lake

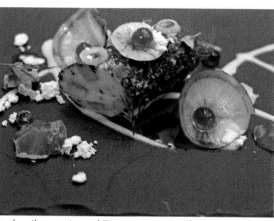

In the silvery-mirrored Trump International Hotel and Tower, find this signature restaurant on its namesake floor. Walk between the glassed-in wine cellars to enter this dramatic dining room, which puts the Tribune and Wrigley buildings at your fingertips. The ceiling soars to an enormous Swarovski crystal chandelier that hangs like an inverted wedding cake over a curving back wall of African rosewood and projected images to convey the menu's theme. Servers don three-piece suits and are always well-versed in the frequently changing offerings.

The educational and entertaining prix-fixe may be mapped out as the "Express Line" (11-course) or "All-day Pass" (20-course) options. Yet this is no gimmick; Chef Thomas Lents crafts each dish to tell a story. A single cube of ice is the pedestal for beef and oyster tartare topped with a poached quail egg, oyster leaf, chive blossoms, toast points, and a truffle coin. The "Irish contribution" is a spin on fish and chips, using fried cod and potato croquettes with lime and caper aïoli. The kitchen's take on Sinclair's "Jungle" combines Wagyu deckle, heart, horseradish, and micro-vegetables.

Desserts can be mouthwatering odes to extinct candy bars.

E4 (locator)

# Sumi Robata Bar

 Japanese

 **C2**

## 702 N. Wells St. (at Huron St.)

**Phone:** 312-988-7864
**Web:** www.sumirobatabar.com
**Prices:** $$

Lunch Mon – Fri
Dinner Mon – Sat
 Chicago (Brown)

There's a degree of authenticity to this traditional *robata* bar and that includes the discreet entrance, although a spacious patio ultimately lets you know you're not in downtown Tokyo. Sit at the counter to best appreciate their specialty— the Japanese art of grilling. For a good value lunch look no further than the bento boxes, but come at night and you'll be able to try a variety of grilled items where the natural flavors shine through, whether that's Wagyu beef or crab. You can also try more unusual cuts that you may hitherto have avoided, such as chicken heart or tail.

The service is smiley, helpful, and sincere. The guys behind the counter have a more serious countenance—well, good grilling is a serious business.

# Sunda

 Fusion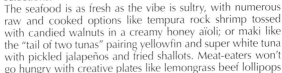

**D3**

## 110 W. Illinois St. (bet. Clark & LaSalle Sts.)

**Phone:** 312-644-0500
**Web:** www.sundachicago.com
**Prices:** $$

Lunch & dinner daily

Grand (Red)

The Sunda shelf, an underwater outcropping that stretches along the coastline of Southeast Asia, connects the countries that provide culinary inspiration for this enormous River North lounge and restaurant. The beautiful people are naturally attracted to the clubby vibe Sunda radiates, complete with thumping music and a wide range of cocktail and sake selections.

The seafood is as fresh as the vibe is sultry, with numerous raw and cooked options like tempura rock shrimp tossed with candied walnuts in a creamy honey aïoli; or maki like the "tail of two tunas" pairing yellowfin and super white tuna with pickled jalapeños and fried shallots. Meat-eaters won't go hungry with creative plates like lemongrass beef lollipops and oxtail potstickers.

# Topolobampo ✿

**D3**

**445 N. Clark St.** (bet. Hubbard & Illinois Sts.)

**Phone:** 312-661-1434
**Web:** www.rickbayless.com
**Prices:** $$$

Lunch Tue – Fri
Dinner Tue – Sat
Grand (Red)

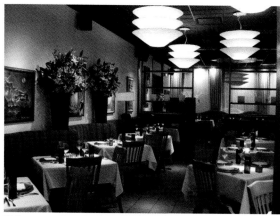

This crown jewel of the Rick Bayless empire is situated in the same home as Frontera Grill, and merely steps away from Xoco. Inside, a subtle renovation has left the dining room calmer, more removed from the front area's fiesta. Terra-cotta tiles, stucco walls, and colorful paintings bring a clear Mexican feel to the entire space. Servers are friendly, upbeat, and very capable of handling the non-stop crowds.

Lunch is always nice and an easier reservation, but dinner brings the deliciously full experience of all the authentic color, texture, and contrast of upscale Mexican cuisine. Enticing starters include fresh masa tortillas folded over organic cheddar with thinly sliced wild mushrooms, onion, and inky bits of *huitlacoche* with tomatillo salsa. The *sopa Azteca* is one of the best versions in the country and an absolute must, made with pasilla broth, chicken, crispy tortillas, avocado, local cheese, and *crema*.

Desserts may feature a contemporary take on *crepas de cajeta*, shaped like a burrito and filled with ripe plantain, bittersweet chocolate, and *cajeta* alongside caramelized plantain ice cream and toasted meringues. Don't miss their superbly rich *café de olla*, presented in a French press.

# Tortoise Club

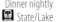

American

**E4**

### 350 N. State St. (bet. Kinzie St. & the Chicago River)

**Phone:** 312-755-1700
**Web:** www.tortoiseclub.com
**Prices:** $$$

Lunch Mon – Fri
Dinner nightly
State/Lake

Every city needs a restaurant with the word "club" in the title—somewhere reassuringly old-school where you'd take your future father-in-law if you want to marry his daughter. Tortoise Club fits the bill perfectly. If it was just a few years older, it would be called an institution because it also harks back to more dissolute times; order a Negroni at lunchtime here and no one will bat an eyelid.

The place has an unapologetically masculine look thanks to the mahogany paneling and dark leather seating. It has a lounge bar with nightly live jazz and a familiar menu of American classics, from big plates of seafood to great steaks. Where it differs from many similar spots is that here the service is sprightly and sincere and the welcome is warm.

# Travelle

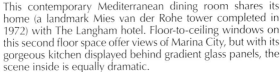

Mediterranean

**E4**

### 330 N. Wabash Ave. (bet. Kinzie St. & the Chicago River)

**Phone:** 312-923-7705
**Web:** www.travellechicago.com
**Prices:** $$$

Lunch & dinner daily

Grand (Red)

This contemporary Mediterranean dining room shares its home (a landmark Mies van der Rohe tower completed in 1972) with The Langham hotel. Floor-to-ceiling windows on this second floor space offer views of Marina City, but with its gorgeous kitchen displayed behind gradient glass panels, the scene inside is equally dramatic.

Sink into creamy, glove-soft leather seating to partake in creative tastes of falafel dressed with pickled onion and a swipe of *vadouvan*-tinged yogurt; or crisp-skinned striped bass plated with roasted cauliflower, shaved raw celery, and toasted hazelnuts before being finished off with a drizzle of pomegranate molasses. Travelle's take on baklava is stacked with Nutella and zinged by balsamic pearls and lemon gelée. One word: yum!

# Union Sushi + Barbeque Bar

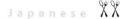

**C2**

J a p a n e s e   🍴🍴

### 230 W. Erie St. (at Franklin St.)

**Phone:** 312-662-4888
**Web:** www.eatatunion.com
**Prices:** $$

Lunch Mon – Fri
Dinner nightly
🚇 Chicago (Brown)

The slogan of this big, bustling restaurant is "Uniting Japanese culinary tradition with a distinctly American persona," which roughly translates to "Japanese food with a party hat on." The cocktails are good, the noise levels are high, and there are more tattoos in the room than a Yakuza convention.

The menu will take forever to read so just go directly to their two specialties—the assorted sushi rolls, some of which use black rice, and meats and fish expertly cooked over an open flame on the seriously hot *robata* grill. The ingredients are good and the flavor combinations don't get silly. Just remember that sharing is the key to keeping that final check in check, especially as the T-shirted staff are masters of upselling with an iPad.

# Untitled

**D4**

C o n t e m p o r a r y   🍴🍴

### 111 W. Kinzie St. (bet. Clark & LaSalle Sts.)

**Phone:** 312-880-1511
**Web:** www.untitledchicago.com
**Prices:** $$

Dinner Mon – Sat

🚇 Merchandise Mart

The unmarked speakeasy-style entrance to Untitled hides a wonderland below Kinzie Street—a warren of rooms both intimate and grand. A handsomely stocked whiskey library with more than 400 selections makes it a must-visit for serious tipplers and music lovers alike; in true supper club fashion, a rotation of musicians from jazz and blues to standards and soul graces the stage a few nights a week.

The well-appointed menu takes its cues from the surroundings, featuring a revue of shareable plates, charcuterie, and raw bar offerings. Salmon belly tartare glistens with pearls of smoked roe, and house-cured *guanciale* makes pan-seared striped bass and creamy white beans a bit more decadent. Gild the lily with a tuile-topped spoonful of classic chocolate mousse.

# Vermilion

 E3

## 10 W. Hubbard St. (bet. Dearborn & State Sts.)

**Phone:** 312-527-4060
**Web:** www.thevermilionrestaurant.com
**Prices:** $$

Lunch Mon – Fri
Dinner nightly
Grand (Red)

 Andy Warhol would feel right at home among these silver-painted brick walls, high-fashion black-and-white photographs, metallic chairs, and curtains. The cool lounge atmosphere is best for dressed-up evenings or a celebratory Latin-tinged cocktail at the bar.

Two expansive menus—one vegetarian, the other carnivorous—encompass Indian-inspired tapas and street foods. If feeling overwhelmed by the choices, stick to the chef's specialties or go for the prix-fixe and let the kitchen decide. Meaty delicacies include spice-rubbed Mysore lamb chops with pink pickled onions. *Gobi* Portuguese lets tart tomatillo chutney and crunchy eggplant offset sweet coconut gravy and tender cauliflower. *Shahi tukra* pleases the palate with crisp fried semolina cakes drenched in caramel sauce.

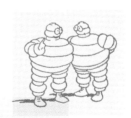

Chicago ▲ River North

Sunday brunch plans?
Look for the 🛏 !

# Streeterville

Bounded by the strategically set Chicago River, swanky Magnificent Mile, and sparkling Lake Michigan, Streeterville is a precious quarter in the Windy City, housing hotels and high-rise residences alongside offices, universities, and museums. If that doesn't bespeak cultural diversity, the sights and smells at Water Tower Place's **foodlife** is indisputable testimony. Located on the mezzanine floor of the shopping mall, this simple food court has been elevated to an art form. A veritable "United Nations of food courts," foodlife draws a devoted following to its 14 different kitchens that whip up everything from Chinese potstickers and deep-dish pizza, to crispy fried chicken. One such

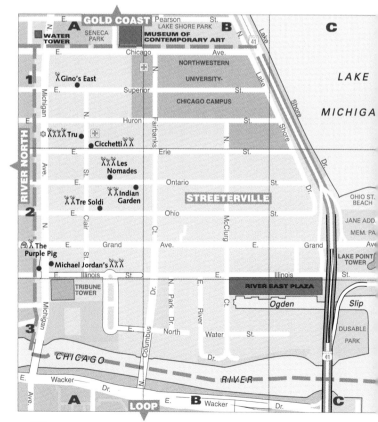

tenant, **Wow Bao**, is known to dole out some of the best steamed veggie- and meat-filled buns in town. In fact, they were so popular that four locations soon sprouted downtown. Unlike other food courts, you're given a card that can be swiped at as many stalls as you choose. Once you've had your fill, bring the card to the cash registers to receive your balance, and *voila*—a single bill to pay!

Hopping skyscrapers, the **John Hancock Center** is another iconic tower known to many as a "food lover's paradise." Lucky locals can

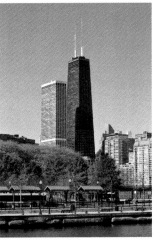

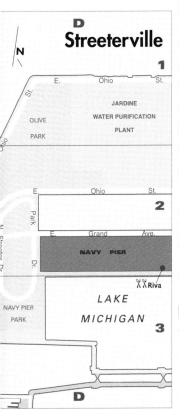

choose to dine with fine wine at **Volare Ristorante Italiano**; while bachelors in business suits may shop for groceries with sky-high prices to match the staggering view at **Potash Brothers**. For those whose tastes run more toward champagne and cocktails rather than cheeseburgers and crinkle-cut fries, there's always the **Signature Lounge**, located on the 96th floor of the John Hancock Center. An idyllic setting for delicious nightcaps, the Signature Lounge also presents incredible brunch, lunch, dinner, and dessert menus that employ some of the freshest and finest ingredients around town. While their creative cocktails may result in sticker shock, one peek at the sparkling cityscape will have you...at hello.

## ART & CULTURE

The Museum of Contemporary Art is located next to Lake Shore Park, the city's outdoor recreational extravaganza. Well-renowned for housing the world's leading collection of contemporary art, patrons here

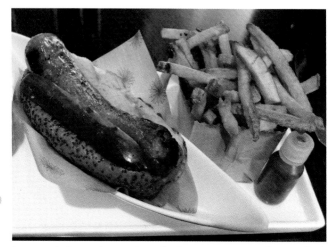

know to balance the gravitas of the setting with fresh nourishment at cute and casual **Puck's** (Wolfgang, naturally) **Café**. But, it's also the peppers and potatoes that lure folks to the farmer's market, held at the museum every Tuesday from June through October. Choose to bookend a home-cooked meal with some dark chocolate decadence at **Godiva Chocolatier**—a beautiful boutique carrying everything from chocolate-covered strawberries and truffles, to gourmet biscuits, chocolate bars, and snacks.

The world convenes at Chicago's lakefront **Navy Pier** for a day of exploration and eats. Showcasing lush gardens and parks in conjunction with shops and dining stalls, families usually flock to **Bubba Gump Shrimp Co.** for its convivial vibe and shrimp specials. But, locals looking for live music with their carnitas and margaritas may head to **Jimmy Buffett's Margaritaville Bar & Grill** (named after the rockstar himself). For stellar snacking in between meals, venture towards **Garrett Popcorn Shops**, which promises to have you hooked on sweet-and-salty flavors like CheeseCorn and Macadamia CaramelCrisp. The choices are plenty and you can even create your own tin here. After, move on to more substantial chow like an all-natural Chicago-style dog (slathered with mustard, onion, relish, sport peppers, tomatoes, and celery salt) from **America's Dog**. This classic destination showcases an impressive range of city-style creations from Houston, New York, and Philadelphia, to Detroit, Kansas City, and San Francisco. Meat-lovers who mean business never miss **M Burger**, always buzzing with business lunchers, tourists, and shoppers alike. It should be renamed "mmm" burger simply for its juicy parcels of bacon, cheese, and secret sauce. Even calorie counters may rest easy as the all-veggie "Nurse Betty" is sure to sate. For a bit more intimacy and a lot more fantasy, **Sayat Nova** is superb. Highlighting a range of *kibbe* alongside more exotic signatures like *sarma* or meat- and veggie-filled grape leaves bobbing in a light garlic sauce, this Middle Eastern marvel keeps its options limited but fan following infinite.

Locals know that Chicago is big on breakfast—so big that they can even have it for dinner at Michigan Avenue's **West Egg**. This convivial café-cum-coffee corridor serves three meals a day, but it is their breakfast specials (choose between pancakes, waffles, or other "eggcellent" dishes) that keep the joint jumping. Finally, the Northwestern Memorial Hospital complex is another esteemed establishment that dominates the local scene. Besides its top medical services, a parade of dining gems (coffee shops, lounges, and ethnic canteens) catering to their lineup of staff, students, and visitors looms large over this neighborhood and lake.

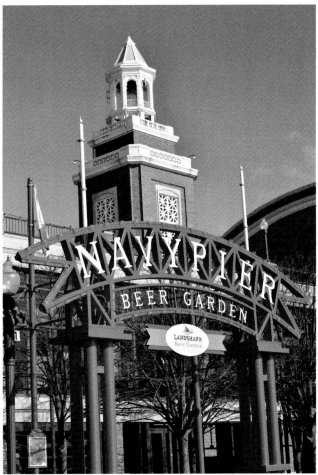

# Cicchetti

Italian

 **A1**

### 671 N. St. Clair St. (at Erie St.)

**Phone:** 312-642-1800
**Web:** www.cicchettirestaurant.com
**Prices:** $$

Lunch & dinner daily

Grand (Red)

As this breezy spot proves, Venetians don't eat tapas—they nibble delicately on *cicchetti*. Bellinis and cocktails spiked with Italian spirits set the mood, whether in the handsome bar area or under towering ceilings braced by exposed wood beams. And with a host of sophisticated dishes, the menu keeps both budget-oriented and splurge-ready guests happy. Though many plates are meant for sharing, bowls of pasta and *secondi* make hearty main meals. Buttery polenta offsets charred baby squid in a zippy purée of black garlic, black pepper, and squid ink; while tangy tomato sauce and fried sage play counterpoint to Barolo-braised short rib ravioli. Tiramisu comes in sundae form, appearing as a gelato with Fernet Branca menta fudge sauce and Amarena cherries.

# Gino's East

Pizza

 **A1**

### 162 E. Superior St. (bet. Michigan Ave. & St. Clair St.)

**Phone:** 312-266-3337
**Web:** www.ginoseast.com
**Prices:** $$

Lunch & dinner daily

Chicago (Red)

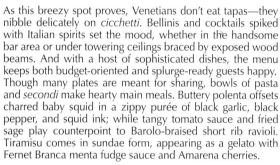

Pizza pilgrims continue to make the trek to the original location of this renowned local deep-dish chain, where a 45 minute wait is the norm. However, solo diners may rest assured as they can order personal pies from a walk-up counter. The walls, scribbled with years of graffiti, are nearly as iconic as the high-walled pies themselves, whose crusts gets their signature crunch from cornmeal and searing-hot metal pans rife with two inch-high sides.

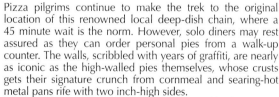

Filled with heaps of mozzarella and toppings like the "Meaty Legend" lineup of spicy pepperoni, Italian sausage, and both Canadian and regular bacon before getting sauced, it's hard to eat more than two wedges here. Nonconformists can of course opt for thin-crust pies, gussied-up by add-ons like roasted red peppers.

# Indian Garden

XX

**247 E. Ontario St. (bet. Fairbanks Ct. & St. Clair St.)**

| | |
|---|---|
| **Phone:** | 312-280-4910 |
| **Web:** | www.indiangardenchicago.com |
| **Prices:** | $$ |

Lunch & dinner daily

 Grand (Red)

Frequent diners know it as "The IG," but first-timers will appreciate the copious lunch buffet as much as the doctors, med students, and locals. These faithful droves routinely make the trip up a few flights of stairs to get their *pakora* and tandoori fix on, among kitschy but ornate touches like richly colored fabrics and wafting incense.

Though the à la carte menu offers Northern Indian dishes brought to the table in shiny copper vessels, the lunch buffet covers all bases with vegetarian, chicken, and lamb items. Staples like *saag*, *dal*, naan, and basmati rice are freshly made. *Bhuna gosht* mixes succulent lamb with tomatoes, onions, and spices; while *lassi* or masala tea provide refreshment along with a decent selection of wine, beer, and cocktails.

# Les Nomades

XXX

**222 E. Ontario St. (bet. Fairbanks Ct. & St. Clair St.)**

| | |
|---|---|
| **Phone:** | 312-649-9010 |
| **Web:** | www.lesnomades.net |
| **Prices:** | $$$$ |

Dinner Tue – Sat

Grand (Red)

A distinctively scalloped awning on a quaint brownstone sets Les Nomades apart in the heart of Streeterville. The warren of elegant old-world dining rooms within remains hushed with the murmur of couples clinking martinis in etched cocktail glasses or quietly chatting with owner Mary Beth Liccioni in the second-floor tea salon.

Downstairs, Executive Chef Roland Liccioni's four- and five-course prix-fixe options showcase classic French dishes with global touches (think: chicken dumplings and sliced shiitakes floating in crystal-clear duck consommé flavored with a hint of star anise). The kitchen employs a heavier hand with main course preparations—whether in *loup de mer* with truffled vermouth sauce, or slow-roasted veal- and lamb-loin over classic pommes purée.

# Michael Jordan's

Steakhouse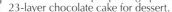

**505 N. Michigan Ave. (bet. Grand Ave. & Illinois St.)**

**Phone:** 312-321-8823                                    Lunch & dinner daily
**Web:** www.mjshchicago.com
**Prices:** $$$                                              Grand (Red)

Leave your dated 1993 Bulls jersey in the closet for a meal at this swanky steakhouse, tucked just off the lobby of the InterContinental Hotel. Leather and velvet accents telegraph an upscale vibe, and references to His Airness are subtle— from oversized sepia photographs of basketball netting to a 23-layer chocolate cake for dessert.

A glass of Amarone with dry-aged Porterhouse are always a slam-dunk, but the kitchen also turns out pleasing modern twists on steakhouse classics. Chicago's famous Italian beef sandwich gets an upgrade with smoked ribeye and aged provolone. Similarly, the traditional wedge salad is presented as a halved small head of baby romaine, layered here with creamy Wisconsin blue cheese and thick slabs of crispy bacon.

# The Purple Pig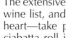

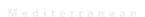 Mediterranean

**500 N. Michigan Ave. (at Illinois St.)**

**Phone:** 312-464-1744                                    Lunch & dinner daily
**Web:** www.thepurplepigchicago.com
**Prices:** $$                                              Grand (Red)

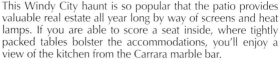

This Windy City haunt is so popular that the patio provides valuable real estate all year long by way of screens and heat lamps. If you are able to score a seat inside, where tightly packed tables bolster the accommodations, you'll enjoy a view of the kitchen from the Carrara marble bar.

The extensive small plates menu is primed for pairing with the wine list, and unusual cuts of meat—like a panini with pork heart—take precedence. Inspired by a Chicago beef, this ciabatta roll is moistened with jus, stuffed full of pork, and dressed with sweet peppers and spicy-tangy giardiniera. A plethora of charcuterie, fried bites, and spreads like whipped feta with cucumbers guarantees all who sip and sup here leave with a full belly and wine-stained mouth.

# Riva

🍴🍴

**D2**

### 700 E. Grand Ave. (on Navy Pier)

**Phone:** 312-644-7482          Lunch & dinner daily
**Web:** www.rivanavypier.com
**Prices:** $$

If a stroll along Navy Pier works up an appetite, follow your nose (and stomach) past the Ferris wheel to Riva, a nautically themed escape from the carnival atmosphere. The upstairs dining room is a visual feast, with colorful murals above the open kitchen and sweeping lakeshore views; while a casual café downstairs serves drinks and light bites.

Though the menu swims with seafood, Prime steaks and Italian-inspired dishes like pear-and-cheese agnolotti offer variety. Caper-studded Louis sauce augments a single plump cake of jumbo lump crab with a crisp side of Asian slaw. A fillet of Atlantic salmon is placed atop a vibrant plate and paired with cherry tomato fondue, a handful of quartered Brussels sprouts, and bite-sized potato *gnocchetti*.

# Tre Soldi

🍴🍴

**A2**

### 212 E. Ohio St. (bet. Fairbanks Ct. & St. Clair St.)

**Phone:** 312-664-0212          Lunch & dinner daily
**Web:** www.tresoldichicago.com
**Prices:** $$               🚇 Grand (Red)

Set a few steps above street level, Tre Soldi's tomato-red awning and floor-to-ceiling windows beckon Michigan Avenue shoppers and business lunchers. Inside, splashes of red-and-white allude subtly to those classic red-sauce joints complete with checkered tablecloths, but glossy ceramic-tiled columns and Italian stone floors up the ante.

Rome and its surroundings inspire the menu and all-Italian wine list. Local Slagel Family Farm's beef becomes carpaccio, shingled on the plate and drizzled with tangy mustard aïoli, fresh parsley, and celery leaves. Thin-crust pizzas strewn with quality ingredients like *cavolo nero*, featuring caramelized onions and pecorino, are large enough to share. Finish with dark chocolate-hazelnut tarts, perfectly balanced by apricot jam.

# Tru

**A1**

Contemporary

XXXX

### 676 N. St. Clair St. (bet. Erie & Huron Sts.)

**Phone:** 312-202-0001
**Web:** www.trurestaurant.com
**Prices:** $$$$

Dinner Mon – Sat

Chicago (Red)

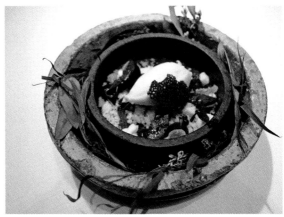

Fine dining at Tru has a strong air of formality that extends from the service team to the moneyed, well-dressed clientele. Beyond the discreet exterior, find an intimate lounge with a spotlit, vivid blue sculpture. A wall of branches and net curtains divide the cavernous space; white walls adorned with Warhol lithographs lend a luxe-gallery feel. Leather and velvet banquettes surrounding well-spaced tables are popular for quiet meetings or romantic interludes.

The variety of dining options begins with an excellent three-course prix-fixe, extending all the way up to a deep-pocketed caviar menu. However, the aptly named "The Experience" menu fulfills its literal promise of exploring Chef Anthony Martin's very modern kitchen. Superlative talent is abundantly clear in the smooth and creamy artichoke soup with chive-oil dressing, fresh cod roe, and a fine wafer of crisped skin. Succulent frog legs are the center of an impeccable presentation of fresh favas, earthy-sweet chanterelles, and a foamy herbed velouté sauce garnished with edible flowers. Solid desserts include a combination of white chocolate, milk chocolate, and *sudachi*-flavored mousse.

Splurge on the extraordinary wine pairings.

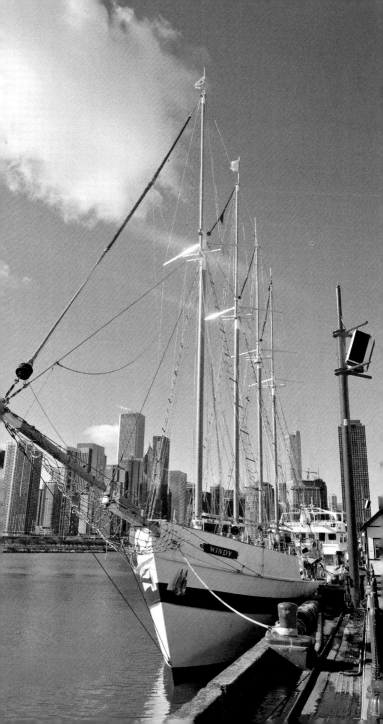

# West Loop

## GREEKTOWN · MARKET DISTRICT

Once home to warehouses and smoke-spewing factories, the West Loop is arguably the most booming part of Chi-town, whirring with art galleries, lofts, nightclubs, and cool, cutting-edge restaurants. Young residents may have replaced the struggling immigrants of yore; nevertheless, traces of ethnic flavor can still be found here. They certainly aren't as dominant as before—what a difference a century or two can make—but nearby **Taylor Street** continues to charm passersby and residents alike with that timeless, slightly kitschy feel. It is delis, groceries, and food galore!

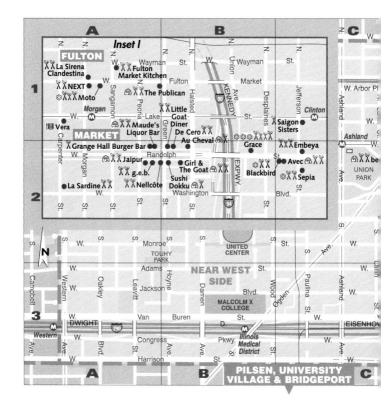

## A MEDITERRANEAN MARVEL

For tasty, Mediterranean-inspired munching, make your way to Greektown where everybody's Greek, even if it's just for the day. Shout "opa" at the **Taste of Greece** festival held each August, or while away an afternoon at the always-packed **Parthenon**. Its moniker may not signal ingenuity, but the menu is groaning with gyros, signature lamb dishes, and even flaming *saganaki,* displaying serious showmanship. Sound all too Greek to you? Venture beyond the Mediterranean and into "Restaurant Row" along Randolph Street, where culinary treasures hide among beautiful, fine dining establishments. Whet your appetite with everything from sushi to subs—this mile-long sandwich breed is a best seller bursting with salty meats at **J.P. Graziano's**. Don't let their long lines deter you; instead, take your smoky temptation to **West Loop Salumi** and let their platters of glistening cured treats do the trick. If all else fails, round-up say 1,000 of your closest friends for a Middle-Eastern meze at one of the Moroccan spots nearby.

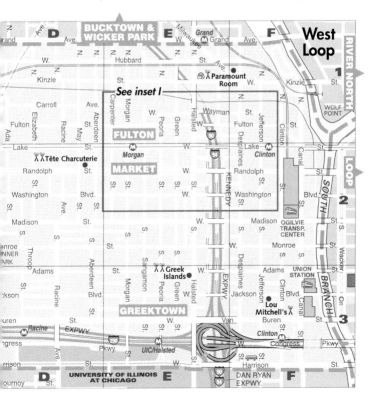

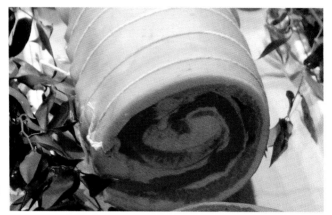

Wash down West Randolph's exquisite eats with intricately crafted sips at **The Aviary**. This bar in West Fulton Market is the brainchild of Chef Grant Achatz, and boy is it a charmer. Noted as much for its expert bartenders and their spherical concoctions as for its tedious reservation process (this is a Kokonas business, after all!), The Aviary is also highly devoted to product freshness and flavor. For even more of a scene, head downstairs to **The Office**, a super secret and super exclusive bar, before settling in for an intimate dinner at Next's private dining space, **The Room**. Some carousers may choose to continue the party at **CH Distillery**, which is known to cull the finest spirits in-house and couple them with such simple small plates as potato pancakes, to more lavish bites like red caviar atop pumpernickel blinis. Nerd alert: the name CH is a double-entendre indicating the molecular formula for ethanol as well as Chicago's abbreviation. Rather whip it up than wolf it down? Beef up your kitchen skills at the **Calphalon Culinary Center**, where groups can arrange for private hands-on instruction. After mastering the bœuf Bourguignon, get in line at **Olympic Meat Packers** (also known as Olympia Meats), or walk into **Peoria Packing**, a veritable meat cooler where butchers slice and dice the best cuts to order. Foodies also make the rounds to Paul Kahan's **Publican Quality Meats**, another carnivorous mecca, for their mind-boggling array of specialty eats, matched only by the equally spectacular setting. Think: intimate cocktail gathering-meets-extravagant dinner party.

For artisan food paradise savvy gourmands gather at **Dose Market**, a pop-up bazaar featuring the finest in food and chefs (as well as their own secret ingredients). Meanwhile, treasure hunters troll the stalls at **Chicago French Market**, an epicurean hub and multi-use arena catering to a variety of palates. Red meat fiends love **Fumaré Meats and Deli** for traditionally smoked cuts; Creole food fans stop by **Lafayette** for Louisiana bayou favorites like crawfish pie or shrimp étouffée; while health-nuts can't get enough of **RAW**, a grab-n-go vegan spot committed to providing the healthiest food money can buy. Moving beyond the market, even the most die-hard dieters need a lil' sugar from nearby **Glazed and Infused**, an early member of the current donut craze, before spicing things up at the flagrantly sexy **RM Champagne Salon**.

## BEER & THE BALLGAME

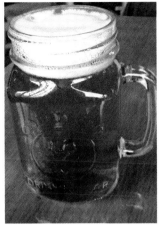

Hoops fans whoop it up at Bulls games at the United Center, also home to the Blackhawks. Depending on the score, the most exciting part of the night is post-game, binging with buddies over beer and bar food. **The Aberdeen Tap**, for instance, is a neighborhood hangout where everybody knows your name as well as the impressive selection of beers on tap. They boast over 65 brews, so be sure to take your more finicky friends to **Rhine Hall**, a boutique brandy distillery run by a father-and-daughter duo. Finally, those who prefer a little brawl with their beer are bound to fall for **Twisted Spoke**, a proverbial biker bar with tattoos and 'tudes to match. The music is loud and drinks are plentiful, but it's all in good testosterone- and liquor-fueled fun.

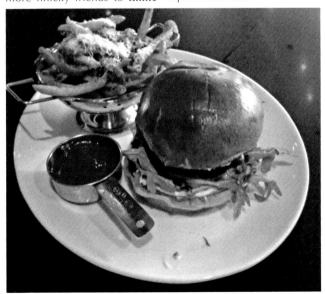

# Au Cheval

American ✗

**B2**

### 800 W. Randolph St. (at Halsted St.)

**Phone:** 312-929-4580
**Web:** www.auchevalchicago.com
**Prices:** $$

Lunch & dinner daily

🚇 Morgan

This corner bar on Randolph Street's restaurant row may be dim, but it's got a few glittering edges. The reel-to-reel in the doorway lends a retro feel, but the rest is decidedly cushy. Late-night revelers prefer to sit at tufted leather booths or savor beers at the zinc-topped bar, rather than endure a wait for a table in the raucous space. Bartenders work just as hard as line cooks until the wee hours.

The kitchen puts a highfalutin spin on simple bar eats. In-house butchers craft 32-ounce pork Porterhouses for sharing; foie gras for folding into fluffy scrambled eggs; and house-made sausages for bologna sandwiches that go well beyond a kid's wildest dreams. Thin griddled cheeseburger patties are perked up by maple syrup-glazed peppered bacon.

# Avec

American ✗✗

**C2**

### 615 W. Randolph St. (bet. Desplaines & Jefferson Sts.)

**Phone:** 312-377-2002
**Web:** www.avecrestaurant.com
**Prices:** $$

Lunch Sun
Dinner nightly
🚇 Clinton (Green/Pink)

"Share and share alike" has been Avec's philosophy since it opened many years ago as one of the culinary standard-bearers on this sweep of West Randolph. From its wooden-planked communal seating to the succession of small plates that arrive as the kitchen fires them, this is a high-decibel hangout. A strict no-reservations policy can make prime-time waits brutal.

The town would riot if the bacon-wrapped, chorizo-stuffed dates; or "deluxe" focaccia sandwiching melted taleggio and truffle oil ever left the menu. But, other delights come and go with the seasons: crisp-skinned wild striped bass reaps flavor from green garlic *bagna cauda* and pickled fiddlehead ferns; just as *bottarga di muggine* brings a saline snap to English pea-and-ricotta crostini.

# bellyQ

 **C2**

Asian ✕✕

### 1400 W. Randolph St. (at Ogden Ave.)

**Phone:** 312-563-1010
**Web:** www.bellyqchicago.com
**Prices:** **$$**

Lunch Sun
Dinner nightly
 Ashland (Green/Pink)

This end of West Randolph Street might be quiet, but it's always a party inside bellyQ. The volume and energy are high throughout the lofty, concrete-heavy space with tabletop hibachi booths and industrial metal seating. A wall-length horse-themed screen separates the restaurant from casual sister spot Urban Belly, which shares the open kitchen. As imagined by prolific Chef/owner Bill Kim, the Asian barbecue experience at BellyQ takes its form in a number of genre-melding shareable plates. A side of *bibimbap*-style sticky rice is crunchy and tender, tossed with glistening slices of Chinese sausage and generously sprinkled with *togarashi*. Chewy chunks of brownie in vanilla soft-serve are drizzled with caramel-balsamic-soy "Seoul sauce" for a savory twist.

# De Cero

 **B2**

Mexican ✕✕

### 814 W. Randolph St. (at Halsted St.)

**Phone:** 312-455-8114
**Web:** www.decerotaqueria.com
**Prices:** **$$**

Lunch & dinner Tue – Sat

 Morgan

As a *muy* popular member of restaurant row, De Cero takes the traditional taqueria and turns it on its feet…with spice! Lively music keeps the energy level high, though low lighting lends a cozy vibe to the sleek wood-dominated space. Two rooms, each equipped with a bar, make it easy to get started with a strawberry-mint margarita or Mexican beer.

This hip spot's name roughly translates to "from scratch," and it shows. Tacos are made with hand-pressed corn tortillas and ordered individually, letting diners sample a range of fillings including rich duck confit and spicy corn salsa. Ample chunks of carnitas with habanero salsa and julienned radish are other favorites. Jalapeño-marinated skirt steak tortas are pressed to order and ooze with melting *Chihuahua*.

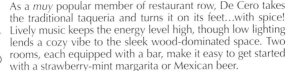

# Blackbird ❀

Contemporary ✗✗

**C2**

### 619 W. Randolph St. (bet. Desplaines & Jefferson Sts.)

| | | |
|---|---|---|
| **Phone:** | 312-715-0708 | Lunch Mon – Fri |
| **Web:** | www.blackbirdrestaurant.com | Dinner nightly |
| **Prices:** | $$$ | 🚇 Clinton (Green/Pink) |

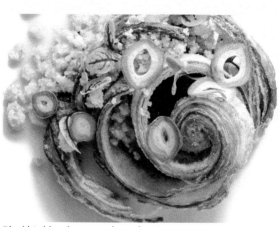

Blackbird has been on the radar since its 1997 opening, in a warehouse building that flaunts the neighborhood's industrial past. Inside, the bright and sleek room mixes high-backed gray banquettes with dark wood chairs and a glossy white counter bar. The service staff is more numerous than cohesive.

This contemporary kitchen seems to find inspiration everywhere it looks. Expect openers like finely chopped beef tartare studded with wheat berries—a brilliant addition that adds heartiness and a toothsome note to the unctuous meat. The dish is artfully topped with shaved breakfast, watermelon, and Spanish radishes and tendril-like oxalis stems. Wood-grilled sturgeon attains new heights here, set in a sloping bowl of ham hock broth with knobs of roasted fingerling potatoes, and a petite dollop of osetra caviar. Finish with a "fall coupe" presented as two scoops of wonderfully tart, slightly sweet, and creamy-smooth apple sherbet in a glass tumbler with savory pastry, whipped cream, and toasted walnuts.

Delicious, creative, and downright beautiful, their prix-fixe lunch is among the best deals of the city. That said, midday burgers are just as popular among the well-to-do crowds.

# Embeya

  Fusion XXX

### 564 W. Randolph St. (at Jefferson St.)

**Phone:** 312-612-5640
**Web:** www.embeya.com
**Prices:** $$

Lunch Mon – Fri
Dinner nightly
Clinton (Green/Pink)

Chef Thai Dang makes his vision clear at Embeya: floor-to-ceiling windows put the entire restaurant on display, letting passersby soak up its intriguing sculptural elements. Blown-glass bouquets of light fixtures hang above communal tables, and wooden screens in intricate cutout patterns divide the airy dining room.

The pan-Asian menu is a product of the chef's Vietnamese heritage combined with skillful Chinese and French techniques. A skin-on sea bass fillet paired with fermented black bean sauce is balanced by sautéed sweet red peppers and green beans. Briefly seared scallops cleverly mirror slices of ripe Asian pear in a tart *calamansi* broth. Tofu-almond custard is dusted with mint chiffonade and fresh lemon zest for a light and bright finale.

# Fulton Market Kitchen

Contemporary XX

### 311 N. Sangamon St. (at Wayman St.)

**Phone:** 312-733-6900
**Web:** www.fultonmarketkitchen.com
**Prices:** $$$

Dinner Mon – Sat
Morgan

Fulton Market Kitchen practically epitomizes the term "feast for the eyes." The interior nearly explodes with color, featuring a series of contemporary art pieces that might include graffiti murals or quirky wood-and-steel assemblages. Fixtures like paint-dripped tables repurposed from bowling alleys and old barn doors complement the eye-popping display.

A cocktail list with sections like "Renaissance" and "Pop Art" and a menu divided into "canvases" carries the art theme further, with ingredients sourced from both global and local markets. A small canvas of ravioli is an intense starter with a melt-in-your-mouth foie gras and duxelle filling, and tender lamb hints at the flavors of North Africa with crisp marinated cucumber, creamy feta, and fresh mint.

# g.e.b.

XX

**A2**

### 841 W. Randolph St. (bet. Green & Peoria Sts.)

**Phone:** 312-888-2258        Dinner Tue – Sat
**Web:** www.gebistro.com
**Prices:** $$       Morgan

It's not likely you'll see peripatetic MasterChef Graham Elliot working the line at g.e.b. any time soon, but his namesake retains the pizzazz it brought years ago as a newcomer to the West Loop. Dramatic backlighting, colorful mosaics, and modern stained glass brighten the narrow, high-ceilinged space. The kitchen hums along in time to music bouncing off polished concrete floors.

Simple comfort food goes upscale with the kitchen's cleverly deconstructed dishes. A breakfast-for-dinner twist on salmon becomes a perfectly seared fillet atop a dilled cream cheese "schmear;" an everything bagel tuile and onion jam drive the point home. Chicken noodle soup becomes pillowy mousseline-filled agnolotti on a bed of sunchoke purée and roasted carrots.

# Girl & The Goat 😊

XX

**B2**

### 809 W. Randolph St. (bet. Green & Halsted Sts.)

**Phone:** 312-492-6262        Dinner nightly
**Web:** www.girlandthegoat.com
**Prices:** $$       Morgan

The revolving door never stops turning as Girl & The Goat's party keeps going. Even on a Monday night, guests linger for hours, shouting over the din at at this sceney but always friendly stunner. Appropriately rustic wooden pillars and beams connect a warren of seating areas, from elevated platforms to banquettes to dim private corner nooks.

A pick-your-own-protein adventure, the menu is organized by ingredient with a dedicated section for goat. Paper-thin goat carpaccio is dusted with fried capers, beads of smoked trout roe, and olive-maple vinaigrette. Red currants brighten the luxe meatiness of wood-fired scallops with subtly smoked uni cream. The kitchen will even send out mini portions of menu items for solo diners—a truly thoughtful touch.

# Grace ✿ ✿ ✿

**B2**

Contemporary 🍴🍴🍴🍴

**652 W. Randolph St. (bet. Desplaines & Halsted Sts.)**

**Phone:** 312-234-9494     Dinner Tue – Sat
**Web:** www.grace-restaurant.com
**Prices:** $$$$     🚇 Clinton (Green/Pink)

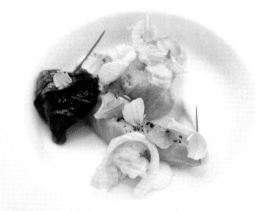

Ask a passing foodie to name one of Chicago's most elegant and sophisticated restaurants and they'll probably say Grace. This room is as handsome as it is urbane and provides a supremely comfortable environment for those spending an evening discovering the culinary wizardry of Curtis Duffy.

You'll be presented with a choice between two seasonally changing menus: "Fauna" or, for vegetarians, "Flora." Opt for the wine pairings and you're done on the decision making for the night. Trying to keep track of the ingredients of each dish will nullify the benefit of the wine so instead just marvel at the clever presentation and dig in—because taste is what this food is all about. The dishes are intricate and elaborately constructed, with herbs playing an integral part rather than merely being a garnish. Occasionally your taste buds will get a little slap, perhaps with the odd Thai or Vietnamese flavor, and the courses will fly by.

This style of cooking is very labor-intensive and if you want to learn more, then take advantage of their offer of a post-prandial kitchen tour.

231

# Grange Hall Burger Bar

A2

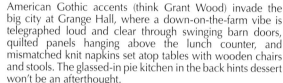

American 🍴

### 844 W. Randolph St. (bet. Green & Peoria Sts.)

**Phone:** 312-491-0844
**Web:** www.grangehallburgerbar.com
**Prices:** 💰💰

Lunch Tue – Sun
Dinner Tue – Sat

🚇 Morgan

American Gothic accents (think Grant Wood) invade the big city at Grange Hall, where a down-on-the-farm vibe is telegraphed loud and clear through swinging barn doors, quilted panels hanging above the lunch counter, and mismatched knit napkins set atop tables with wooden chairs and stools. The glassed-in pie kitchen in the back hints dessert won't be an afterthought.

Choose your own adventure when building a burger, starting with a six- or nine-ounce grass-fed beef patty and adding toppings like Midwestern cheeses, smoked bacon, jalapeños, or homemade pickles. If a wedge of strawberry rhubarb pie or Bourbon-spiked milkshake is calling your name (especially when freshly churned ice cream is involved), go easy on those hand-cut farmhouse chili fries.

# Greek Islands

E3

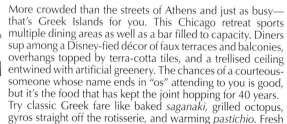

Greek 🍴🍴

### 200 S. Halsted St. (at Adams St.)

**Phone:** 312-782-9855
**Web:** www.greekislands.net
**Prices:** 💰💰

Lunch & dinner daily

🚇 UIC-Halsted

More crowded than the streets of Athens and just as busy—that's Greek Islands for you. This Chicago retreat sports multiple dining areas as well as a bar filled to capacity. Diners sup among a Disney-fied décor of faux terraces and balconies, overhangs topped by terra-cotta tiles, and a trellised ceiling entwined with artificial greenery. The chances of a courteous—someone whose name ends in "os" attending to you is good, but it's the food that has kept the joint hopping for 40 years.

Try classic Greek fare like baked *saganaki*, grilled octopus, gyros straight off the rotisserie, and warming *pastichio*. Fresh seafood doesn't disappoint: fish are grilled whole, filleted, and dressed simply with herbs, a few glugs of olive oil, and a squeeze of lemon.

# Jaipur

Indian 🍴🍴

**A2**

## 847 W. Randolph St. (bet. Green & Peoria Sts.)

**Phone:** 312-526-3655                    Lunch & dinner daily
**Web:** www.jaipurchicago.com
**Prices:** $$                                        Morgan

Business execs expecting the ubiquitous lunch buffet will be sorely disappointed by Jaipur—that is until they realize this popular weekday spot serves an affordable full-service lunch special that brings the buffet to your table in a parade of hammered copper *katoris*. In the evening, locals fill every sleek, nail-studded chair in the refined dining room as they await plates of boldly flavored Indian cooking.

The broad menu features a lengthy selection of fresh, authentically treated favorites, most of which are available as part of the bountiful lunch special. Staples on the buffet and à la carte menu may include *aloo papdi chaat;* a rich chicken korma; spiced carrot soup; and scarlet-red tandoori chicken, served with garlic naan.

# La Sardine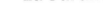

French 🍴🍴

**A2**

## 111 N. Carpenter St. (bet. Randolph St. & Washington Blvd.)

**Phone:** 312-421-2800                    Lunch Mon – Fri
**Web:** www.lasardine.com                Dinner Mon – Sat
**Prices:** $$                                        Morgan

 In a neighborhood packed to the gills with gastronomic innovation, La Sardine may be the most daring option of all, flaunting hearty French bistro food in a warm, rustic setting. The time-tested combination of wheezing accordion music, white linens, tile floors, and pastoral murals make it all the rage among diners craving the familiar—a $25 lunch prix-fixe doesn't hurt either.

Onion soup is straightforward yet sublime, with pungent cheese melting over a moist crouton and oozing down the side of a large ramekin; while fluffy gnocchi *Parisienne* with fresh peas and sweet corn purée help Chicagoans dream of summer and fields of gold. Other standards include a homemade sausage of the day, like the sprightly pheasant offering, served with warm potato salad.

# La Sirena Clandestina

**A1**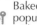

Latin American

### 954 W. Fulton Market (at Morgan St.)

**Phone:** 312-226-5300 — Lunch Sun – Fri
**Web:** www.lasirenachicago.com — Dinner nightly
**Prices:** $$ — Morgan

A relaxing Caribbean vibe breezes its way northward to Fulton Market and settles within La Sirena Clandestina's aquamarine walls. Languidly spinning fans, light filtered through antique etched glass panels, and an international selection of sippable rum and mezcal all conspire to bring guests' blood pressure down a notch or two.

Baked empanadas rotate through a series of fillings, but these popular pockets never leave the menu. Whether stuffed with venison ragù or ricotta, hazelnut, and butternut squash, they're exceptional. Handfuls of Manchego add decadence to plump bomba rice studded with fiery pickled jalapeño rings, toasted pepitas, and buttery white corn. Classic *alfajore* shortbreads filled with dulce de leche and sea salt are a memorable sendoff.

# Little Goat Diner

**B2**

American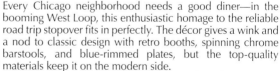

### 820 W. Randolph St. (at Green St.)

**Phone:** 312-888-3455 — Lunch & dinner daily
**Web:** www.littlegoatchicago.com
**Prices:** $$ — Morgan

Every Chicago neighborhood needs a good diner—in the booming West Loop, this enthusiastic homage to the reliable road trip stopover fits in perfectly. The décor gives a wink and a nod to classic design with retro booths, spinning chrome barstools, and blue-rimmed plates, but the top-quality materials keep it on the modern side.

A morning-to-night menu of amped-up diner favorites can be had no matter the hour: craving a shrimp cocktail at 7:00 AM? Five jumbo fried shrimp wrapped in *somen* noodles are ready to go. The Goat Almighty burger lives up to its name with fatty beef brisket, saucy pulled pork, and a ground goat patty. Before hitting the road, grab a cup of Stumptown—and maybe a s'mores cookie—from LG Bread, the next-door bakery and coffee bar.

# Lou Mitchell's

### 565 W. Jackson Blvd. (bet. Clinton & Jefferson Sts.)

**Phone:** 312-939-3111        Lunch daily
**Web:** www.loumitchellsrestaurant.com
**Prices:**        Clinton (Blue)

At the top of Chicago's list of beloved names is Lou Mitchell. This eponymous diner is by no means an elegant affair, but thanks to its delicious omelets and iconic crowd, it has been on the Windy City's must-eat list since 1923. Don't panic at the length of the lines: they are long but move fast, and free doughnut holes (one of the restaurant's signature baked goods) make the wait go faster.

Back to those omelets: they may be made with mere eggs, like everyone else's, but somehow these are lighter and fluffier, almost like a soufflé, stuffed with feta, spinach, onions, or any other ingredients of your choice. They arrive in skillets with an Idaho-sized helping of potatoes. Save room, because everyone gets a swirl of soft-serve at the meal's end.

# Maude's Liquor Bar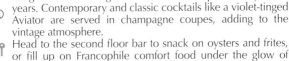

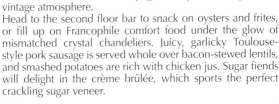

### 840 W. Randolph St. (bet. Green & Peoria Sts.)

**Phone:** 312-243-9712        Dinner nightly
**Web:** www.maudesliquorbar.com
**Prices:** $$       Morgan

Don't be fooled by the aged patina of this sexy boîte: though a few items like the overstuffed curio cabinet and salvaged French metal chairs are true antiques, this chicly disheveled hang has been hiding out on West Randolph for only a few years. Contemporary and classic cocktails like a violet-tinged Aviator are served in champagne coupes, adding to the vintage atmosphere.

Head to the second floor bar to snack on oysters and frites, or fill up on Francophile comfort food under the glow of mismatched crystal chandeliers. Juicy, garlicky Toulouse-style pork sausage is served whole over bacon-stewed lentils, and smashed potatoes are rich with chicken jus. Sugar fiends will delight in the crème brûlée, which sports the perfect crackling sugar veneer.

# Moto ✿

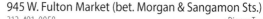

Contemporary ✕✕✕

**945 W. Fulton Market (bet. Morgan & Sangamon Sts.)**

Phone: 312-491-0058
Web: www.motorestaurant.com
Prices: $$$$

Dinner Tue – Sat

🚇 Morgan

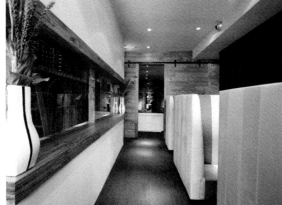

Moto stands amid loading docks and empty warehouses. Close by you can hear the sound of approaching post-industrial regeneration.

If you're lucky you'll get one of the suede booths by the entrance, but more than likely you'll be led downstairs to the bright but windowless room where the focus of your attention will probably be your plate rather than your date—however hard you might try.

Around 15 "courses" are presented in the no-choice set menu, although allergies and dislikes are discussed prior to arrival. In the culinary equivalent of a crystal ball, you're first presented with a miniaturized version of the meal to come: just a single flavor of each course; it's clever and sets the tone. The look of the dishes is quite something else—there are things in boxes and glasses, on top of thyme and charcoal; there may even be an ocean or forest scene. The service team explains each dish in detail and there's no doubt the kitchen has all the techniques down pat, from pickling to dehydrating. However, the best dishes are often the simplest as sometimes there are too many flavors battling for supremacy.

# Nellcôte

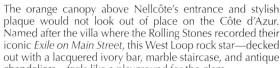

 **A2**                 Italian   XX

### 833 W. Randolph St. (at Green St.)

**Phone:** 312-432-0500                  Lunch Sat – Sun
**Web:** www.nellcoterestaurant.com          Dinner nightly
**Prices:** $$                                   🚇 Morgan

The orange canopy above Nellcôte's entrance and stylish plaque would not look out of place on the Côte d'Azur. Named after the villa where the Rolling Stones recorded their iconic *Exile on Main Street*, this West Loop rock star—decked out with a lacquered ivory bar, marble staircase, and antique chandeliers—feels like a playground for the glam.

Vases of dried lavender evoke scents of the Mediterranean, as do the kitchen's creations, which feature homemade ravioli filled with favas, a poached egg, and Parmesan broth. A hearty and succulent Berkshire pork chop with sweet roasted yams and spicy grated horseradish needs no sides; whereas black pepper semifreddo between chocolate shortbread is memorable when paired with red wine-poached pears.

# NEXT

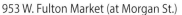

**A1**                 Contemporary   XX

### 953 W. Fulton Market (at Morgan St.)

**Phone:** 312-226-0858                  Dinner Wed – Sun
**Web:** www.nextrestaurant.com
**Prices:** $$$$                                🚇 Morgan

Welcome to dinner as theater, where the only thing more radically varied than each new theme is the quality of the food. Next's conceit is reinvention. It may open the year as, say, a culinary homage to the "Bocuse d'Or" competition—and a superlative roster of French dishes that honor the namesake chef. Four months later, it shutters to re-emerge as a pretty good "Steakhouse" serving a very rare ribeye and elevated country-club tributes. Finally, it may offer a "Chinese: Modern" menu that combines bold experimentation and innovative technique, if not the depth of flavor that a chef's lifetime to dedication to the cuisine might attain.

This is a very unusual place with a masterfully adept (and adaptable) kitchen, but the experience just isn't for everyone.

# Paramount Room

Chicago ▲ West Loop

Gastropub

 **F1**

### 415 N. Milwaukee Ave. (bet. Hubbard & Kinzie Sts.)

**Phone:** 312-829-6300
**Web:** www.paramountroom.com
**Prices:** $$

Lunch & dinner daily

Grand (Blue)

Though a few blocks north of the hot-and-heavy Fulton Market food scene, Paramount Room holds its own on this road less-traveled, thanks to elevated pub grub and a superior beer list. This soaring multi-level tavern lets you choose your style of hangout between a massive mirrored and patina-ed bar, cozy banquettes, high window perches, or a sultry semi-private lounge.

A plump burger made from 100 percent Wagyu beef on a toasted sweet brioche bun exemplifies the quality of ingredients across the menu; when crusted with salty bacon and coupled with crisp-tender green beans plus kicky *sriracha*, it makes for a very luscious meal. With "no crap on tap" as the beer motto, it's almost criminal not to wash down this hearty patty with a Belgian tripel.

# The Publican

Gastropub

**A1**

### 837 W. Fulton Market (at Green St.)

**Phone:** 312-733-9555
**Web:** www.thepublicanrestaurant.com
**Prices:** $$

Lunch Sat – Sun
Dinner nightly
Morgan

The phrase "meat market" has many connotations at The Publican: everything about this bustling Fulton Market spot is communal, from the sprawling U-shaped table that dominates the space to the penned-in booths lining the perimeter to the sink outside the washrooms. That said, the ubiquitous pig-centric décor gives a more straightforward idea of what you'll find on the menu.

As expected, pork takes precedence here with rillettes, platters of paper-thin aged ham slices, and house-made blood sausage to pair with one of the superlative beer selections. Weekend brunch gets in on the game with thickly sliced Publican bacon basted with Burton's maple syrup, or savory mushroom-and-chard French toast topped with roasted tomato and a fried egg.

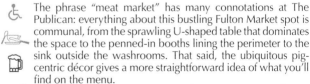

# Saigon Sisters

 **Vietnamese**

**C1**

## 567 W. Lake St. (bet. Clinton & Jefferson Sts.)

**Phone:** 312-496-0090
**Web:** www.saigonsisters.com
**Prices:**

Lunch Mon – Fri
Dinner Mon – Sat
 Clinton (Green/Pink)

The sign of a great restaurant is when the owner is on-site, and such is the case at this local hot spot, where Mary Nguyen Aregoni is as gregarious and welcoming as her staff. Named after Mary and sister, Theresa Nguyen, the lofty space belies its compact size with huge glass windows and high ceilings. Simple banquettes and wood tables are a perfect canvas for the vibrant Vietnamese cuisine that comes speeding out of the kitchen.

Lunch is busy with business types ordering the likes of a fragrant, satisfying, and clear *pho* floating with soft noodles, bean sprouts, jalapeños, and cilantro. Meanwhile, noodles stir-fried with thinly sliced hoisin-glazed pork, char-grilled red pepper, and sliced avocado are a dream team of flavor and texture.

# Sushi Dokku

**Japanese**

**B2**

## 823 W. Randolph St. (at Green St.)

**Phone:** 312-455-8238
**Web:** www.sushidokku.com
**Prices:** $$

Lunch Fri
Dinner Tue – Sat
 Morgan

Creatively adorned nigiri is the featured attraction at this hip sushi-ya that's all wood planks, stainless steel, chunky tables, and hefty benches.

Just one piece of Sushi Dokku's supple cuts showcasing quality and technique is not enough—thankfully each nigiri order is served as pairs. Among the terrific selection, enjoy the likes of hamachi sporting a spicy mix of shredded Napa cabbage, daikon, and red chili; or salmon dressed with a sweet ginger-soy sauce and fried ginger chips. South Pacific sea bream is deliciously embellished with a drizzle of smoky tomato and black sea salt. Those who wish to branch out from sushi should go for *tako yaki* (crispy fried octopus croquettes), grilled hamachi collar, or a brownie-crusted green tea-cheesecake.

239

# Sepia ✿

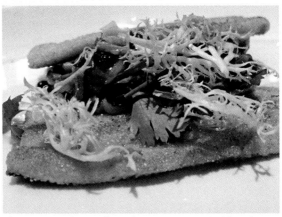

American 🍴🍴

**123 N. Jefferson (bet. Randolph St. & Washington Blvd.)**

| Phone: | 312-441-1920 | Lunch Mon – Fri |
| Web: | www.sepiachicago.com | Dinner nightly |
| Prices: | $$$ | 🚇 Clinton (Green/Pink) |

This consistently excellent destination is set inside a former 19th century print shop that does a fine job mixing original details with modern touches. Here, muted tones in the exposed brick walls and custom tile flooring complement newer elements like floor-to-ceiling wine storage and dramatic smoky-shaded chandeliers that drip with crystals. Though the décor may travel through time, Chef Andrew Zimmerman's cuisine is firmly grounded in the 21st century.

Whether your visit is for lunch or dinner, Sepia always offers a seriously impressive meal. Celery soup may be a commonplace offering, but this version is far from banal. The silky purée is enticingly arranged with tiny cubes of compressed apple, chopped toasted hazelnuts, and paper-thin ciabatta croutons. Entrées have a solid American footing but enjoy some playful tweaking, as in crispy cornmeal-crusted trout served over a salad of black-eye peas with bits of pecans and candied bacon.

The dessert station turns out equally impressive work, including a block of chocolate sponge cake. Moist, dark as ebony, and plated with a scoop of coconut-vanilla sorbet and dried fig compote, it is both delightful and (surprise!) completely vegan.

Chicago ▶ West Loop

C2

240

# Tête Charcuterie

 French

**D2**

**1114 W. Randolph St. (bet. Aberdeen & May Sts.)**

**Phone:** 312-733-1178                                       Dinner Mon – Sat
**Web:** www.tetechicago.com
**Prices:** **$$**                                                      Morgan

No greater respect can be shown to a former meatpacking warehouse than by converting it into a restaurant specialising in charcuterie. This most ancient of culinary arts is joyfully celebrated here in all its forms—there are cured meats, wonderful glistening terrines, rich pâtés, and plump homemade sausages. This is roll-your-sleeves-up food that will put hairs on your chest.

The enthusiasm of the on-view kitchen team is palpable. Curing is done in-house and there's a separate Sausage Room where they create their own varieties, which range from a French *boudin blanc* to a Moroccan inspired merguez. But don't think they can't show a light touch when required: the 'spring garden' served *en cocotte* is one of the prettiest things you'll see.

# Vera

 Spanish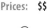

**A1**

**1023 W. Lake St. (at Carpenter St.)**

**Phone:** 312-243-9770                                          Dinner nightly
**Web:** www.verachicago.com
**Prices:** **$$**                                                      Morgan

Pimentón de la Vera, one of the most powerful spices in Spanish cuisine, also provides partial inspiration for this first-come, first-served wine bar in the West Loop dining corridor. (The other homage? Chef/owner Mark Mendez's grandmother.) Exposed brick walls and walnut floors are typically lovely, but do little to soften the din of a happy hour crowd after a few glasses of sherry.

Classic tapas as well as ham and cheese flights comprise the menu, along with larger plates like a piled-high paella with rabbit, duck, and chorizo. Shell out a few extra dollars for crusty bread to sop up the garlicky, lemony olive oil that bathes their plump head-on shrimp. Grilled rounds of octopus are sweet and smoky thanks to a liberal dose of good old pimentón.

# Where to **Eat**

Indexes

# Alphabetical List of Restaurants

# Restaurants by Cuisine

## Belgian

| | | | |
|---|---|---|---|
| Vincent | | X | 37 |

## Chinese

| | | | |
|---|---|---|---|
| Cai | | XX | 76 |
| Homestyle Taste | 😋 | XX | 173 |
| Lao Beijing | | X | 79 |
| Lao Hunan | 😋 | X | 80 |
| Lao Sze Chuan | 😋 | X | 80 |
| MingHin | | XX | 82 |
| Phoenix | | X | 82 |
| Yum Cha | | XX | 165 |

## Contemporary

| | | | |
|---|---|---|---|
| Acadia | ✿ | XxX | 74 |
| Ada St. | | X | 44 |
| Alinea | ✿✿✿ | XxxX | 143 |
| Atwood | | XX | 162 |
| Blackbird | ✿ | XX | 228 |
| Boka | ✿ | XxX | 145 |
| Bottlefork | | X | 188 |
| Café des Architectes | | XxX | 89 |
| Celeste | | XX | 190 |
| deca | | XX | 91 |
| EL Ideas | ✿ | XX | 172 |
| Elizabeth | ✿ | XX | 23 |
| 42 Grams | ✿✿ | XX | 24 |
| Fulton Market Kitchen | | XX | 229 |
| g.e.b. | | XX | 230 |
| Girl & The Goat | 😋 | XX | 230 |
| Goosefoot | ✿ | XX | 26 |
| Grace | ✿✿✿ | XxxX | 231 |
| Lobby (The) | ✿ | XxX | 197 |
| Mindy's Hot Chocolate | | XX | 58 |
| Moto | ✿ | XxX | 236 |
| NEXT | | XX | 237 |
| Nightwood | 😋 | XX | 175 |
| North Pond | ✿ | XX | 150 |
| Pump Room | 😋 | XX | 95 |
| Schwa | ✿ | X | 64 |

| | | | |
|---|---|---|---|
| Senza | ✿ | XX | 132 |
| Sixteen | ✿✿ | XxxX | 206 |
| sola | | XX | 133 |
| Trenchermen | | XX | 68 |
| Tru | ✿ | XxxX | 220 |
| Untitled | 😋 | XX | 210 |
| Wood | 😋 | XX | 135 |

## Deli

| | | | |
|---|---|---|---|
| Bourgeois Pig Cafe | | X | 144 |
| Eleven City Diner | | X | 78 |
| Frances' Deli | | X | 147 |

## English

| | | | |
|---|---|---|---|
| Pleasant House Bakery | | X | 176 |

## Ethiopian

| | | | |
|---|---|---|---|
| Demera | | XX | 22 |
| Ras Dashen | | X | 33 |

## Filipino

| | | | |
|---|---|---|---|
| Isla | | X | 27 |

## French

| | | | |
|---|---|---|---|
| Bistro Campagne | | XX | 21 |
| Bistronomic | | XX | 88 |
| Bistrot Zinc | | XX | 89 |
| Brasserie by LM | | XX | 76 |
| Brindille | | XxX | 189 |
| Chez Joël | | XX | 170 |
| Cyrano's Farm Kitchen | | XX | 191 |
| Everest | ✿ | XxX | 163 |
| La Petite Folie | | XX | 81 |
| La Sardine | | XX | 233 |
| Le Bouchon | | X | 56 |
| Les Nomades | | XxX | 217 |
| Maude's Liquor Bar | 😋 | XX | 235 |
| Mon Ami Gabi | | XX | 149 |
| Paris Club | | XX | 200 |
| Tête Charcuterie | | XX | 241 |

## Fusion

| | | | |
|---|---|---|---|
| Belly Shack | 🤝 | ✕ | 47 |
| Embeya | | ✕✕ | 229 |
| Mott St. | 🤝 | ✕ | 59 |
| Sunda | | ✕✕ | 207 |
| Takashi | ✿ | ✕✕ | 66 |

## Gastropub

| | | | |
|---|---|---|---|
| Bangers & Lace | | ✕ | 46 |
| Dawson (The) | 🤝 | ✕✕ | 52 |
| Dusek's (Board & Beer) | 🤝 | ✕ | 171 |
| Farmhouse | | ✕ | 192 |
| Gage (The) | | ✕✕ | 162 |
| Gilt Bar | 🤝 | ✕✕ | 194 |
| Hopleaf | 🤝 | ✕ | 27 |
| Longman & Eagle | ✿ | ✕ | 108 |
| Owen & Engine | | ✕✕ | 61 |
| Paramount Room | 🤝 | ✕ | 238 |
| Pl-zeň | | ✕ | 176 |
| Publican (The) | 🤝 | ✕✕ | 238 |
| Three Aces | | ✕ | 178 |

## German

| | | | |
|---|---|---|---|
| Radler (The) | | ✕ | 112 |

## Greek

| | | | |
|---|---|---|---|
| Greek Islands | | ✕✕ | 232 |
| Taxim | | ✕✕ | 67 |

## Indian

| | | | |
|---|---|---|---|
| Chicago Curry House | | ✕✕ | 77 |
| Cumin | 🤝 | ✕ | 52 |
| Indian Garden | | ✕✕ | 217 |
| Jaipur | 🤝 | ✕✕ | 233 |
| Mysore Woodlands | | ✕✕ | 30 |
| Paprika | | ✕ | 31 |
| Raj Darbar | | ✕ | 152 |
| Sabri Nihari | | ✕✕ | 34 |
| Vermilion | | ✕✕ | 211 |
| Viceroy of India | | ✕✕ | 36 |

## Indonesian

| | | | |
|---|---|---|---|
| Rickshaw Republic | | ✕ | 153 |

## International

| | | | |
|---|---|---|---|
| Bar Pastoral | | 🍽 | 123 |
| Beatrix | 🤝 | ✕✕ | 187 |
| Boarding House (The) | | ✕✕ | 188 |
| Bread & Wine | | ✕ | 103 |
| Red Door | | 🍽 | 62 |

## Italian

| | | | |
|---|---|---|---|
| Anteprima | | ✕ | 20 |
| a tavola | | ✕✕ | 45 |
| A10 | 🤝 | ✕✕ | 75 |
| Azzurra EnoTavola | 🤝 | ✕ | 46 |
| Baffo | | ✕✕ | 186 |
| Balena | 🤝 | ✕✕ | 144 |
| Bar Toma | | ✕✕ | 88 |
| Briciola | | ✕✕ | 49 |
| Cafe Spiaggia | | ✕✕✕ | 90 |
| Ceres' Table | 🤝 | ✕✕ | 124 |
| Cicchetti | | ✕✕ | 216 |
| Coco Pazzo | | ✕✕ | 191 |
| Due Lire | | ✕✕ | 22 |
| Frasca | | ✕✕ | 127 |
| Merlo on Maple | | ✕✕ | 92 |
| Nando Milano Trattoria | | ✕✕ | 60 |
| Nellcôte | | ✕✕ | 237 |
| Nico Osteria | | ✕✕ | 93 |
| Ombra | | 🍽 | 30 |
| Osteria Langhe | | ✕✕ | 110 |
| Osteria Via Stato | | ✕✕ | 200 |
| Pelago | | ✕✕✕ | 94 |
| Phil Stefani's 437 Rush | | ✕✕ | 201 |
| Piccolo Sogno | | ✕✕ | 61 |
| Pizzeria da Nella | | ✕ | 152 |
| Prosecco | | ✕✕✕ | 202 |
| Riccardo Trattoria | 🤝 | ✕✕ | 153 |
| Rosebud | | ✕✕ | 177 |
| RPM | | ✕✕✕ | 204 |
| Siena Tavern | | ✕✕ | 205 |

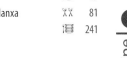

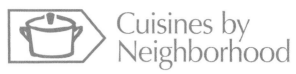

# Cuisines by Neighborhood

Indexes ▲ Cuisines by Neighborhood

259

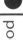

Indexes ▲ Cuisines by Neighborhood

# Starred Restaurants

*W*ithin the selection we offer you, some restaurants deserve to be highlighted for their particularly good cuisine. When giving one, two, or three Michelin stars, there are a number of elements that we consider including the quality of the ingredients, the technical skill and flair that goes into their preparation, the blend and clarity of flavours, and the balance of the menu. Just as important is the ability to produce excellent cooking time and again. We make as many visits as we need, so that our readers may be assured of quality and consistency.

A two or three-star restaurant has to offer something very special in its cuisine; a real element of creativity, originality, or "personality" that sets it apart from the rest. Three stars – our highest award – are given to the choicest restaurants, where the whole dining experience is superb.

Cuisine in any style, modern or traditional, may be eligible for a star. Due to the fact we apply the same independent standards everywhere, the awards have become benchmarks of reliability and excellence in over 20 countries in Europe and Asia, particularly in France, where we have awarded stars for 100 years, and where the phrase "Now that's real three-star quality!" has entered into the language.

The awarding of a star is based solely on the quality of the cuisine.

❀ ❀ ❀

## Exceptional cuisine, worth a special journey

One always eats here extremely well, sometimes superbly. Distinctive dishes are precisely executed, using superlative ingredients.

❀ ❀

## Excellent cuisine, worth a detour

Skillfully and carefully crafted dishes of outstanding quality.

❀

## A very good restaurant in its category

A place offering cuisine prepared to a consistently high standard.

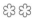

# Bib Gourmand

This symbol indicates our inspectors' favorites for good value. For $40 or less, you can enjoy two courses and a glass of wine or a dessert (not including tax or gratuity).

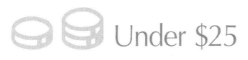
# Under $25

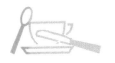

# Brunch

# Late Dining

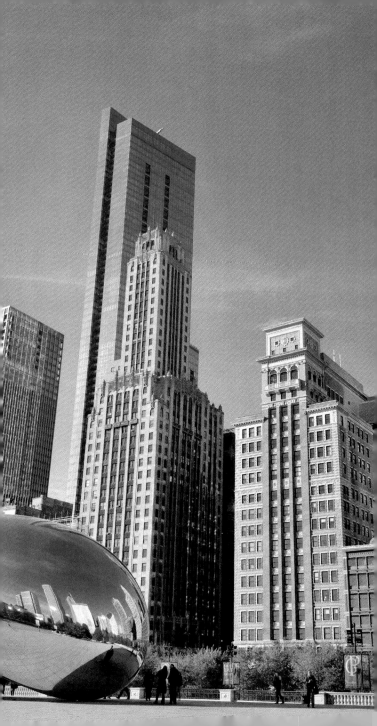

# Credits

# Notes

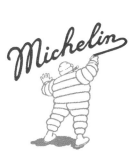

# **Michelin** is committed to improving the mobility of travellers

## ON EVERY ROAD AND BY EVERY MEANS

**Since the company came into being** – over a century ago – Michelin has had a single objective: to offer people a better way forward. A technological challenge first, to create increasingly efficient tires, but also an ongoing commitment to travelers, to help them travel in the best way. This is why Michelin is developing a whole collection of products and services: from maps, atlases, travel guides and auto accessories, to mobile apps, route planners and online assistance: Michelin is doing everything it can to make traveling more pleasurable!

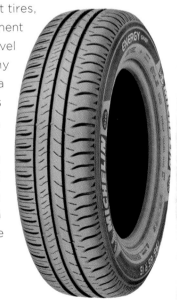

# → Michelin Apps

Because the notions of comfort and security are essential, both for you and for us, Michelin has created a package of six free mobile applications—a comprehensive collection to make driving a pleasure!

→ **Michelin MyCar** • *To get the best from your tires; services and information for carefree travel preparation.*

→ **Michelin Navigation** • *A new approach to navigation: traffic in real time with a new connected guidance feature.*

→ **ViaMichelin** • *Calculates routes and map data: a must for traveling in the most efficient way.*

→ **Michelin Restaurants** • *Because driving should be enjoyable: find a wide choice of restaurants, in France and Germany, including the MICHELIN Guide's complete listings.*

→ **Michelin Hotels** • *To book hotel rooms at the best rates, all over the world!*

→ **Michelin Voyage** • *85 countries and 30,000 tourist sites selected by the Michelin Green Guide, plus a tool for creating your own travel book.*

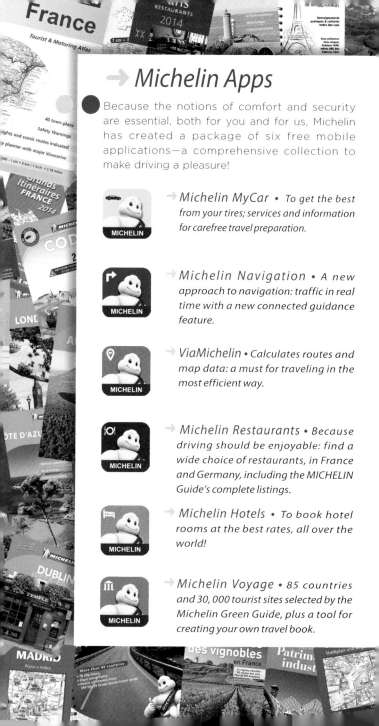

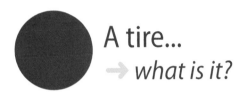

# A tire...
## → what is it?

**Round, black,** supple yet solid, the tire is to the wheel what the shoe is to the foot. But what is it made of? First and foremost, rubber, but also various textile and/or metallic materials... and then it's filled with air! It is the skilful assembly of all these components that ensures tires have the qualities they should: grip to the road, shock absorption, in two words: 'comfort' and 'safety.'

**1 TREAD**
The tread ensures the tire performs correctly, by dispersing water, providing grip and increasing longevity.

**2 CROWN PLIES**
This reinforced double or triple belt combines vertical suppleness with transversal rigidity, enabling the tire to remain flat to the road.

**3 SIDEWALLS**
These link all the component parts and provide symmetry. They enable the tire to absorb shock, thus giving a smooth ride.

**4 BEADS**
The bead wires ensure that the tire is fixed securely to the wheel to ensure safety.

**5 INNER LINER**
The inner liner creates an airtight seal between the wheel rim and the tire.

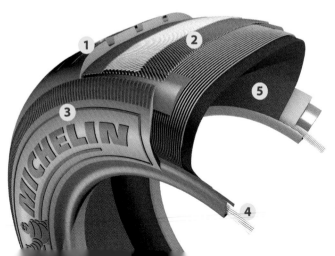

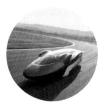
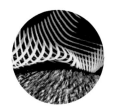
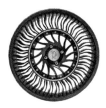

# Michelin
## → *innovation in movement*

**Created and patented** by Michelin in 1946, the belted radial-ply tire revolutionized the world of tires. But Michelin did not stop there: over the years other new and original solutions came out, confirming Michelin's position as a leader in research and innovation.

## → *the right pressure!*

**One of Michelin's priorities** is safer mobility. In short, innovating for a better way forward. This is the challenge for researchers, who are working to perfect tires capable of shorter braking distances and offering the best possible traction to the road. To support motorists, Michelin organizes road safety awareness campaigns all over the world: "Fill up with air" initiatives remind everyone that the right tire pressure is a crucial factor in safety and fuel economy.

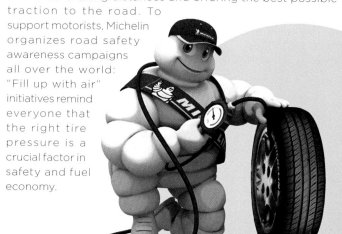

# The Michelin strategy:
→ *multi-performance tires*

**Michelin is synonymous** with safety, fuel saving and the capacity to cover thousands of miles. A MICHELIN tire is the embodiment of all these things – thanks to our engineers, who work with the very latest technology.

Their challenge: to equip every tire – whatever the vehicle (car, truck, tractor, bulldozer, plane, motorbike, bicycle or train!) – with the best possible combination of qualities, for optimal overall performance.

Slowing down wear, reducing energy expenditure (and therefore $CO_2$ emissions), improving safety through enhanced road handling and braking: there are so many qualities in just one tire – that's Michelin Total Performance.

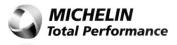

**MICHELIN**
**Total Performance**

Every day, **Michelin** is working towards sustainable mobility

OVER TIME, WHILE RESPECTING THE PLANET

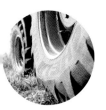 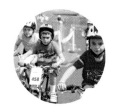 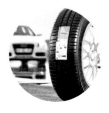

# Sustainable mobility
## → *is clean mobility... and mobility for everyone*

**Sustainable mobility** means enabling people to get around in a way that is cleaner, safer, more economical and more accessible to everyone, wherever they might live. Every day, Michelin's 113,000 employees worldwide are innovating:

• by creating tires and services that meet society's new needs.

• by raising young people's awareness of road safety.

• by inventing new transport solutions that consume less energy and emit less $CO_2$.

## → *Michelin Challenge Bibendum*

**Sustainable mobility** means allowing the transport of goods and people to continue, while promoting responsible economic, social and societal development. Faced with the increasing scarcity of raw materials and global warming, Michelin is standing up for the environment and public health. Michelin regularly organizes 'Michelin Challenge Bibendum', the only event in the world which focuses on sustainable road travel.

**MICHELIN**
**CHALLENGE BIBENDUM**

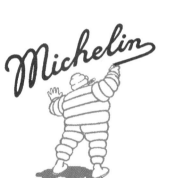